Vicky Vaselewski

NUTRITION ESSENTIALS FOR MENTAL HEALTH

A Norton Professional Book

NUTRITION ESSENTIALS FOR MENTAL HEALTH

A Complete Guide to the Food-Mood Connection

LESLIE E. KORN

FOREWORD BY JAMES LAKE, MD

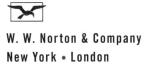

W. W. Norton & Company
New York • London

This book proposes to educate the reader about the role of diet and nutrition in mental health. It is not intended to replace medical treatment for serious illness, or to replace or approximate formal training and licensure.

For information about permission to reproduce selections from this book, write to Permissions, W. W. Norton & Company, Inc., 500 Fifth Avenue, New York, NY 10110

For information about special discounts for bulk purchases, please contact W. W. Norton Special Sales at specialsales@wwnorton.com or 800-233-4830

Manufacturing by Maple Press
Book design by Molly Heron
Production manager: Christine Critelli

Library of Congress Cataloging-in-Publication Data

Names: Korn, Leslie E.
Title: Nutrition essentials for mental health : a complete guide to the food-mood connection / Leslie E. Korn ; foreword by James Lake, MD.
Description: First edition. | New York : W.W. Norton & Company, [2016] | "A Norton professional book." | Includes bibliographical references and index.
Identifiers: LCCN 2015035638 | ISBN 9780393709940 (hardcover)
Subjects: LCSH: Mental health–Nutritional aspects. | Nutrition–Psychological aspects.
Classification: LCC RC455.4.N8 K67 2016 | DDC 616.89/0654–dc23
LC record available at http://lccn.loc.gov/2015035638

W. W. Norton & Company, Inc.
500 Fifth Avenue, New York, N.Y. 10110
www.wwnorton.com

W. W. Norton & Company Ltd.
Castle House, 75/76 Wells Street, London W1T 3QT

1 2 3 4 5 6 7 8 9 0

I give my heartfelt gratitude to my husband, Rudolph Rÿser. He brings immense joy and laughter to my life, which always salves the rigors of completing a book. He steps in when I ask without hesitation to edit, give guidance, prepare great meals, and share unflagging optimism. He is more than half of my overflowing cup.

Contents

Acknowledgments

I am fortunate to benefit from family and friends who have been immensely support-ive throughout the writing of this book. They were willing to read chapters to test the coherence and relevance of my ideas, to test recipes, and to lead the cheer. Having friends in "the field" helps. Jill Charney and Marilyn Piper took time from their busy lives to offer valuable suggestions that helped me improve this book. Marlene Brem-ner, my longtime assistant, always holds a steady oar to my projects, tracking all the minutiae, while offering important editorial suggestions. I am grateful to Dr. James Lake for his supportive reading of the text and contribution of the Foreword; and to Dr. Nicholas Gonzalez, Gray Graham, and Dr. Ethan Russo for their generous shar-ing of perspectives and analysis that expanded my own. Susan Butterworth gener-ously offered suggestions on motivational interviewing and nutrition behavior change. I am thankful to my two editors at Norton: Andrea Costella Dawson, who first invited me to write the book and skillfully guided its initial development, and Benjamin Yarling, whose consistent support and enthusiasm has made the whole pro-cess a pleasure. I am grateful to have been guided to the path of healing through nutrition when I lived for many years in the jungle of Mexico beginning in 1973 and at first fell ill with all kinds of tropical illnesses. Village women fed me plants and foods to nourish my recovery and became lifelong friends, colleagues, and comadres. I have learned much of what I know about mental health nutrition from my clients (both north and south of the border), who have courageously questioned the mental health status quo and sought my support for their health and healing.

Foreword

> The doctor of the future will give no medication, but will interest his patients in the care of the human frame, diet and in the cause and prevention of disease.
>
> —Thomas A Edison

In the face of widespread and often inappropriate prescribing of powerful psychotropic medications, accumulating research evidence supports the use of a range of non-pharmacological approaches for the prevention and treatment of depressed mood, anxiety, dementia, substance abuse, and other common mental health problems. Diet, exercise, and stress management fall under the broad heading of 'lifestyle" changes and, among these, diet is certainly the *most important*. Dr. Korn's new book is an important contribution to the growing dialog in the medical community and the general public on the role of nutrition in health and mental health. *Nutrition Essentials for Mental Health: The Complete Guide to the Food-Mood Connection* provides a comprehensive account of the evidence for nutrition in maintaining optimal mental health and treating many common mental health problems. Dr. Korn offers clear, simple strategies that will guide you in helping clients think about foods that are better suited to their unique biochemical constitutions and mental health needs. The book provides a comprehensive, step-by-step review of the vital links between what we eat, how our brains function—*or don't*—and our capacity to *think and feel*. The book is a *tour de force* of the complex dynamic relationships that exist between the digestive process, the body, and the brain, beginning with the simple acts of chewing and swallowing and progressing through the complex phases of digestion and elimination. Dr. Korn introduces an important emerging concept in Western medicine called the "human microbiome," according to which health and mental health are viewed in relation to the *microbiome-gut-brain axis* (Foster & McVey Neufeld, 2013). The microbiome is essentially an ecosystem of symbiotic bacteria and a host of other microorganisms residing in the healthy gut. Recent studies demonstrate that the microbiome plays a critical role in brain development, behavior, and mental health throughout the life span. Bacteria in the microbiome activate neural pathways and central nervous system signaling systems that play a role in mood regulation, memory, and cognition. Recent research findings show that the gut microbiota are influenced by stress, diet, and a host of other factors in the environment, supporting Dr. Korn's thesis that interventions based on dietary change and stress management are vitally important for prevention and treatment of common mental health problems.

Epidemiological data on relationships between diet and prevalence rates of depressed mood, dementia, and other common mental health problems support the central role of nutrition in the world's major healing traditions from earliest historical times. Almost half of studies on nutrition and mental health published between 1971 and 2014 reported significant positive relationships between diet and depressed mood (Opie, O'Neil, Itsiopoulos, & Jacka, 2014). A large population study revealed an alarming correlation between an increased prevalence rate of Alzheimer's disease in developing countries and multiple lifestyle factors related to increasing globalization such as smoking, alcohol consumption, and the Western diet (i.e., high daily calories consumed and high consumption of animal fat in the diet; Grant, 2014). These results are consistent with the findings of a 36-month prospective trial in which healthy adults who followed a Mediterranean diet experienced a reduced rate of cognitive decline compared to individuals following a Western-style diet with fewer vegetables and high animal fat (Gardener et al., 2014). In keeping with the latest research findings, changes in diet are frequently "prescribed" as a central part of treatment in Chinese medicine and Ayurveda, on the assumption that without addressing *imbalances* in the body and mind at a basic level, there may be little hope for changing the factors that manifest as illness. The ancient wisdom of recommending dietary changes for improved health and well-being is reflected in a quote attributed to Hippocrates, the father of Western medicine, who said, "Let food be thy medicine, thy medicine shall be thy food." In addition to the increased attention to the role of diet in maintaining optimal mental health, research findings from placebo-controlled studies support the use of high-potency nutrient supplements in the treatment of specific psychiatric disorders. For example, foods rich in B vitamins such as whole grains and leafy green vegetables may be especially beneficial for mood regulation. Several B vitamins are essential cofactors that facilitate the synthesis of neurotransmitters that play a central role in mood regulation. Individuals with mental health problems who may be at risk of a nutritional deficiency because of their dietary preferences should be encouraged to take appropriate doses of vitamins, minerals, or other supplements that are known to be beneficial for their mental health problem. As Dr. Korn explains, medical problems and mental illness often occur together; however, causal relationships between particular physical ailments and mental health are often difficult to discern. When a mental health problem is addressed with dietary changes that result in optimal nutrition, medical problems often improve. Sound nutrition advice should always comprise a cornerstone of a comprehensive integrative treatment plan. Even in cases where prescription psychotropic medications are a necessary part of treatment, simple changes in nutrition provide important "add-on" benefits to medications by optimizing levels of micronutrients critical for healthy brain functioning.

Various chapters cover the importance of nutritional assessment in mental health care, the best foods and nutrients for mental health, food allergies, sensitivities and special diets, and practical strategies for supporting optimal brain health when weaning off of psychotropic medications. Chapter 3 on nutritional assessment should be required reading for all mental health professionals. In this chapter, Dr. Korn provides a template for evaluating each patient's unique history; identifies pertinent medical, social, and family issues that affect nutrition; and explains how to assess clients for blood sugar handling, food allergies and sensitivities, inflammation, oxidative stress, mitochondrial energy production, and the methylation pathway, all of which play critical roles in health and mental health.

Nutrition Essentials for Mental Health: The Complete Guide to the Food-Mood Connection is a powerful new synthesis of the role of nutrition in mental health. In these pages clinicians will discover many valuable clinical pearls and insights to guide them when advising their patients about practical, safe, effective, and affordable strategic approaches to eating and taking supplements for optimal health and well-being, as well as for preventing and treating common mental health problems. By examining the relationship between *what we eat* and how our bodies and brains function, Dr. Korn addresses complex problems of mental health prevention and treatment at the *most fundamental level*. Optimal nutrition and the strategic uses of supplements should be included as a necessary and *central* component of integrative treatment addressing depressed mood, anxiety, bipolar disorder, substance abuse, attention-deficit/hyperactivity disorder, schizophrenia, cognitive decline, and dementia. This book should be required reading for all psychiatrists and psychologists and, more importantly, for medical students and residents in psychiatry, family medicine, internal medicine, and pediatrics, where education on nutrition has been historically lacking.

James Lake, MD, is the former chair of the International Network of Integrative Mental Health and the author of *Textbook of Integrative Mental Health Care* (New York: Thieme, 2006).

References

Foster, J. A., & McVey Neufeld, K. A. (2013). Gut-brain axis: How the microbiome influences anxiety and depression. *Trends in Neurosciences, 36*(5), 305–312.

Gardener, S. L., Rainey-Smith, S. R., Barnes, M. B., Sohrabi, H. R., Weinborn, M., Lim, Y. Y., … Martins, R. N. (2014, July 29). Dietary patterns and cognitive decline in an Australian study of ageing. *Molecular Psychiatry.* [Epub ahead of print]

Grant, W. B. (2014). Trends in diet and Alzheimer's disease during the nutrition transition in Japan and developing countries. *Journal of Alzheimers Disease, 38*(3), 611–620.

Opie, R. S., O'Neil, A., Itsiopoulos, C., & Jacka, F. N. (2014, December 3). The impact of whole-of-diet interventions on depression and anxiety: A systematic review of randomised controlled trials. *Public Health Nutrition,* 1–20. [Epub ahead of print]

NUTRITION
ESSENTIALS
FOR
MENTAL
HEALTH

CHAPTER 1

Why Does Nutrition Matter in Mental Health?

Diet Essential: *Mood follows food: Eat breakfast.*

There is no doubt that nutrition affects mental health. Poor nutrition leads to and exacerbates mental illness. Optimal nutrition prevents and treats mental illness. Note the word "optimal" for nutrition to prevent and treat illness. One's diet cannot be just "good" or provide the basics to survive; it must be nutrient dense and tailored to the needs of the individual who may have been missing the basic ingredients for optimal brain function since life in the womb.

Where there is mental illness, there is poor diet. Where there is mental illness, there is a long history of digestive problems. By adding the lens of nutrition, diet, and digestion to your clinical toolbox, you will forever change your approach to client care and enhance the efficacy of all your other methods.

I have written this book to take you step by step through all the essentials required for integrating nutritional therapies into mental health treatment. Even if you do not apply all of these approaches yourself, you will know about these therapies for referrals and collaborative work. Importantly, this book is designed for you the clinician to try the methods, techniques, and recipes on yourself so that you enhance your own well-being and stamina.

Changing thoughts, beliefs, behaviors, and habits happens slowly in therapy. Changing nutritional beliefs and behaviors is no different. But results are assured. This book is not ideological; it is practical. It is intended to provide concrete steps to modify beliefs and behaviors for healthful results.

Some people respond better to psychodynamic therapy methods, while others need and respond better to cognitive-behavioral therapy (CBT) or solution-focused methods. Similarly, some people function better as carnivores while others function better as vegetarians. Knowing who you are and what your body needs is the art and science of mental health nutrition. But what is incontrovertible is that nutrition matters and it is the most important missing link to mental health in society today.

In this chapter and the ones to follow, I will help you guide each client through each stage of dietary and nutritional change. While I will suggest some first steps, much like a jigsaw puzzle, you can start almost anywhere and begin to form the pattern that leads to improved health.

WHAT IS THE STANDARD AMERICAN DIET?

The standard American diet (SAD) makes us sad! This too-frequently prescribed diet consists of overly processed foods containing refined sugars in fruit juices and sugary drinks, and highly refined rice, pastas, and flours used in breads and bakery goods. These processed products are loaded with chemicals and synthetic preservatives, hormones, antibiotics, and food colorings that are known to alter our mood. This type of diet is a prime contributing factor resulting in health complaints for many clients. The SAD leads to chronic inflammatory states and sets the stage for neurotransmitter imbalances. Much of it is "fake food" with dozens of chemical ingredients created in the laboratory and not on the farm or in nature. Such so-called foods are designed to survive on the shelf for months at a time—thus reducing costs to the manufacturers. The SAD diet makes us SAD because it does not provide the nutrients our brain and body need to function well. That some of us survive (though rarely thrive) on a SAD diet is just the luck of the draw, and for some people illness comes in childhood or not until middle age, but it comes invariably, just as a car without the right fuel eventually sputters to a stop.

There are many reasons why people do not receive the nourishment their minds/bodies need. Many experience chronic poverty or injury-related economic loss that precludes access to high-quality, nutritious food. Some do not know what good nutrition is and are vulnerable to advertisements or medical myths. People may suffer deficits in self-care leading to poor nutrition; or they may have been hospitalized for extended periods during which they have been served poor-quality food cheaply acquired and prepared by the hospital. Still others who are addicted to substances such as alcohol, cocaine, or methamphetamines do not eat well or even enough at all, and what they do eat is not metabolized properly. Pharmaceutical medications, alcohol, and many commercially produced drugs deplete important nutrients needed by the body. One of the most important influences on mental health resulting from a poor or nutritionally deficient diet is the inflammatory response. Inflammation is now understood to underlie most mental illness, including depression. Decreasing inflammation is so fundamental to healing that a separate discussion is necessary.

Inflammation and Mood

Escalating inflammation in the body and brain is one of the major consequences of the SAD. Chronic low-level inflammation contributes to depression and cognitive decline.

Some Factors Causing Inflammation in the Body

- Stress
- Poor-quality foods
- Physical inactivity
- Obesity
- Smoking
- Increased gut permeability
- Lack of sleep
- Toxic exposures
- Vitamin D deficiency

Everyone is familiar with the inflammation that occurs as a result of an injury, for example a fall leading to a bruise or cut. The tissue becomes red and swollen, and it is often painful. This is the body's natural immune response, helping us to heal from injuries and infection. Similar inflammation also occurs systemically throughout the body but is often invisible. If this inflammatory response within the body is chronic, cell immune secretions remain turned on all the time. These cells produce proteins called *cytokines* that contribute to depression and to the breakdown of nerve cells. People who experience major depression have increased levels of inflammatory cytokines that, in turn, negatively affect neurotransmitter function. Certain foods such as refined sugars trigger these inflammatory cytokine responses in the body. These foods are called "dietary stressors." Other foods, like fresh berries and herbs like turmeric and ginger, can "quench the fires" of inflammation. Stimulating the anti-inflammatory cytokines can improve depressed mood and increase treatment response to conventional antidepressant medication by counterregulating production of pro-inflammatory cytokines. Stress is also a cause of inflammation and depression. Relaxation decreases the inflammatory response. The elimination of sugar helps to stabilize mood and also reduces cytokine production and thereby reduces systemic inflammation. This is one of the first steps to take with all clients, whether they are depressed or not: reduce stress, eliminate inflammatory foods, and increase anti-inflammatory foods.

WHAT ARE TRADITIONAL, AUTHENTIC DIETS?

One of the points I will emphasize throughout this book is the concept of "traditional nutrition and foods." These are foods, diets, and preparation methods that have been used by our ancestors for millennia. They are foods that have evolved to optimize nourishment. In modern society, food and diet are often dissociated from authentic cultural traditions. There is social pressure to conform and relinquish healthy cultural traditions upon arrival in the United States among immigrants and native populations as well. We are, however, experiencing revitalization across modern SAD societies of reclaiming local, fresh, nutrient-dense, and optimally prepared traditional foods made relevant to our needs for the 21st century. Although these foods and methods remain inaccessible to many, especially the economically impoverished, this need not be the case. In this book I explain low-cost approaches to mental health nutrition. As you will see, food is much more than nourishment: Food is medicine. Food is nutrition. Food is ceremonial. Food is sacred. Food is culture and tradition. Food is an anchor to culture and personal well-being. Food is the direct link between the environment and human health. It is the avenue by which a healthy environment can provide complete nutrition and a sense of integration and wellness. Yet for many of our clients food is inaccessible, food is addicting, food is fraught with memories of harsh discipline or fights, or food is linked to the inner fight for a certain look or body, as occurs with body dysmorphia and eating disorders. In these cases food becomes a metaphor as well as a substance that requires the integration of nutrition and counseling in order to decondition negative associations and beliefs, and to regulate affect that hampers health. The mental health clinician is ideally suited to this integrative partnership with the client.

The traditional nutrition—also called authentic nutrition—approach to mental health suggests that in order to achieve health and well-being, mentally and physically, we should eat the types of foods similar to the foods our ancestors ate. This means foods free of refined sugars and grains, with no synthetic preservatives or food coloring, and minimally processed. These foods should be prepared in their natural state. Traditional or authentic foods are low glycemic, anti-inflammatory, and rich in omega-3 fatty acids. Depending on the region of the world, these foods may include a low to moderate or even high complex carbohydrate, moderate-protein, moderate-to high-fat diet. Antioxidant-rich fruits and vegetables of all colors, and fiber sources also known as prebiotics may include bark flour, psyllium, chia, cactus, bran, and oatmeal. Fermented foods such as kimchi, sauerkraut, and fresh natural yogurt and kefir provide probiotics for digestion, colon health, and detoxification.

There is a tremendous diversity of foods, and we have the ability to adapt and use many foods from our neighbors as well as ancestors. Some of our ancestors ate a diet of fresh blood and raw milk (and still do); others ate lots of blubber and fish and only a few carbohydrates in the forms of berries and roots during the summer months. Traditional diets obtain dietary fats from fish, birds, plants, and wild game. Wild animals have only one-tenth the fat of farmed cattle, include natural essential fatty acids, and they also do not have the harmful antibiotics and hormones that disrupt endocrine function and gut health. Not until 16th-century colonization and 20th-century development brought refined flours, sugars, and soy protein as substitutes for their traditional diets did the Inuit located in the Arctic region suffer suicide, depression, and heart disease. The diet of people in late 19th-century Scotland included oats, turnips and potatoes, leeks, cabbage and kale, bitter greens like nettles, sorrel, sulfur-rich garlic, butter and cheeses, fish, shellfish and seaweed, game, and wild berries (Czapp, 2009). This diet today would serve the needs of many people of Scotland and other northern European areas very well. Oats (steel cut, not instant) and the straw from green oats, called oat straw, are medicinal nourishing foods that have powerful anxiolytic properties that I recommend for anxious clients.

Before the 16th century, wheat, beef from cattle, milk, and pork did not exist in the western hemisphere. Therefore, these foods may not be the most beneficial for peoples indigenous to the western hemisphere. By contrast, peoples in India evolved in a warmer climate with subtropical foods and an emphasis on more vegetables and carbohydrates. The peoples of tropical Mesoamerica, Africa, and India have accessed fats from nuts, plants, ducks, insects, and turkeys, and they have depended upon many more vegetables, fruits, and grains endemic to their regions. Weston Price, in the course of his global travels in traditional societies, asked the question: "Who is the healthiest among peoples on the planet?" While looking for an answer, he found that they all consumed moderate amounts of saturated and monounsaturated animal fats, suggesting that our modern fears of saturated fats are among the paradigmatic myths of modern medicine. He and other researchers also failed to find any society that was *vegan*, suggesting that veganism is a modern dietary invention and while there is much emotional and spiritual merit in veganism, there is little evidence for any biological merit.

Traditional diets vary widely; for example, the authentic Inuit diet may include up to 75% dietary fat, much of it saturated and thus anti-inflammatory, whereas an Indian diet might include nutrients from larger amounts of plant proteins—nuts and legumes—cooked in the rich anti-inflammatory spices like turmeric, cinnamon, and ginger.

Authentic foods are those foods and medicines that naturally evolved over time within a specific human culture. These foods bring balance to the body, mind, and spirit. How does one integrate authentic foods, traditional foods, and whole foods today while living in rural or urban settings? What are the options and ideas for using food as a delicious source of nutrition and medicine?

As a general rule we all benefit when the majority of daily food intake includes whole foods that are nutrient dense and freshly prepared. Some proportion of daily food should include both raw and cooked foods, and ideally some wild foods. Food that is obtained from cans or other packages should be minimized. Many foods are best eaten with minimal processing to ensure maximum nutrition and health benefits, while some require cooking, especially long cooking at low heat. The enzymes required for natural health and proper digestion are richest in raw foods. Slow cooking in water, boiling, salting, broiling, pickling, roasting, baking, drying, steaming, fermenting, and some smoking are the essential processing methods that ensure maximum nutrition. Frying should be limited to special occasions. By preparing fresh foods, one can control the preparation, including the amount of salt and commercial fats used, in order to maintain optimal nutritional value. Fresh foods are also free of harmful preservatives.

One of the most important elements to successful mental health nutrition is that there is no one diet for everyone. Hence the ancient wisdom, "One man's meat is another man's poison." For nutrition to be effective, diet must be tailored to the metabolism of each individual. Nutritional needs are determined biochemically at the individual level. This is genetically based and is culturally and environmentally linked to our ancestry. Aligning our "fuel" with the rate at which we can burn it enhances efficiency and performance. A consistent use of fuel inappropriate for the individual body leads to decline.

Eating according to your individual type means identifying what kind of body you have and how it digests and metabolizes food, or "fuel." The rate at which you digest carbohydrates is called the "rate of glucose oxidation." This rate governs the amount of carbohydrates, proteins, and fats your body requires for your "fuel mixture." Our bodies are determined by our cultural and genetic heritage, which developed in the environment where our ancestors evolved. Just because your people moved out from Africa 400 years ago doesn't mean that your metabolism is that much different than your ancestors. If your ancestors migrated from England to the United States 200 years ago, it doesn't mean that you can now function as a vegetarian. We carry the history of our ancestors and in particular our parents in our genes, and that determines our metabolism. If your people are from Greece and thrived on a Mediterranean diet rich in plant proteins and you have children with an individual from Greenland, your child will have a dominant metabolism and may need to eat either like someone from Greece or Greenland or perhaps will be able to enjoy a mixture.

INDIVIDUALIZED NUTRITION

One of the ways I inform my clients about an individualized approach to diet and nutrition is to use the metaphor of a car. Different types of vehicles require different kinds of gas. For example, if I put 87-octane fuel into a car that takes only diesel, I can destroy the engine. Some cars do better with lower octane and some higher octane; the right fuel ensures the smooth running of the vehicle. This does not always mean that a vehicle will not run, but more so that it will not run optimally in the way it is meant to. This concept is analogous to our own "engine." Each of us has an engine that requires a different mix of "fuel." Fuel in the form of food is made up of protein, carbohydrates, and fats. The correct fuel mix, meaning the correct ratio of protein, carbohydrates, and fats for the individual, will ensure smooth healthy functioning. This concept, which is based in science, thus puts to rest all the confusion about the various diets that are out there and also the confusion about research on diets, all of which can show both positive effects and negative effects. It is not the diet that determines well-being, but the individual's alignment with the dietary "fuel." Hence, there is no one right diet for everyone. If we continue this analogy between cars, fuel, and the combustion that moves it forward with human fuel, such as food, then what we are looking at scientifically is called *oxidation*. Oxidation is the rate at which we burn carbohydrates, or glucose. Some of us burn carbohydrates more quickly, and some burn them more slowly.

To begin identifying your nutritional type, you may carry out either or both tests in Box 1.1.

Box 1.1
Identifying Your Nutritional Type

Niacin Test: Take 50 mg of niacin on an empty stomach. Niacin has little or no effect on a slow oxidizer, mild effect on the mixed or balanced oxidizer. and a strong flush on the fast oxidizer.
Vitamin C Test: Take 8 grams of vitamin C over an 8-hour period (1,000 g every hour). The fast oxidizer will not feel well, the slow oxidizer will have little or no response, and the balanced oxidizer will not have much of a response.

Most clients are unfamiliar with the science of nutrition or of physiology. I continue the use of the metaphor in order to explain what is happening to their body/mind: Daily, one has to ensure the engine (the brain-stomach) has the proper fuel mix (carbohydrates, proteins, and fats). If it is too low-octane, there's backfiring (fermentation and gas). If it is too high, it goes unused and is a waste, leaving waste deposits (gout). At periodic intervals one has to change the oil filter (flush the gallbladder), tune the engine (take a rest), do a lube (ingest fish oils or hydrate), and of course wash the car (detoxify). Simple images, but oftentimes our clients are dissociated from their bodies—that is, separated from its functions and actions—and can better understand anatomical and physiological mechanism through metaphor. When I ask a client the last time she flushed her gallbladder—and she never has—or suggest there is not enough fire in the gallbladder to digest the food (spark the engine), it becomes clear that often people take care of their cars more than their bodies.

A car may perform well when it is new (young), but as it reaches the 50,000-mile mark (40–50 years) it begins to break down—if it hasn't already. The clutch goes, the brakes give out, and under extreme stress, such as cold wet winters, the bottom rusts out (adrenal foundation) sooner and the paint (skin) cracks.

People can be divided into three general body categories: the *fast oxidizers*, whose blood pH tends toward a little more acid and are carnivores; the *slow oxidizers*, whose blood pH tends to be more alkaline and do better on more plant proteins; and the *mixed or balanced individuals* who do well with a mix of carbohydrates, proteins, and fats. What foods/fuel mix we require is determined by our genetics, just like the color of our eyes, our height, or our blood type. We are a product of our parents' rates of oxidation, also called metabolism. If we are eating food that does not burn efficiently based on the need of our engine, then we will not function optimally and this also underlies not only physical but mental health problems/illness.

Types of Oxidizers

What kind of food supports the fast oxidizer? These individuals do well with a high-protein, high-fat diet to slow down their rate of oxidation and to stabilize their blood sugar. They will also do well on the purine foods, such as organ meats, sardines, and anchovies. Their ideal ratio is 50% protein, 20% carbohydrates, and 30% fat. They will benefit from fruits and vegetables more so than grains. Slow oxidizers do best with 25% protein, 60% carbohydrates, and 15% fats. They may do best on animal protein like chicken, turkey, pork, fish, and eggs. The balanced/mixed oxidizers will burn efficiently using 30% protein, 40% carbohydrates, and 30% fats. No one does well on refined sugar and refined wheat flour. When one eats well 90% of the time, an occasional "refined" food will not be harmful.

Thus, the fast metabolizer is what we would call a carnivore, the slow metabolizer would be on the vegetarian spectrum, and the mixed will benefit from a range of foods. Keep in mind that we are talking about a spectrum. Later, when we explore the use of the food diary, one of our basic principles is asking our clients what makes them feel best and what makes them feel worse, and this is applied to diet as well as behavior.

A diet that is rich in plant proteins, fruits, nuts, seeds, legumes, and grains provides a superior foundation for mental health nutrition and will benefit nearly everyone. Nuts and seeds, especially nut butters, and the grains quinoa and millet are good sources of protein along with well-soaked and well-cooked beans. Depending upon one's individual biochemistry, one can continue as a vegetarian or will benefit from adding fish (pesco), milk (lacto), eggs (ovo), and various forms of poultry and meats. The key to a successful plant-based diet is ensuring a diversity of proteins to provide the complement of amino acids necessary for neurotransmitter function.

People who are depressed, lethargic, anxious, or prone to panic and also following a vegetarian or vegan diet will most likely improve by including animal proteins into their meals. In these cases it is common that the individual is not aligned with her or his true dietary needs. It is often in these cases that an individual is a vegetarian for spiritual, emotional, or environmental reasons; however, genetically she or he is not a true vegetarian and, indeed, may be a fast metabolizer. If the person is willing, I ask her or him to eat animal protein three times daily for 7 days and then we can assess changes in mood.

Table 1.1 reviews the nutritional types, and food ratios are discussed further in Chapter 5.

TABLE 1.1

Nutritional Types: Ideal Percentages of Food Intake

Type	Protein	Carbohydrates	Fat
Fast oxidizer	50%	20%	30%
Slow oxidizer	25%	60%	15%
Mixed oxidizer	30%	40%	30%

GOOD FOOD IMPROVES MOOD

Mood follows food, and mood swings follow blood sugar swings. Refined carbohydrates, such as sugar and white flour, cause blood sugar to rise sharply and then drop; hence the quick pick-me-up when we grab sugar followed by the just-as-quick letdown within an hour or two as glucose levels drop and fatigue and irritability return. Thus, the first two dietary steps that are required to help clients with low mood or mood lability is to begin nutritional change by decreasing and eliminating refined carbohydrates and sugars from their diet, while increasing the intake of quality protein. Many people will first be "withdrawing" from their addiction to refined carbohydrates.

People under chronic stress are vulnerable to reactive hypoglycemia, which can occur as a result of an excessive release of insulin following a high (refined) carbohydrate meal. Primary hypoglycemia can occur when there is an inadequate supply of carbohydrates. High or low blood glucose levels affect mental functioning. The resulting drop in blood glucose leads to a drop in mood, irritability, anxiety, nervousness, craving of sweets, panic, crying, fainting, motor weakness, personality changes, headaches, visual disturbances, confusion, and shakiness. Some of the symptoms that are mistaken for mental health symptoms are anxiety, worry, inability to focus, irritability, restlessness, insomnia, temper tantrums, hyperactivity, and depression. Problems associated with hypoglycemia also include foggy thinking because the brain is not receiving as much blood sugar as it needs to function properly.

Cortisol is responsible for raising blood sugar levels, but under chronic stress, cortisol is low and cannot raise those levels, resulting in the symptoms of irritability, shakiness or feeling like rubber, or dizziness. The time it takes for these symptoms to occur is usually about 2 to 5 hours after eating. In addition to high carbohydrate meals, smoking cigarettes may increase severe hypoglycemia by two-and-a-half times. Carbohydrate intake should be about 100–130 grams per day. Insulin resistance, which often is the precursor to type 2 diabetes, co-occurs with functional hypoglycemia. People who are insulin resistant feel sleepy after they eat because excess insulin promotes excess serotonin in the brain (Kharrazian, 2013). This also explains why people often eat high-sugar foods or starchy carbohydrates in order to calm down.

When assessing for mood changes and inattention in both children and adults, it is important to rule out reactive hypoglycemia, food allergies, or other medical conditions. Many children with apparent attention problems who regularly go off to school with sugary cereals and milk for breakfast would have more sustained and focused energy simply by eating more protein for breakfast. Research demonstrates a significant relationship between unhealthy diet and poor mental health in children and adolescents (O'Neil et al., 2014). Indeed, I recommend always evaluating (and changing) a child's diet prior to mental health treatment. It will also obviate the need for medication. Hypoglycemia is almost always apparent in cases of alcoholism, which is also where sugar (alcohol) is being consumed in high quantities. Hypoglycemia is commonly seen in people with schizophrenia, drug and food addictions, and people with obesity. Many people who suffer from hypoglycemia are also deficient in essential fatty acids (EFAs). Symptoms include dry skin, dry hair, adrenal insufficiency, and poor functioning of the pancreas, liver, and gallbladder.

Without reducing the intake of refined carbohydrates such as sugar, balancing mood will remain out of reach for the mood disordered, and one may never know why. Hypoglycemia refers to low blood glucose, which is often associated with poor adrenal function. People under stress are vulnerable to reactive hypoglycemia because stress negatively affects the regulation of blood glucose. Most patients who do not eat a healthy diet and binge on carbohydrates have hypoglycemia and do not know it. Many vegetarians experience it, since they often do not consume enough proteins to stabilize their blood sugar. Hypoglycemia contributes to mood lability and inattention. This condition is often misidentified as the rapid cycling of bipolar disorder or attention-deficit/hyperactivity disorder (ADHD). Without eliminating hypoglycemia as a cause of mood cycling, an accurate diagnosis cannot be made. Children and adults with severe mood swings and irritability experience significant improvement when the hypoglycemia and carbohydrate addiction are addressed.

People who fall asleep but awaken 3–4 hours later and cannot get back to sleep may also experience nighttime hypoglycemia and will feel better when eating some protein and carbohydrates just before going to bed.

A diet that is low in carbohydrates with a low or moderate protein intake and lots of fats is beneficial for those with insulin or leptin resistance, but only until the resistance improves and weight, blood pressure, sugar, and cholesterol have normalized. Carbohydrates can be increased in the diet once this improvement is seen. Carbohydrates can then be reduced as needed if symptoms return. Despite the fact that glucose is a major fuel for the brain, low-carbohydrate diets have not been found to affect cognitive function negatively (Brinkworth, Noakes, Buckley, Keogh, & Clifton, 2009).

In general, everyone functions best by eating three to six meals a day, including snacks, and most people would benefit by eliminating refined carbohydrate consumption and combining vegetable carbohydrates with healthy, high-quality fats like butter, avocado, coconut, nuts, and eggs. Eating organic starchy and nonstarchy vegetables as the primary source of carbohydrates is optimal. Eating small amounts of high-quality protein, fat, and vegetables every 3 hours is an essential dietary approach to recovery from hypoglycemia (see Appendix A for General Guidelines for a Hypoglycemic Diet).

DIGESTION AND MENTAL HEALTH

The intestinal tract, or the gut, is often called the "second brain" because it is a major source of neurotransmitter production in the body. Thus, it is not surprising that people with chronic digestive problems are often anxious and depressed. The healthy bacteria, known as probiotics, help to lower the stress response by regulating GABA, the relaxation neurotransmitter via the vagus nerve. Probiotics may be bought in capsule or liquid form in a health food store and are also found in fermented foods.

Fermented foods are among the best foods for both intestinal and brain health. All traditional diets have some form of fermented foods. The health benefits of yogurt and kefir, among other fermented foods, derive from their beneficial bacteria. Fermented foods' value is well known in traditional cultures everywhere, as they are used to restore and maintain the bowel "garden," where the bacterial flora grow. Where fermented foods are not available, yogurt and sauerkraut can be made at home easily and inexpensively and are a wonderful food preparation and "science" experiment to share with children.

Another common practice of our ancestors involves making gelatin-rich meat broths that contain collagen and amino acids that are easy to assimilate and help brain function. Freshly made bone and vegetable broth is the first food to choose as a staple in helping people recover from mental illness. Yet many people no longer cook or prepare foods, relying instead on packages, microwaves, and fast foods. Among the initial steps to explore with clients is how to integrate food preparation, both raw and cooked, into their lives.

When discussing diet and nutrition, I usually use a food, mood, and exercise diary, which asks clients to keep detailed track for three days of what they eat, how they feel, and when they move or exercise. This diary is a valuable tool for revealing clients' self-care routines—or lack of them—and can greatly enhance awareness of what one eats and how it affects energy and mood. But, however the conversation begins, recognizing that mood is a mind-body experience and not just based on personal history or mental processes, can be crucial in increasing clients' sense of self-efficacy and broadening their perspective on the many pathways to change.

I have organized the book with attention to what I consider the most important diet essentials. It is not an exhaustive list; however, adhering to these main essentials will help clients on their path of recovery.

Diet Essentials

1. *Mood follows food: Eat breakfast.* Do not allow yourself to become hungry. Eliminate refined carbohydrates. When your blood sugar drops, so does your mood. Eating protein stabilizes your mood. Eating only carbohydrates allows you to feel energized at first, and then relaxation or even fatigue may set in. Eating fats provides a sense of feeling full.

2. *Nourish the first brain and the second brain.* The brain is made up of 60% fat. It needs enough good quality fat, proteins, and carbohydrates (sugar) to function. To improve mood, focus, attention, and memory, eat plenty of good fats like butter, eggs, avocados, walnuts, and coconut oil, and eliminate all poor-quality fats and trans-fats, like French fries and fats (partially hydrogenated oils) added to canned and packaged foods. The "second brain" is the digestive system, the "gut" where food is digested and absorbed. Nourish the second brain with fiber and fermented foods. It also generates the healthy bacteria and neurotransmitters that support efficient brain chemistry.

3. *Eat only when relaxed.* Digestion occurs when the autonomic nervous system is switched on. The juices containing digestive enzymes flow in a state of relax-

ation. Eating under stress is like putting a pot of food on the stove to cook, not lighting the fire, and letting it sit there for two days; it bubbles, ferments, and becomes gaseous.

4. *Symptoms tell a story of nutritional and emotional challenges.* Our role is to listen to the story and, together with the client, make the story coherent and actionable.

5. *Where there is mental illness, there is always a history of digestive problems.* Use nutrition to balance the five essential factors that underlie mental illness: circadian rhythms, blood sugar and functional hypoglycemia; food allergies and sensitivities; inflammation; oxidative stress and mitochondrial function; and inadequate methylation.

6. *Eliminate exposure to additives, preservatives, hormones, toxic pesticides, and fertilizers on food.* Mental health is affected negatively by dietary exposure to food toxins and allergens. Use wild foods and organic foods. If you cannot obtain these foods all the time, focus your attention on organic eggs and meat products and detoxify your fruits and vegetables.

7. *No single diet is right for everyone.* Each person has a different cultural-genetic heritage and therefore a different metabolism. Some peoples like the Inuit require mostly meat and fish, whereas people from India do well on a predominance of legumes, vegetables, fruits, and grains. Most people require a mix. However, that mix of food can vary greatly. Know your ancestral and genetic heritage and try to eat for your individual metabolic type.

8. *Eat all the colors of the "brainbow."* Eat whole, nutrient-dense foods from the whole color spectrum to obtain your nutrients. Prepare fresh foods daily.

9. *Diet is essential, but not sufficient.* A healthy diet is essential for mental health; however, it is not generally sufficient to treat mental illness. To treat mental illness, it is essential to choose a healthy diet along with regular use of vitamins, minerals, fats, and glandulars.

10. *Choose healthy foods and nutrients over alcohol and drugs to alter consciousness.* Foods and nutrients, alcohol, and drugs can all alter consciousness. Distinguish between altering consciousness for health or for addiction. Understand what is being altered in order to gain control over an addiction. Transform addiction into positive states of consciousness, linked to ceremonial and group activities.

11. *Integrate behavioral change strategies with the principle of nutritional substitutions.* Personal change takes place by integrating positive activities (habits) first and then eliminating negative habits (activities). Identify one positive

change behavior and its corresponding negative habit at a time. Substitute healthier foods that will satisfy the same needs.

NUTRITIONAL QUESTIONS AND CONCERNS CLIENTS BRING TO US AND HOW WE CAN RESPOND

Our clients bring a range of questions and concerns about their physical and mental well-being. Many clients want advice and support to either improve the efficacy of their medications, reduce the dosage, or eliminate or stay off medications. Among the questions my clients have presented are the folllowing:

Q. My primary care provider has suggested that I take medication because I am depressed, but I would prefer not to. Are there any nutritional alternatives that I could consider?

A. Commonly a client with depression, anxiety, or insomnia has been advised to take medication, and for any number of reasons she does not want to. She may not want to because she doesn't believe in medications, she may be afraid of them, maybe she has tried them in the past with negative side effects, or she may have cultural or philosophical reasons why. Our first response is to understand what she would like to do to address her symptoms and what her fears and concerns are about medication. My goal is to prioritize nonpharmaceutical approaches to addressing her symptoms, and my first response is to instill hope that she can manage these symptoms and even eliminate them when combining psychology and nutritional interventions. Throughout this book we explore in a step-by-step process both initial and more complex explorations that are isomorphic to our clients' personalities and their stated needs.

Q. The school and teacher sent a letter saying that they strongly encourage us to get a consultation for medication for our 8 year old, who they deem as having ADHD. We would rather explore other options at this point. Can you tell me what they are and how to begin a nutritional program?

A. Parents of children with symptoms of ADHD are commonly advised by the school system that their child needs medication. In this type of consultation we have an opportunity to explore dietary influences on behavior, the research on nutritional supplementation, and explore self-care behaviors and exercise routines. This will also intersect with our clinical expertise on learning styles and family stressors that may contribute to oppositional or hyperactive behavior (which may also be misdiagnosed or require reframing) as part of a comprehensive treatment approach. Above all my goal is to instill in the parents the hope and belief that their child can come into balance without the use of medications.

Q. I have been taking antidepressant and antianxiety medication for 12 years. I want to stop using these medications, but every time I stop I feel worse. Can you help me?

A. Oftentimes we work with people who are already on medication and want to come off the medications, and they want to know if nutrition can help them do that. No matter where a client is on her journey toward health, she will benefit from education about the role of food and diet in mental health. For example, I might begin a discussion about the role of refined foods and their effect on mood, or the effects of protein on neurotransmitter synthesis. As I am exploring some basic concepts about alternatives to medication, I can begin to discuss the self-care that is required to come off and stay off of medication, and again, I can encourage her that many thousands of other people have been able to successfully withdraw from and stay off medication.

Q. I have been eager to stop taking my medication, and I started taking some nutritional supplements and herbs that my friend told me worked the same way. Do you know about St. John's wort and 5-HTP and tryptophan?

A. Clients may reveal that they are combining a variety of prescription and nonprescription medications that may have harmful drug-nutrient-herbal interactions. They may also share what may appear to be radical dietary practices. Reviewing specifically what they are taking and exploring these interactions as well as identifying what practices they are adhering to and why sets the stage for informed decision making and improved efficacy. It also prevents unintended side effects.

Q. I have been through several rounds of CBT treatment for my eating disorder and while it has helped a lot, I still find myself craving certain foods. And if I don't eat that food I just end up hurting myself in another way. Do you think there may be certain foods that I am "allergic" to or addicted to that are making my disorder worse?

A. Clients in recovery from eating disorders and *body dysmorphia* may also have a history of self-harming behaviors and traumatic stress, all imbalances that respond very powerfully to nutrition and mental health when they are understood and treated together as co-occurring symptoms.

Q. I am under a lot of stress at work, and I am still 10 years away from retirement. I just don't have the mental focus and my memory seems to be failing me. I have been trying different nutrients I read about on the Internet, but I am not sure if they are working. What do you think would work best?

A. Increasingly, as the population ages, we are providing support to people with cognitive decline who are interested in staving off the negative effects of aging. They may ask about whether the research they have been reading on the Internet about *Gingko biloba* and turmeric is reliable. This provides an opportunity to explore their concerns. It may also lead to a referral for neuropsychological testing. It provides the therapist with an opportunity to share evidence-based research on prevention and treatment of cognitive decline.

Q. I am feeling a lot of pressure from my spouse to lose weight. But honestly I feel fine and I exercise several times a week and my blood tests look good. I am wondering what you think about my assessment, and if we might plan on a couples session to educate my spouse?

A. Many people are concerned with weight loss, especially if we work in the fields of behavioral medicine, hypnotherapy, and fitness. Likewise, clinicians can be susceptible to the belief system that even a little excess body fat is unhealthy. Friends, partners, and coworkers may also put pressure on our clients to lose weight or collude with them around unrealistic weight loss goals. However, there is growing evidence that having some excess body fat is actually healthier than a deficit of body fat. Thus, exploring a client's concerns about weight provides an opportunity to understand the meaning of their body weight, their sense of well-being, and their current nutritional habits, and it allows us to work with them to craft an overall wellness approach that focuses more on conditioning and well-being than numbers on a scale. This may also lead to family and couples work on these issues and can become a family nutritional wellness plan that honors each individual's unique needs. However, a discussion of body weight may also lead us to work with providers to conduct lab tests on thyroid or other hormone levels, address menopause or andropause, and further understand the intersection of physical well-being and mental health.

Unless you have identified with a specialty niche practice in mental health nutrition, clients may not discuss their questions without prompting. This is the value of the assessment process we explore in Chapter 3. In these cases, we may raise questions about nutrition as we work with a client to increase awareness about the connection between good nutrition and mental health. As I explore throughout this book, there are complex interrelationships between mental and physical health; indeed, it would be difficult to identify any mental health illness that did not have a physical symptom associated with it. Thus, we are on the front-line of educating our clients and helping them understand those relationships. Yet understanding the relationships between nutrition and mental health is only part of the process; carrying our change behaviors through self-care is the other necessary component.

Our clients often have chronic illnesses and seek help for depression or grief associated with functional illness. For example, depression resulting from chronic pain, traumatic brain injury, or diabetes is common and clients may experience problems enacting self-care. Often these clients have a difficult time with self-care because they feel they are being deprived of pleasures associated with food. Our work in nutrition and psychology can support these clients to reframe their illness and also help them find pleasure in new food choices. John's story is emblematic of the role nutrition plays in many of our clients' health (see Box 1.2).

Box 1.2
John's Story

John was 38 years old, recently divorced, and living alone. He arrived to therapy saying that he was always tired and moody. He had been diagnosed with ADHD since childhood and, more recently, bipolar disorder. He drank a lot of sodas, and sometimes he would not eat in the morning, or sometimes he just ate a donut with his coffee and creamer. He often grabbed a processed meat sandwich and French fries for lunch. He was taking three medications for blood pressure, cholesterol, and depression, and he used benzodiazepines to sleep. He worked as a supervisor and found himself increasingly snapping at his employees. He had the beginnings of a potbelly, his blood glucose levels were borderline high, and he was drinking beers at night to relax, though he often woke in the middle of the night if he did not medicate ahead of time. He expressed concern that he was using alcohol to self-medicate. He said he was always hungry and did not feel satisfied no matter what he was eating.

Together we reviewed John's dietary habits step by step and prioritized the kinds of foods he liked and disliked. We did a comprehensive medication history, symptom history, and a Food-Mood diary.

John was able to identify the same times of day that his mood and energy lowered, and these were also the times he became irritated at work. I identified hypoglycemia as a contributing factor to his mood lability. His chronic stress both at work or more recently due to his divorce, and the years leading up to it, had depleted his energy and taxed his adrenal function, which regulates glucose metabolism. He was using both stimulants and sedatives. He was able to concentrate and became more focused. Once he was less depressed, he felt more motivated to get a little exercise to increase his stress management. He started taking B vitamins, glucose tolerance factor, and fish oil. I suggested that he have one glass of red wine at night but earlier in the evening with his meal.

John's diet had deteriorated since his divorce due to stress, and he had never been responsible for preparing his food before. I educated him about the basic connections between food and mood and suggested that a change in his diet would also help his focus and attention. John's diary illuminated for him the patterns of his food and mood relationship. We began by identifying three positive changes he could institute in his diet and behaviors, and three behaviors or foods he would relinquish. He really liked bacon and eggs, and steaks, and thought he should not eat them due to his cholesterol levels. But I assured him he would benefit from eating those foods daily if he liked. And I proposed a 4-week plan after which we would assess his diet options. He agreed to include one fresh salad from a salad bar (but not use the bar salad dressings) and one piece of fruit daily and to begin cooking for himself by obtaining a Crock-Pot to prepare meat and potatoes. He agreed over the next 1 month to eliminate the donuts. I also suggested that he take a B-complex vitamin along with minerals. Fish oil would help his blood pressure and cholesterol, and help him focus, and supplemental taurine and magnesium would help lower his tension and blood pressure, and help him sleep. If he chose to drink one beer (instead of red wine), it would be a dark one, made with either hops or oats because it was richer in minerals.

By the end of the first week John began to feel more stable emotionally, had more energy, and was more satisfied with his diet. He was able to stop eating donuts but still was drinking more coffee. John also began taking nutrients and by week 2 felt more hopeful and in control. He was choosing some new restaurants to eat at, which is where he ate salad and proteins and whole grains and began inviting people to join him for some meals. By the end of the first month he was making a stew once a week at home. He eliminated sugar and reduced his coffee to two cups a day and he began to feel more stable. When he came in 3 months later he had dropped 10 pounds, was feeling much better, sleeping better, had begun dating, and said he now wanted to begin to reduce his medications.

SCOPE OF PRACTICE, LAWS, AND COMPETENCY

When integrating nutritional therapy into your practice, you will want to answer three questions. (1) The *scope of practice* of your discipline and whether it prohibits or can include the integration of providing nutritional therapies. This also intersects (2) *legal issues*; every state has different laws about the types of nutritional advice a professional or layperson can provide a client. Then, finally, consider your level of (3) *competency* to provide different types of nutritional counseling and therapies. For example, to suggest that a client stop smoking, or eat healthy fats, or stop drinking too much coffee to improve anxiety requires a basic level of competency. It requires a greater level of competency and confidence to suggest that a client use 300 mg of magnesium along with 450 mg of lactium (an anxiolytic milk protein) to decrease anxiety. In this scenario, one has a basic level of psychoeducation to impart to reduce anxiety. The next steps require knowledge of state laws as well as competency to make recommendations for nutrient recommendations. A third level of competency would be required if this same client has been on benzodiazepines for years and wanted to withdraw and use alternatives to the medication.

Scope of Practice

Mental health practitioners can integrate nutritional therapy at three levels of practice: psychoeducational, collaborative, and autonomous. The most basic and accessible level is where nutrition becomes a component of *psychoeducation* about wellness and self-care strategies. Much of what I talk about in this book falls within this area. Every clinician can feel competent in her or his ability to educate a client about the basic role of nutrition and the choices she makes to improve mental health.

Psychoeducation

Nutrition as psychoeducation involves making linkages between how and what clients eat and drink and the effect on their mental wellness. The Food-Mood diary and clinician checklist described in Chapter 3 help to explore basic self-care patterns and provide simple change steps. A review of a client's diary might lead to exploring how much caffeine a client is drinking in relation to her reports of anxiety and insomnia, or if she is eating breakfast or three or more meals a day, or eating enough protein or good-quality fats. Exploring food addictions is also within the scope of psychoeducation behaviors, along with healthy recipes and engaging family in food gathering and preparation. It might also include educating a family about the role of nutrition in ADHD or integrating these self-care strategies into group therapy for survivors of sexual abuse. At this level, nutrition-as-psychoeducation includes coaching for success and setting the stage for a deeper exploration that may lead to a collaborative relationship or a referral.

Collaboration

As we move along the spectrum of integrating nutritional therapies into mental health treatment, we move into an area where we may have more complex knowledge about the next steps a client may take, but we may not be licensed to evaluate, recommend, or prescribe based on that knowledge, or implementation may be beyond our current level of competency. This will then require a *collaborative relationship* with a more advanced nutritional professional or a professional who is licensed to design nutritional programs or to prescribe. For example, a client who we work with may want to stop his medications. We may have knowledge of the role of nutrition and the use of amino acids and fish oils, but if we are not the prescriber, we will want to coordinate our dietary and nutrient suggestions with the prescriber as we cocreate a withdrawal schedule and nutrient plan. Or perhaps we have a client who is depressed and also has type 2 diabetes and is on a variety of medications, including sleep medication. We believe that she will benefit from taking fish oil and a nutrient mix containing magnesium and glucose tolerance factor, but that these combinations will also synergize the benefits of medications and possibly lead to lowering blood sugar too much. Thus, we would coordinate and collaborate with the prescriber or another professional.

Autonomous Practice

The final area of scope is where we practice as an autonomous mental health nutrition professional. This will occur when a combination of competency, credentials, and state laws allows the clinician to fully integrate nutritional therapies into mental health counseling. Engaging in the scope defined at levels 1 and 2 may require additional training, certification or licensure, or years of clinical experience may lead to this stage.

As an autonomous practitioner you will include all or most aspects of nutritional therapies, including assessment and evaluation, ordering and analysis of nutritional laboratory tests, program design including prescriptive plans for treatment and medication withdrawal, and coaching for success, all of which are detailed in this book. However, because of client needs during the acute phase of withdrawal from medications, I always recommend a collaborative team approach, and I explore this in more depth in Chapter 8.

Similarly nutrition professionals may decide to obtain training and licensure in a mental health discipline.

Legal Issues

The practice of nutritional therapy in the United States is governed legally by each individual state. The Center for Nutrition Advocacy maintains an up-to-date database on the legal right to practice nutrition in each state. Because this is often changing, it is wise to explore the limitations for each state.

As a general rule, states define practice in this variety of ways:

- It is illegal to perform individualized nutrition counseling unless licensed or exempt. Effectively only registered dieticians (RDs) are eligible for licensure.
- It is illegal to perform individualized nutrition counseling unless licensed or exempt. There is a non-RD pathway for licensure.
- It is legal for all to perform individualized nutrition counseling; effectively, only RDs are eligible for government recognition and thus may be the only practitioners eligible for insurance reimbursement.
- It is legal for all to perform individualized nutrition counseling, though there may be limitations on insurance reimbursement eligibility (Center for Nutrition Advocacy, 2014).

Competency

Competency occurs in relationship to scope of practice and legal issues. Once you have determined the extent of practice allowed in your state, the next step is to explore your own competency. This book provides information that can be categorized into two broad areas. One comes under what we call "psychoeducation" or self-care education, which is basic nutrition and diet knowledge that anyone could share. The second category requires more knowledge and training, often involving the prescription of specific dietary regimens or nutritional protocols. However, the lines are blurred, and it is up to clinicians to understand where their competency is, as well as what is allowed under the license or certification they are practicing. Where the knowledge is of the second category, prescriptive, it is still useful to you as the clinician because you will be able to understand the state of the art in the field, with a working language that will enable you to effectively collaborate with nutritional experts on behalf of your client.

Because laws and requirements for practice vary state to state, there are also a variety of training programs, both online and onsite, as well as hybrid. At the end of this book I provide several resources for study that offer training, certification, and graduate degree programs. Investigating the quality and focus of each program along with its alignment with current state laws will be essential. The integration of nutritional therapy into mental health treatment is the revolution that is currently underway. There are significant opportunities for the clinician who specializes in this subject; however, even at a minimum, integrating basic nutritional education into a client's self-care program will reap benefits.

Competency Through the Inner Laboratory

There are two intersecting aspects that lead to competent care: the kind that derives from advanced training and clinical experience and the competency that comes from self-knowledge and experience. As mental health clinicians, we undertake some form of psychotherapy or counseling in order to engage the methods we ourselves will practice and to explore our own inner life in order to better serve our clients. This same principle should be applied to our work in nutritional therapies when advising clients about strategies for improving well-being. This suggests that we enter into our own health and healing using ourselves as a laboratory to explore the methods and practices that we propose. While we may not need to undertake every method, or eat every food or nutrient we will suggest, we should have an ongoing self-care plan rooted in healthy nutrition, supplementation, and detoxification.

This also provides an important self-care method for coping with the stressors of mental health practice, and it provides insight into the challenges our clients will face as they undertake change. Just as mental well-being is a lifelong process, so is changing nutritional behavior a dynamic experience that should be responsive to changing requirements of the life cycle.

The level of disclosure of one's own nutritional practice with a client will be a reflection of one's theoretical orientation. We will at times serve as a therapist, role model, guide, and coach. As a general rule, I think it is helpful to let the client know that we are on a path of health that incorporates nutritional change and the ways in which it has been helpful, without necessarily disclosing a lot of specific details or reasons for specific methods or nutritional protocols, just as we wouldn't reveal what medications we might be taking.

WHY GOOD FOOD PREPARATION AFFECTS MENTAL HEALTH

Diet Essential: *Prepare fresh foods daily.*

Preparing fresh food is an act of self-nourishment, emotionally as well as physically. The stressors of trauma, modern life, and advertising cause us to dissociate from the simple self-care rituals that invigorate us. Many of the suggestions throughout this book are about overcoming the conditioned responses that result from the incessant message that what we put into our bodies doesn't matter to mental health. Food gathering, preparation, and sharing is a ritual that, when done well, leads us into the parasympathetic state of relaxation and provides the endorphin rush of attachment and connection. This is often a lost ritual, though we do still gather for holidays or special events. Infusing each step of the nutritional process with a ritual or mindful process enhances relationships and digestion and well-being. The rituals of food preparation and sharing are rhythmic and repetitive, requiring integration of both the right and left hemispheres of the brain. It helps us to realign within our own nervous system and to synchronize with the nervous systems of others. This social connection is where mental health nutrition begins.

One of the basic themes to consider throughout this book is that good, "real" food is medicine and "fake" food is toxic to brain health. The second theme is that many foods are psychoactive; that is, they alter consciousness and, like all things that alter consciousness, some foods may be beneficial or detrimental to mental well-being. The altering of consciousness is not the problem; it is the choice of substance and its effects that become problematic. Hence, my approach is to suggest choosing one's "food-as-drugs" wisely, with awareness, and finding the best "substitutions" to enhance mental health and "withdraw" from the dangerous "food drugs." For example, one of the adages I teach my clients is: "Coffee is a drug, not a beverage." So use it like a drug—to achieve a desired, beneficial effect, not like an overconsumed beverage that causes negative side effects.

Real Comfort Food

If food is not satisfying and at times even comforting, dietary changes will not be sustained.

We often turn to food to comfort stress or unpleasant emotions, which is not inherently a bad thing. It is the fact that we turn to unhealthy, high-carbohydrate, high-sugar, processed foods for comfort. We can use food as part of a self-comforting strategy if we do it with awareness and make choices that will enhance our health rather than put us into a soporific state. There is nothing wrong with wanting and having comfort foods, but the key is not to eat them to excess and to explore if they become more than the occasional strategy.

What are comfort foods? Comfort foods are probably different for everybody, but in general they are usually high-fat, high-sugar, refined carbohydrate foods. These sugars and fats release opioids in the brain, similar to the way narcotics do, creating a pleasure response. Even thinking about these foods can trigger these brain reactions, just like imagining juicing a lemon will stimulate salivary flow.

Our definition of comfort food often comes from our childhood and what our parents gave us to calm us down in times of distress, or these foods may be associated with love; it might be sugary foods like donuts, cookies, and refined carbohydrates. In my family it was chicken fat on rye bread sprinkled with lots of salt. Others may have enjoyed white rice or white pasta with butter and salt, tapioca pudding, or Froot Loops and milk. White foods in general seem to be common comfort foods—think potatoes, bread, sour cream, bananas, and sugar. Comfort food may provide a nostalgic feeling related to cultural or familial traditions. Culturally related comfort foods have made a comeback in restaurants specializing in comfort foods.

Often we go to comfort food when we haven't had a chance to prepare healthy foods. What might you prepare in advance to preempt the need for comfort but to satisfy and nourish yourself?

Principle of Substitutions

We crave foods for a variety of reasons: We need the nutrients they offer, and the body provides a message to eat that food. People often remark that they get a craving for beef, for example. We also crave foods that we are allergic to; these foods function like a drug. Wheat and gluten are highly allergenic to people for whom it triggers opioid-like reactions. We crave food that reminds us of a certain time in our life, linked to people we have loved and lost, or comfort foods that are linked to our country of origin or holiday times. We also crave foods to alter consciousness; for comfort and anxiety reduction (carbohydrates and fats), and energy and focus (proteins and dopamine-rich coffee). Foods we crave provide chemical reactions that the brain/mind wants and needs. The key is to understand one's unique "craving" profile and interpret the foods one craves and when, to understand the (emotional) biochemistry of the foods, and to find substitutions that address these needs but are healthier and without the side effects. This is the "principle of substitutions" (see Table 1.2), which means that you can find an alternative food to provide the same effect, by substituting a healthy food or substance for a less healthy one.

Comfort food examples may include grilled cheese, mashed potatoes, pancakes, bread, pizza, macaroni and cheese, frozen lasagna, spaghetti and meatballs, Danish coffee cake, fried chicken, fast food, pie, donuts, Chinese food, egg rolls, frosting, and chocolate. Each culture also has its own comfort foods; these include fish and chips, custard, pies, puddings, soups and stews, bangers and mash in Great Britain, *pierogi* from Poland, *kvas*, borscht from Russia, baked beans, meatloaf, macaroni and

TABLE 1.2

Substituting Unhealthy Comfort Foods With Healthy Options

Unhealthy Comfort Foods	Healthy Substitutions
Bread or sweets	Sweet potatoes
Sugary treats	Smoothie sweetened with stevia
Chocolate with sugar	Unsweetened cocoa powder with stevia/homemade stevia-sweetened chocolate candy
Cane sugar	Honey or maple syrup
Honey	Stevia
Coffee	Black tea, decaffeinated coffee, herbal coffee substitutes (roasted dandelion root, ramon nut [bread nut]), green tea, chai, or Turmeric-Rooibus Brain Chai (see recipe in Chapter 6)

cheese, fish sticks, pot pies, and chicken noodle soup in the United States. Many of these foods can still be part of a healthy "comfort" self-soothing plan by changing some of the ingredients. For example, making mashed potato (or mashed sweet potato) with ghee and sea salt; baked sweet potato fries dipped in homemade mayonnaise; gluten-free macaroni and cheese; homemade pizza with gluten-free crust, homemade sauce, and topped with vegetables and organic sausage; healthy homemade almond-chocolate treats; and coconut black rice pudding.

Essential First Steps

Now you are ready to start making changes to feel better physically, mentally, and emotionally, and to have more fun in the kitchen.

Even before a formal assessment, I work with clients to answer the following questions as a start to our discussions about their current nutritional self-care behaviors and to explore with them some initial questions:

- How many of my meals am I preparing?
- How many meals a week are "fast food?"
- How am I preparing my meals?
- Which foods make me feel good?
- Which foods make me feel bad?
- How do foods alter my consciousness?
- What foods do I like but don't often prepare?

- Who are my allies for change in the family?
- Who are my allies for change among my friends?

Another exercise to begin with is to make a food substitution list as provided in Table 1.3. The change process can be slow, so be gentle with yourself and your clients. Follow where your interest and energy takes you, and while a pinch of discipline is always useful, you don't need to have too heavy a hand. Most of our clients are already too hard on themselves; so gentle self-compassion is the key to long-term success . And above all, "trust your gut" as you embark on this adventure. We explore in the next chapter how the "gut" affects everything from the food we digest, to what nourishes our brain and body, as well as our emotional well-being.

Essential Next Steps
- Manage blood glucose levels.
- Eat breakfast, lunch, dinner, and a snack before sleep.
- Decrease stimulant foods if anxious.
- Reduce or eliminate sugar/refined foods.
- Eliminate "enriched" foods.
- Identify comfort foods.
- Plan healthy nutritional "substitutions."
- Consider your own "laboratory of competency."
- Explore state- and discipline-specific requirements for nutritional practice.

TABLE 1.3
Exercise: Make a Food Substitutions List

Building on our concept of substituting healthy foods for unhealthy ones but still satisfying our needs, try this exercise. Using two columns, make a list of the foods that comfort you in the left column. As you review the list, make a list of healthy substitutions for these foods in the right column. For example:

Comfort Foods You Enjoy	Healthy Substitutions
Wheat toast with butter and jam	Baked potato with all the fixings
Chocolate bar with sugar	Hot cocoa sweetened with stevia and real whipped cream
Fast-food French fries	Fries baked in olive oil and topped with cilantro mayonnaise dip

CHAPTER 2

The Second Brain: Trust Your Gut

Diet Essential: *Nourish the first and second brain.*

The discovery of the "second brain," also known as the enteric nervous system, has confirmed our experience that the "gut" communicates with our first brain. This second "brain" controls the digestive system via a complex network of over 100 million nerves and chemicals that send messages to the central nervous system, and this "brain" allows us to feel in our "guts." When we say: "I just feel in my gut that is right," or "my gut is telling me no," that sensation is the second brain communicating. Feeling and sensation are part of its function, and it is linked to our emotional lives and intuition. The majority of fibers in the vagus nerve carry messages from the digestive system to the brain. The feeling of "butterflies in the stomach" describes the physiological stress we experience in the gut. This "second brain" is a term coined by Gershon (1998). It controls the breakdown and absorption of foods, elimination of waste, and the rhythms of peristalsis that move food along the digestive tract. It takes food particles and transforms them into little chemical messengers that support our emotional and cognitive life. The revolution that has occurred is that we now know that it is this second brain that makes these little messengers, the neurotransmitters, and supports bacteria that help regulate brain function.

An important discovery of the last 30 years relevant to the second brain and mental health is the endocannabinoid (eCB) system. This system figures in mental health, nutrition, and especially, in pain and the addictions. Note the middle word root "canna" and you will note it is related to the word *cannabis*. This system was identified as functioning in the first and second brain when scientists first began to identify the parts of the brain that responded to cannabis, or marijuana. The eCB system is involved in all aspects of mental and physical health: the microbiome and gut permeability, the stress response, appetite, obesity and eating disorders, the experience of pain (McPartland,

Guy, & Di Marzo, 2014), and the "bliss states." The neurologist Russo (2004) proposes a concept called clinical endocannabinoid deficiency syndrome, which may contribute to migraine, fibromyalgia, irritable bowel syndrome, and psychological disorders. Knowledge of this system is also central to understanding why people with schizophrenia and posttraumatic stress disorder (PTSD) may use cannabis to self-medicate, and the ways in which medical cannabis represents a growing option for less toxic medical treatments for mental illness and chronic physical diseases.

Digestion occurs in a state of relaxation. Stress can slow down or stop the digestive process. When the nervous system goes into a "freeze, fight, or flight" response, it impairs digestive muscle contractions, reduces the secretion of digestive enzymes, and redirects blood flow away from the digestive organs where it is needed and instead floods the extremities and muscles with blood, which are now poised for an emergency.

Stress wreaks havoc on the digestive system, causing esophageal spasms (hiccups), a rise in stomach acid (heartburn), nausea, diarrhea, and constipation. It exacerbates the symptoms of digestive disorders like inflammatory bowel disease, stomach ulcers, and celiac disease (Iliades, 2014).

Chronic stress is also connected to allostatic load, which refers to the cumulative effects of the "wear and tear" on well-being. Allostatic load is of special importance to the second brain because the social stressors of poverty and discrimination, as well as environmental toxins, affect the ability to metabolize food, especially glucose. For example, the stress of poverty is linked to the stress of malnutrition and poor-quality nutrition on child and adult development. These stressors also include less access to quality nutrition at a time when even greater needs are placed on the mind and body for nourishment. Environmental toxins in poor urban centers are linked to higher rates of diabetes, and environmental toxins in the food supply are associated with earlier puberty in girls, which has a domino effect on risk factors like depression and sexual abuse. Incorporating socioeconomic context and the complex interplay of ethnicity and stress on mental health and nutritional status is essential to the nutritional change model I discuss throughout this book in order address affordability and health disparities.

Hormones are also an important part of the digestive process and function to regulate appetite and digestive juices. Nerves connect the brain, spinal cord, and digestive organs and release chemicals that stimulate either contraction or relaxation of the gastrointestinal (GI) tract muscles. Hunger hormones are produced and released by the stomach and small intestinal lining.

The first brain relies on the right mix of glucose and fat. If you do not consistently eat the correct combination of glucose and fats, you deprive the brain of its optimal fuel, frequently leading to hypoglycemia and ongoing cravings and hunger. Meals low in protein and fat and high in carbohydrates raise blood sugar, but they also drop sugar levels precipitously, sending the brain on a rollercoaster. These high glycemic meals impair satiety hormones and cause an increase in hunger hormones (Baum et al., 2006), which leads to overeating. These types of high-carbohydrate meals also result in fatigue. This pattern is common in people with mood lability, and they respond well to a diet low in carbs, high in animal and plant protein, and moderate in fat and vegetables. The "power lunch" refers to eating a lunch of protein and vegetables (no grains or alcohol) when negotiating an important contract or business exchange and gaining a mental edge by staying alert and awake without the sedating effects of grains and starchy carbohydrates.

STRESS AND DIGESTION

In order for digestion to function smoothly, one needs to be relaxed when eating. There is a long-time association between stress and digestive upset. This is mediated by the autonomic nervous system (ANS). Under normal circumstances the parasympathetic mode of the ANS is the autopilot that "automatically" drives the overall function of the digestive system, from the release of digestive enzymes and juices to peristalsis and elimination. In mental health we have long observed the relationship between anxiety and digestive problems. We once believed that anxiety drove the digestive problems, and thus we teach relaxation exercises that are helpful. This makes sense, as the parasympathetic system, our relaxation response, needs to be "on" for digestion to occur smoothly. However, we now know that the effect of the gut, or the digestive system, on anxiety and emotions in general is bidirectional due to the vast network of chemical messengers, the neurotransmitters that are produced in the gut. Mindfulness exercises such as the one provided in Box 2.1 help clients engage their relaxation response and enhance their awareness.

Box 2.1
Exercise to Teach Clients: Chewing the Raisin

To enhance parasympathetic nervous system function and relaxation, I guide a client through a series of mindfulness exercises beginning in the office and ask the client to complete the others at home and to share with other family members. Begin by reading aloud, allowing enough time to reflect on each observation and sensation:

Hold a raisin and observe it as though you are the first person to ever touch a raisin and you are investigating for the first time. See the raisin in all of its detail; observe every part of it—the wrinkles, the way the light shines on it. Touch the raisin and explore the texture and sensation. Smell the raisin and inhale its aroma; take note of how this fragrance may stimulate your stomach or mouth. Gently and slowly place the raisin in your mouth and, before chewing, take time to notice how it feels on your tongue and any other sensations you notice. Prepare to chew the raisin by slowly finding out how to position it for chewing. Chew the raisin a couple of times and notice what happens when you do, really tasting it in all of its subtle complexities. Before swallowing, notice how the texture of the raisin changes as you chew it. When you are ready, think about swallowing the raisin and experience the intention of swallowing. Then swallow the raisin. Afterward, see if you can feel the raisin as it moves to your stomach. Observe how you feel after this exercise in mindful eating.

Neurotransmitters

Neurotransmitters (NTs) are brain chemicals that communicate information throughout our brain and body. They relay signals between neurons. They affect mood, sleep, concentration, weight, carbohydrate cravings, and addictions, and they can contribute to depression, pain, anxiety, and insomnia when they are not in balance. Research continues to illuminate the ways that foods affect how NTs are made in the gut and how, in turn, this affects the brain and mind. Friendly bacteria play a role in the production of gamma-aminobutyric acid (GABA), the "antianxiety" NT illuminating the complex relationship between the brain and the gut. The gut and the brain regulate eating behavior and appetite by way of NTs. Dopamine and serotonin are the two primary neurotransmitters associated with the regulation of food intake (Bello & Hajnal, 2010; Capasso, Petrella, & Milano, 2010). For example, when people start selective serotonin reuptake inhibitors (SSRIs), or the serotonergic amino acid 5-HTP, they can become nauseated by the increase in serotonin levels in the gut. Stress impairs digestion, and poor digestion affects the neurochemicals that influence mood and well-being. Like the brain, the second brain uses over 30 NTs, and 95% of the serotonin in the body is located in the gut. High levels of serotonin are also linked with irritable bowel syndrome (Hadhazy, 2010).

Impaired digestion of protein means the amino acids are not available to the brain to support NT production, directly affecting mood, sleep, and cravings. The overuse of antibiotics, along with insufficient prebiotics in the diet to prepare the garden of the intestines to grow healthy gut microbiota, impairs the production of

NTs and subsequently causes mood problems like depression and anxiety. Most antidepressants are believed to work by increasing the availability of specific neurotransmitters, but this theory is unproven; they often have side effects, lead to chemical imbalances, have limited efficacy (especially in mild to moderate depression), and become less effective over time. The theory of mood disorders as primarily based in NT imbalance is giving way to a more holistic understanding of multiple influences on mood and cognition of which NT function is only one. Indeed, the groundbreaking work by Kirsch et al. examined the role of the placebo effect on depression and suggested that there is no significant difference between antidepressant effect and placebo effect except in the severely depressed, and for the severely depressed it is "the relationship between initial severity and antidepressant efficacy [that] is attributable to decreased responsiveness to placebo among very severely depressed patients, rather than to increased responsiveness to medication" (2008, p. 266).

In Chapter 7, I explore the use of amino acid therapy as an adjunctive or alternative method of influencing NTs, as a natural approach to antidepressant and anti-anxiety medications. These pharmaceutical-grade amino acids may be compounded according to the specific biochemical needs of the individual to provide the building blocks that support specific NT production.

Essential Behavioral Steps for Relaxed Digestion

- Eat in places that induce relaxation rather than places where one feels stressed.
- Employ rituals such as communal eating, giving thanks, and potlucks; this can also reduce stress and improve digestion.
- Breathe slowly and rhythmically before eating and during the meal.
- Eat with others when possible and without the distraction of the TV or computer.
- Put the fork or spoon down between bites and let it sit for 15–30 seconds or more.
- Chew food 50 times or until almost liquid.
- Set nutrients on the table in the kitchen organized by whether they are to be taken before the meal, during the meal, or after the meal.
- Additionally, smoking, caffeine, and alcohol consumption all impair digestion and affect the stress response. Reducing or eliminating these three major stress factors should be included in goal setting early on with the client.

Mindful eating (see Box 2.2) is an exercise that may be discussed in the office and practiced at home.

Box 2.2
Exercise: Mindful Eating

Observe yourself chewing. Pay attention to the texture and flavors of the food, the smells, and the position of the food on the plate. Embrace the whole of the sensory experience. The production of saliva breaks down the food and tends to enhance the experience of texture and flavors on different parts of the tongue. Chew every bite until it is liquid in the mouth, allowing the food to travel down the throat and into the belly.

HOW FOOD NOURISHES YOUR BRAIN, MIND, AND EMOTIONS

Food is made up of carbohydrates, proteins, fats, water, vitamins, and minerals. Carbohydrates are sugars, starches, and fibers, either simple (as in fruits, vegetables, and sugars) or complex (as in whole grains, starchy vegetables, and beans). The purpose of digestion is to break down these foods into smaller particles so they can be absorbed in the bloodstream and used throughout the body. Digestion releases the nutrients in food so that the body utilizes them. This process takes place in the gastrointestinal tract. Carbohydrates break down into glucose, which supports brain function; proteins, from meat, beans, eggs. and dairy products, are broken down into smaller molecules called amino acids, which are the building blocks of neurotransmitters that also support brain function. Fats provide energy for the body and the brain, which is mostly made up of fats.

Fats are a macronutrient that provides energy and lubrication for the brain and insulation for body organs and the body generally. They are essential for the absorption of nutrients, particularly the fat-soluble vitamins A, D, E, and K. These vitamins require fat for transport to cells. Low-fat diets, for example, may be a poor mental health risk factor due to inadequate levels of these essential vitamins.

There are three main categories of dietary fats that are required for good mental health: saturated fats, monounsaturated fats, and polyunsaturated fats.

Fats

Saturated Fatty Acids

Traditional fats such as butter, coconut, tallow, and suet (from cows and lambs); fat from ducks, geese, chickens, and turkeys; and lard from pigs are all "saturated" fats. They are "traditional dietary fats" since they have been used in cooking for thousands of years before the development of commercially created saturated fats such as shortening and margarine. Natural saturated fats are normally solid at room temperature. This type of fat includes different fatty acids such as butyric acid (found in butter), lauric acid (found in coconut oil and palm oil), myristic acid (found in dairy products), palmitic acid (found in meat and palm oil), and stearic acid (found in meat and cocoa butter). These fatty acids exhibit antibacterial, antifungal, and anti-inflammatory properties that help to protect the body.

It is a medical myth that saturated fats are dangerous. Saturated animal fats (from pasture-fed livestock) provide fat-soluble vitamins A, D, and K2. Eating saturated fats has been shown to lower Lp(a), which is an indicator of heart disease risk. Saturated fats stimulate prostaglandin 3, which is a pain-reducing anti-inflammatory, and exert a protective anti-inflammatory effect mediated via the vagus nerve and cholinergic anti-inflammatory pathways through the activation of cholecystokinin and nicotinic acid receptors (Luyer et al., 2005). If you do not eat enough fats, the body can make saturated fats out of refined carbohydrates. It is this process of high carbohydrates converting to triglycerides that raises triglycerides in the body (not saturated fat consumption). This process is associated with depression and vital exhaustion (Igna, Julkunen, & Vanhanen, 2011).

The Dangers of Trans Fatty Acids

A commercially created form of fat that does not occur in nature is called "trans fat." Trans fats are a contaminant by-product of commercial hydrogenation of vegetable oils. The process of hydrogenation renders liquid vegetable oils as creamy, spreadable substances that are used to make margarines and baking shortenings, but the high temperature needed to produce the products breaks down the vegetable fats and creates trans fats. Preparing foods with hydrogenated oils may result in food containing high levels of trans fats.

Changing diets to include healthy fats for brain function is one positive behavior that is easy to accomplish. The second behavior required is to eliminate the use of unhealthy fats or trans fatty acids. The scientific evidence is strong that trans fats consumed in even limited amounts interfere with the delta-6 desaturase enzyme and other enzymes necessary for the conversion of Omega-3 and Omega-6 to essential fatty acids (to sustain life) necessary for cellular and organ health (Enig, 2000). Essential fatty acids (EFAs) are those fats that are required for body health, cannot be synthesized by the body, and must be obtained from dietary sources.

Most commercially processed foods, such as cookies, margarine, shortening, crackers, chips, salad dressings, and snack foods, contain trans fatty acids from ingredients such as "partially hydrogenated" oils of any kind, as well as deodorized vegetable oils and monoglycerides and diglycerides.

Polyunsaturated Fatty Acids

Polyunsaturated fats (PUFAs) include soybean oil, corn oil, sunflower oil, and fatty fish such as salmon, tuna, herring, mackerel, and sardines. These oils containing PUFAs are normally liquid at room temperature and solid when cooled. Nuts, seeds, fish, and leafy greens also contain polyunsaturated fats. There are two types of essential fatty acids (Omega-3 and Omega-6) that may be derived from polyunsaturated fats. Omega-9 is another, but it is a nonessential fatty acid since the body can convert Omega-3 and Omega-6 to produce Omega-9. It is a valuable fatty acid obtained from avocados and avocado oil. Two absolutely essential Omega-3 fatty acids, eicosapentaenoic acid (EPA) and docosahexaenoic (DHA), must be obtained from dietary sources such as fatty fish and nuts. They are the building blocks for hormones that control immune function, blood clotting, and cell growth as well as components of cell membranes.

The use of polyunsaturated vegetable oils, such as corn, linseed/flax, safflower, soy, and walnut oil, and also those found in margarine and shortening, has increased as people have turned away from using animal fats like lard and butter. Polyunsaturated fats are low in saturated fat and are cholesterol-free, but they become rancid more easily and are more toxic when used for frying and are thus more likely to cause inflammation.

Margarine and shortening also contain hydrogenated polyunsaturated vegetable oils, which contain trans-fatty acids (see earlier). Avoid any products with ingredients preceded by "hydrogenated" or "partially hydrogenated." Polyunsaturated oils are also known to cause sterility and impaired immune function. Notably, liver damage, impaired reproductive health, damage to the lungs, digestive disorders, learning delays, weight gain, and neurological problems are frequently associated with polyunsaturated oil consumption.

Monounsaturated Fatty Acids

Monounsaturated fats (MUFAs) are obtained from vegetable sources such as avocado and avocado oil, olives and olive oil, and tree nuts. MUFAs include palmitoleic acid and oleic acid—oils that are normally liquid at room temperature and solid or semisolid when cold. Olive oil is best eaten raw and not used in cooking. It is well known for its medicinal benefits on the gallbladder and for its rich source of chlorophyll, which detoxifies the intestinal tract. Other healthy foods containing MUFAs are full-fat dairy products and red meat from lamb, beef, and wildlife, such as deer, elk, moose, and bear.

Essential Fatty Acids

Introducing good-quality fats into the diet as both foods and supplements and eliminating poor-quality fats is a primary way to begin a nutritional program of recovery. Essential fatty acids (EFAs) are fats that are essential and must be obtained through foods. They are essential to health and recovery. The Inuit located in or near the Artic Circle, whose diet consists of up to 70% animal fat and protein, showed few signs of mental illness or heart disease prior to the introduction of nonlocal foods to their diet. The primary essential fatty acids are Omega-3 (linolenic acid), Omega-6 (linoleic acid), and arachidonic acid (AA). The brain is made up of 60% fat, called docosahexaenoic acid (DHA). A variety of fish oils from krill, sardines, salmon, and cod can easily be integrated into the diet. A complement of fats from animals, vegetables, nuts, and seeds extracted via a "cold process" should be integrated into a daily diet for health with all other oils, along with the much-maligned egg, rich in choline, for the brain and memory.

Phospholipids are a special type of fat that comprise neuron membranes and support communication between neurons. Think of the layers in lasagna; without the various fillings, lasagna would not taste like much or even do much since the pasta needs the filling to really add the "zest." Such are phospholipids to brain cells. Significant research demonstrates that problems in phospholipid metabolism contribute to major depression, schizophrenia, and bipolar disorder (Eggers, 2012; Horrobin, 2001; Leyse-Wallace, 2008), suggesting a role for both testing and supplementation of eicosapentaenoic acid (EPA) as well as phosphatidyl serine and phosphatidylcholine in these disorders in particular (Eggers, 2012).

Carbohydrates

Carbohydrates are the second category of food nutrients. Carbohydrates function primarily to regulate fat metabolism and thus generate energy for daily living. Protein, fats, and carbohydrates all work together to support the engine of the brain—sugar, glucose, amino acids, and fats, which lubricate and ease connection at the synapses. Too much or too little of different kinds of nutrients creates imbalances that have a negative effect on mood and cognitive function. For example, too much glucose from a diet high in refined carbohydrates is now considered a risk factor for dementia—now referred to as type 3 diabetes. An annual HbA1c test, as explained in Box 2.3, can provide information on Alzheimer's risk due to blood glucose levels.

Box 2.3
Blood Glucose and Alzheimer's Risk

The HbA1c test assesses an average blood glucose level over the previous 3 to 4 months. Because HbA1c is a glycation of the hemoglobin protein, the test is also a marker of protein glycation. When HbA1c levels are elevated, as they are in diabetes, it indicates that proteins including hemoglobin are being glycated. When proteins are glycated, inflammatory cytokines and free radical production is increased, leading to oxidative stress, which is a significant risk factor for Alzheimer's and brain shrinkage.

Carbohydrates are made up of sugar molecules and are either simple or complex. A single sugar molecule is known as a simple sugar, whereas many sugar molecules bonded together in a chain is called a complex carbohydrate, or starch. Sugar is the simplest form of carbohydrate and is found in fruit, vegetables, dairy products, and refined sugar. Complex carbohydrates are either starch or fiber. Starchy vegetables, such as carrots, potatoes, and peas, and grains, such as wheat, rice, barley, and oats, are sources of starch. Starches can also be from refined foods, such as cornstarch, chips, and certain dessert foods. Complex carbohydrates provide necessary fiber in the diet. Grains are a particular type of carbohydrate. Most people will do well on fruits and vegetables, and some will do well with grains, though some clinicians, such as the neurologist Perlmutter (2014), suggest that grains should be avoided altogether because they are detrimental to cognitive function in particular.

Carbohydrates provide the body with the energy that it needs. Carbohydrates require enzymes, such as amylase and lactase, to break down into simple sugars like glucose in order to be used by the body. The salivary glands and the pancreas secrete amylase. Lactase is produced in the small intestines and breaks down lactose, the sugar found in milk and dairy products.

Proteins

Proteins are the third category of nutrients essential to both mental and physical health. They fuel every function of living cells. Proteins are derived from either animal or plant sources, and they must be broken down by digestion into amino acids in order to be used by the body. Animal proteins such as whey, eggs, beef, casein, and fish differ from plant proteins such as soy, pea, hemp, and rice in many ways, including cholesterol and saturated fat levels, digestion rates, allergens, and their amino acid profiles.

Protein Requirements

Everyone has a different need for protein relative to her or his individual biochemistry. Some need more protein than others. However, during times of stress they are more essential; they support growth and repair in the body, which tends to break down under stress. A broad approach to calculating protein needs is to identify the optimal daily ratio of protein that is about 0.5 grams of protein for every pound of lean (muscle) body mass. A person with 20% body fat mass has 80% lean mass. So for someone who weighs 200 pounds, the lean mass is 160 pounds. To determine the protein requirement, divide 160 by 2.2, which converts pounds to kilograms, resulting in 72.7 grams of protein. Protein requirements increase if one is doing vigorous exercise, and women generally need less protein. People who eat the standard American diet tend to overconsume poor-quality protein at nearly twice the amount that is necessary, while vegetarians tend to underconsume proteins. Both approaches are problematic for mental health. Protein from animal foods have better amino acid profiles than plant proteins, meaning they have higher amounts and proportions of the essential amino acids. Another challenge in vegetarian diets is the failure to consistently combine proteins that have complete amino acids, and this leads to deficits in NT synthesis.

It is important to address both quality and quantity when determining protein requirements. Eggs are a perfect protein and provide about 5 grams of protein per egg, the equivalent of a handful of nuts or seeds. Milk and yogurt provide about 10 grams of protein per cup (milk products are best eaten raw and unpasteurized). Beans, cottage cheese, and tofu each provide about 15 grams of protein per cup. Meat, chicken, and fish provide about 25 grams of protein per 3- to 4-ounce serving.

Proteins along with vegetables are also part of the satiety complex. Proteins such as nuts, seeds, and whey, along with greens, cruciferous vegetables, and root vegetables, all promote satiety (Baum et al., 2006), which is important especially when making dietary changes and in hypoglycemia, compulsive and night eating disorder, and bulimia. Raw almonds are an ideal food to eat as a snack or at the start of a meal. This may underlie the wisdom of Ayurvedic medicine that suggests eating 10 raw almonds a day for brain health and relaxation. I can think of no simpler daily habit to support brain health and a relaxed mood.

Protein Deficiency

Insufficient protein intake is not always the problem; rather it is often the inadequate digestion of proteins that causes protein deficiency. Before protein is available for the body to use, it must be broken down into more digestible forms. Insufficient hydrochloric acid is one cause of poor protein digestion, as hydrochloric acid is needed to break protein down into its constituent parts. Without enough hydrochloric acid, proteins are not fully digested, nutrient absorption is reduced, and satiety signals to the brain are impaired. Antacid use is another cause.

Protein deficiency is most likely to occur in people on a strict vegetarian diet who do not consume adequate amounts of plant proteins, or who do not combine them to obtain the complement of all amino acids. Bulimia, fruitarian diets, diets high in refined carbohydrates, and alcoholic liver damage also contribute to protein insufficiency, which in turn affects amino acid and NT levels. Symptoms of protein deficiency include a lack of mental focus, emotional instability, impaired immune function, fatigue, hair loss, and slow wound healing.

FIRST THINGS FIRST—CHEWING AND THE DIGESTION IN THE MOUTH

Diet Essential: *Eat only when relaxed.*

The gastrointestinal (GI) tract is a long system of hollow organs that are joined together, creating an unbroken tube that begins at the mouth and ends at the anus. These organs include the mouth, esophagus, stomach, small intestine, large intestine, rectum, and anus. The liver, gallbladder, and pancreas are additional, solid organs that play essential roles in the digestion of food. Food enters the mouth, is chewed and reduced by saliva, which adds a lubricating antibacterial fluid that helps food travel down the esophagus. From there it travels into the stomach, where powerful stomach acids break it down so it can be further absorbed. The liver and gallbladder digest fats, and when the foods are washed with pancreatic juices rich in enzymes, the food is called chyme. If foods are not fully broken down, they can ferment in the digestive tract. Imagine filling a pot with meat and vegetables and putting it on the stove but neglecting to light the fire to cook it. What would happen? Over a few hours into days it would start to ferment and sour, bubble and smell. This happens in the belly of someone who is not digesting her or his food. The bubbles result from gas, and the sour comes out in bad breath and flatulence.

Digestive enzymes help break down food, much like a fire on the stove prepares food to be eaten. Enzymes break down food into nutrients that the body can absorb. The salivary glands, stomach, pancreas, and the intestines all secrete digestive enzymes. Digestive enzymes are also found mainly in raw foods, and they are especially rich in papaya and pineapple, making some raw foods *de rigueur* of every diet. Low and deficient enzyme levels may be responsible for food intolerances, most commonly to gluten, dairy, legumes, fruits, and vegetables, causing conditions like eczema and celiac disease.

Digestion starts in the mouth with the breakdown of starches by chewing and mixing food with salivary enzymes and finishes in the colon with the excretion of waste. Stress also affects digestion beginning in the mouth. If food is not chewed sufficiently, it can go down the esophagus in large chunks unprepared for further digestion.

Stress can also affect digestion at the esophageal sphincter, where like a drawbridge it may open when it is supposed to close or close when it is supposed to open. Sometimes it relaxes too much and closes on part of the stomach, pushing the stomach up. This is called a hiatal hernia. When the sphincter does not close effectively, this allows stomach acid to rise into the lower esophagus, causing acid reflux or gastroesophageal reflux disease (GERD). There are high rates of GERD in people with PTSD, suggesting the link between anxiety and GERD.

Mouth Digestion

Digestion of food also begins with how it is prepared. As a general rule, cooked foods are more easily digested than raw. Fuel in the form of food goes into the mouth and begins the process of digestion with the mechanical movement of chewing and the secretion of saliva, which breaks down starches.

Under stress, one eats too rapidly and swallows food whole; under stress, the acids and enzymes required to break down food cannot do their job. With food undigested in the belly, pains and gases develop, perhaps medications are used to quell the discomfort, nutrients are malabsorbed, and organs including the brain are malnourished. Eating food slowly allows for the initial breakdown of starches. Starchy carbohydrates require the enzyme amylase. The salivary glands store amylase and secrete it to aid in the digestion of sugars. There are two kinds of saliva—a thin, watery saliva that moistens the mouth and the food, and a thick, mucous saliva that lubricates the food and helps form it into a ball, called a bolus, which can then be swallowed.

The Esophagus and Stomach

The stomach receives the fuel, which should already be predigested by the salivary enzymes. The stomach acid then digests proteins. Proteins are large food molecules that need to be broken down by proteolytic enzymes into their smaller components called amino acids, which in turn are the building blocks of neurotransmitters. Proteins are either animal based (meat, seafood, eggs, dairy) or plant based (beans, nuts, seeds). The muscle of the stomach churns the food up and mixes it with the gastric juices. This is what we call the digestive fire. Without stomach acid, food would not be digested. This is another place where stress can interrupt digestion.

Pepsin is secreted by the stomach and begins the process of protein digestion, and the pancreas secretes trypsin, chymotrypsin, and proteases into the small intestines; the pancreas also secretes proteases. Proteolytic enzymes, also secreted by the pancreas into the small intestines, break down proteins that were not fully digested by the stomach. Proteins and fats are not absorbed when there is a lack of pancreatic enzymes, and this can lead to nutritional deficiencies.

Insufficient gastric acid secretion is known as hypochlorhydria. When food is not broken down because of hypochlorhydria, it moves into the small intestine and colon undigested and the body is not able to make use of it. Absent the ability to break down proteins, the second brain cannot make the NTs such as tyrosine and tryptophan required for healthy neurotransmitter production for the first brain. This condition frequently results in anxiety, depression, pain, chronic indigestion, food allergies, and asthma.

Hydrochloric acid (HCl) is produced by the stomach and contains enzymes that help break down proteins. Gastric acid production decreases with age, and a lack of HCl can cause other digestive problems like small intestinal bacterial overgrowth (SIBO) because of elevated pH levels. SIBO inhibits nutrient absorption and assimilation of the B vitamins folate, B6, and B12, resulting in major depression (Logan & Katzman, 2005), and low HCl in general is associated with increased levels of anxiety. It now becomes ever more clear why, over time, poor digestion means poor mental (and physical) health.

Symptoms of Low Stomach Acid Production
- Feeling full after eating
- Multiple food allergies
- Gas, bloating, belching, burning, flatulence after meals
- Indigestion, diarrhea, constipation

- Undigested food in stool
- Abnormal intestinal flora or chronic Candida infections
- Nausea when taking supplements
- Brittle nails
- Dilated capillaries in the cheeks and nose (not related to alcoholism)
- Iron deficiency
- Adult acne

Hydrochloric acid (HCl) production can be stimulated and increased by the use of supplemental HCl, which also destroys harmful stomach bacteria, and increases nutrient absorption. HCl also requires zinc, copper, iron, magnesium, boron, calcium, selenium, and vitamins B3 and B12 to do its job efficiently, and supplementing with B12 and folate will support HCl production and the absorption of proteins.

The Liver and Gallbladder

While the stomach is adding fire to the mix, the gallbladder is emulsifying the fats needed to elevate mood and decrease stress as well as to maintain artery health and reduce inflammation. The brain is mostly fat in the form of docosahexaenoic acid, and neurons require fats to function smoothly, just like a car needs lubrication. Without access to good fats or the ability to use these fats, the brain does not get the fuel it requires. If the gallbladder is not functioning well, dietary fats or fish oil supplements will be less effective because those nutrients cannot be emulsified and assimilated.

Normally, the liver and gallbladder work together to emulsify fat, just like dish soap breaks down the grease in a frying pan. Bile, which is made up of bile salts, cholesterol esters, and lecithin, emulsifies the fats and separates them into smaller fat globules so they can pass through the digestive system. Contrary to conventional belief that one must follow a low-fat diet with gallbladder problems, a very low-fat diet can cause the gallbladder's "muscle motor" to slow down. This special muscle pushes out bile into the duodenum. When the muscle fails, it leads to a buildup of sludge like a stagnant pond that backs up. Good-quality oils, in particular a regular dose of olive oil mixed with lemon juice, avoids this immobility.

The word *bile* is derived from the Latin *bilis*, meaning anger or displeasure. Traditional Chinese medicine suggests the emotion of anger derives from a congested gallbladder and liver. Sayings like "That takes gall" or "I got my bile up" refer to the longheld belief that a congested liver/gallbladder results in anger and rage. Junk food, refined foods, trans fatty acids, and alcohol abuse contribute to chronic gallbladder congestion, low bile output, gravel, and gallstones. Other symptoms of gall-bladder problems include burping, flatulence, a feeling of heaviness after a meal, shoulder pain, pain under the ribs on the right side or in the back directly behind the diaphragm, and nausea. Awakening with bloodshot eyes after a heavy meal the night before is another sign of gallbladder distress.

Medical practitioners in the United States remove over 750,000 gallbladders annually. Treatable gallbladder disease is at epidemic levels and is at the heart of poor mental health. Poor liver and gallbladder function worsen stress and depression. Some medical researchers suggest that there is a genetic cause for gallbladder disease (and diabetes) within certain cultural groups, especially in American Indians and peoples south of the US border. But there was virtually no gallbladder disease among these peoples prior to the arrival of the "modern" standard American diet. Removal of the gallbladder only aggravates health problems by decreasing the capacity to digest foods and fats. Removing the gallbladder surgically is like throwing out the garbage pail instead of simply emptying it. Surgery for gallbladder conditions should always be avoided except if an individual's life is in immediate danger.

For those who have had their gallbladder removed, replacement supplements should include natural ox bile, betaine, taurine, vitamin C, and pancreatase to support fat digestion and alleviate the frequently persistent digestive difficulties people experience without a gallbladder. Beets and beet tops, which are rich in betaine, are among the best foods for gallbladder function and mental health in general.

Cholesterol as Hormone Precursor

Most cholesterol is made in the liver. Sufficient cholesterol is essential for mental health. Despite the popularized view that cholesterol is dangerous, I want to emphasize that cholesterol is necessary for proper brain and nervous system function, and it is an important part of our ability to use serotonin, thereby preventing depression. People have differing needs for cholesterol; some do well with total cholesterol at 240 and others do well at 180. For those whose cholesterol dips too low for their individual needs, anxiety may follow.

The body maintains a balance of cholesterol by producing more of the substance when insufficient amounts are available from food, and the total body cholesterol level reduces when quantities greater than needed by the body are consumed (Enig, 2000).

Cholesterol is frequently condemned as a major cause of heart disease, but this is untrue. Efforts to reduce cholesterol with diets extremely low in fat and with medications contributes to significant mental distress, including anxiety, muscle pain, and suicide attempts (Perez-Rodriguez et al., 2008). Statin drugs used to lower cholesterol, such as Lipitor, Pravacol, Mevacor, and Zocor, are known to cause significant side effects such as muscle wasting and weakness, heart failure, depression, cancer, and cognitive impairment. Numerous studies have demonstrated that there is no significant relationship between cholesterol intake and heart disease (McNamara, 2014) but rather that people with cholesterol below 200 consistently show lower cognitive functional capacity (Elias, Elias, D'Agostino, Sullivan, & Wolf, 2005). A recent study of 50,000 individuals in Norway found that women with total cholesterol over 200 mg/dL lived longer than those with lower cholesterol (Petursson, Sigurdsson, Bengtsson, Nilsen, & Getz, 2012). People with elevated homocysteine levels have a greater risk of cognitive decline. Low plasma cholesterol (160 mg/dL) may serve as a biological marker of suicidality (Vuksan-Ćusa, Marcinko, Nać, & Jakovljević, 2009) and is linked with depression and increased mortality from accidents and homicides (Leyse-Wallace, 2008).

Cholesterol is a precursor of hormones, the raw material for producing certain fat-soluble vitamins like vitamin D. Cholesterol is the liquid "band-aid" that is released to scout out and repair arterial inflammation frequently caused by trans fats, stress, manufactured foods, contamination from waste, and environmental toxins. The key to managing cholesterol levels is to reduce inflammation, not cholesterol per se. Hormones made by cholesterol are important for blood sugar regulation, mineral metabolism, and our ability to tolerate stress.

Restricting cholesterol in the diet reduces the amount of Omega-3 in the diet, and concurrently DHA levels are reduced. This affects the ratio of Omega-3's to Omega-6's, increasing Omega-6 levels, altering the membranes of brain tissues and increasing one's susceptibility to depression. In fact, in populations where Omega-3 intake is higher, the rates of depression are lower. Indeed, as I explore in Chapter 4, low cholesterol is implicated in autism spectrum disorders.

Cholesterol is also essential for the synthesis of vitamin D, the fat-soluble vitamin. Low levels of vitamin D are associated with chronic pain and depression (Vasquez, Manso, & Cannell, 2004). Cholesterol is also the precursor of glucocorticoids (necessary for blood sugar regulation), mineralocorticoids (essential for mineral balance), ligament strength, blood pressure regulation, and sex hormones. Cholesterol is also the foundation for pregnenolone, which serves as the predecessor to virtually all other steroid hormones (including progesterone, cortisol, aldosterone, and testosterone). Pregnenolone is synthesized in the central nervous system as well as the adrenal glands. Low levels are associated with depression, anxiety, and pain (Marx, 2009). Pregnenolone is also metabolized to allopregnenolone, an anxiolytic. It increases acetylcholine release, which is central to memory and focus and enhances the creation of neurons. Lowering cholesterol decreases the capacity to make pregnenolone. Pregnenolone is also an important ingredient of several brain nutrient support compounds required for brain recovery that I discuss in the next chapter.

Pancreas

The pancreas is an organ that functions as an exocrine and an endocrine gland. The pancreatic juices consist of proteolytic (protein-digesting) enzymes that help to further break down starches, fats, and proteins. As an exocrine gland, the pancreas secretes digestive enzymes into the small intestine that help to break down the chyme that has just left the stomach and entered the duodenum. The pancreatic enzymes secreted into the duodenum include the proteases trypsinogen and chymotrypsinogen, as well as amylase and lipase. Lipase is an enzyme that breaks down fats and is also secreted by the salivary glands. This important enzyme converts fats into compounds useful to the body such as fatty acids and glycerol. As an endocrine gland, the pancreas produces and releases hormones into the bloodstream that help regulate glucose metabolism and blood glucose levels. These hormones include insulin, which lowers blood sugar, and glucagon, which raises blood sugar.

Pancreatic enzymes, including supplemental proteolytic enzymes, improve mental health by reducing inflammation, as explained in Box 2.4.

Box 2.4
Proteolytic Enzymes Reduce Inflammation and Pain

Proteolytic enzymes serve two vital mental health functions:

1. When taken with food, these inexpensive enzymes help to digest food protein and they help to mediate food allergies. Protein-digesting enzymes produced by the pancreas can be further supported by supplementation.
2. When taken on an empty stomach, they "digest" inflammatory cells/proteins and improve immune function, reduce pain, inhibit the formation of fibrin in damaged tissues, and increase circulation to inflamed areas.

Food and supplement sources for these anti-inflammatories are papain (from green papaya), bromelain (from unripe pineapple), and serratiopeptidase (from the silkworm).

The Small Intestine

After food has digested in the stomach, it is released into the small intestine. The small intestine works by peristalsis, the involuntary, undulating, wave-like movements of a muscle that moves food along through the intestines by contracting and relaxing. Under stress, these natural peristaltic rhythms can be disrupted and stop all together, like jamming on the car brakes and backing everything up, or by accelerating and increasing wave action and dumping waste too quickly. Either stress effect leads to discomfort. The small intestines also secrete digestive juices and enzymes so that foods, water, and minerals can be absorbed by the small intestine and passed into the bloodstream, where they are processed further and utilized by the body. It is here that fatty acids and vitamins are absorbed by the lymphatic system, and simple sugars, amino acids, glycerol, some vitamins, and salt are brought to the liver. The essential role of nutrition and intestinal health to mental health is described in Jill's story in Box 2.5.

Box 2.5
Jill's Story

Jill was an accomplished, middle-aged musician who presented with chronic anxious depression, adult acne, and chronic colitis that at times interfered with her work. She was taking antianxiety medication and also medication for colitis. Her diet was very limited because she did not digest food well. She ate no fruits and no raw vegetables and ate a lot of toast and butter and chocolate milk. Her medical history revealed the use of antibiotics as a child, missed school days due to stomachaches, difficulty gaining weight, and acne. She had been tested for celiac disease, but those findings were negative. I referred her to a local naturopathic physician with the request to conduct more extensive testing that analyzed blood, saliva, and feces for food sensitivities to dairy and gluten, gut bacterial levels, and pancreatic enzyme levels. Testing showed there was indeed gluten and dairy intolerance, along with very low levels of digestive enzymes and harmful intestinal bacteria, Clostridium difficile. The naturopath and I consulted and agreed upon a nutritional therapy course of action. We agreed that Jill would benefit from high-dose probiotic supplementation, but if that did not overtake the C. difficile, she suggested a fecal transplant.

Jill eliminated gluten and cow's milk dairy immediately and began making simple meat and chicken broths. After a week she added some root vegetables and leafy greens to the broth and strained them so she could absorb the nutrients, but she still had reduced fiber.

We supplemented her diet with high-dose probiotics because antibiotics would only exacerbate her gut imbalance. However, by eliminating gluten and casein and by introducing probiotic supplementation and bone and mineral broths rich in gut-soothing gelatin, she experienced improvement in 6 weeks. Jill was able to eliminate colitis medication, and at 8 weeks her anxiety decreased and she was able to wean off of all her medications. At 12 weeks her acne, often a symptom of milk sensitivity, had virtually cleared. We continued our work together slowly and included small amounts of raw foods by 6 months. Jill did not miss any more days at work due to digestive problems, and she felt restored and was much happier.

The Microbiome of the Intestines

The intestine, and indeed the whole digestive tract, has come to be known as the *microbiome*. It is like your neighborhood community with people of all kinds: some friendly and some too noisy. Like your neighborhood, your microbiome is a community of a variety of microorganisms, some friendly and others not. A healthy neighborhood predominates with friendly people who cooperate and support each other and effectively manages the troublemakers. So it is with a healthy microbiome: It can tolerate some dissention but too much leads to illness that, if not addressed, can be damaging to the whole neighborhood (digestive system) and then affect the surrounding communities (brain, mental health). Furthermore, bacteria within the gut are manipulative (Alcock, Maley, & Aktipis, 2014) and both influence choices of food based on their needs, but in turn they can also be manipulated by our choice of foods.

Sometimes the bacteria are referred to as flora or microflora; the current term of reference is *microbiota* and the gut garden as a whole is called the *microbiome*, referencing the garden of living microorganisms that influence the whole organism. This microbiome is where the "gut-brain" connection plays on its seesaws, back and forth they communicate, feeding the neighborhood, including the first brain. Healthy intestinal bacteria populate the microbiome "garden" and when in abundance, keep levels of unhealthy bacteria from overpopulating. Healthy bacteria support the secretion and proliferation of neurotransmitters like GABA. Many GABA receptors are located in the stomach and esophagus. Healthy bacteria that populate the gut are essential for stress regulation and GABA, which leads to the reduction of anxiety (Bercik et al., 2011; Bravo et al., 2011).

One of our goals with nutrition is to support the healthy members of the community so the dangerous ones will go elsewhere.

Intestinal or "Gut" Permeability

Let's recall one of the essentials: *Where there is mental illness, there is poor digestion.*

The primary functions of the gastrointestinal tract are digestion and absorption of nutrients. Among the primary purpose of the intestines is to serve as the gatekeeper, a barrier mechanism to keep toxins and proteins out of the bloodstream that do not belong and to allow in those that do. Think of the drain in the kitchen sink. The finer the mesh, the more waste it collects, and the less problematic waste goes down the drain. The larger the mesh, the more particles get through and cause problems because they should not have breached the drain. Hence, the concept of "leaky gut" or intestinal permeability refers to when toxins and allergens breach this barrier.

Excess permeability allows molecules such as certain proteins from foods or toxins to enter the bloodstream, which contributes to allergies, autoimmune disorders, and inflammation. These toxins then travel to the brain and cross over a permeable blood-brain barrier. The blood-brain barrier is designed to protect the brain from unwanted substances and to allow those beneficial substances in that it requires. The blood-brain barrier is like the intestinal barrier subject to permeability that exposes it to toxins.

Symptoms of increased intestinal permeability include abdominal pain, food allergies and intolerances, and cognitive and memory problems. Increased intestinal permeability increases the risk of alcoholism, autism, ADHD, and multiple food and chemical sensitivities (Bland, 2004).

Intestinal permeability is an important problem that is common in all mental illness categories. One of the main reasons gluten and casein intolerance contributes to mental illness, including neurodevelopmental illnesses, is because it increases intestinal permeability (Herbert & Buckley, 2013; Pedersen, Parlar, Kvist, Whiteley, & Shattock, 2014; Whiteley, 2014; Whiteley et al., 2013). The gluten protein called gliadin triggers zonulin, a protein that increases the permeability between cells of the wall of the digestive tract, which leads to system-wide inflammation causing neurological, autoimmune, and mental health problems (Fasano, 2011).

In addition to zonulin and gluten gliadins, intestinal permeability is increased by a variety of factors, including low dietary fiber intake, excess of harmful microbiota, alcohol, age, Crohn's disease, cystic fibrosis, rheumatoid arthritis, ankylosing spondylitis, atopic eczema, HIV, and certain medications, especially NSAIDS and antibiotics. Because autoimmune disease is linked to higher rates of mental illness, and increased intestinal permeability is widely considered to contribute to autoimmune disease, patients with autoimmune disease should be screened for depression and then treatment should focus on improving intestinal permeability.

Stress also increases the intestinal permeability; it can lead to release of mast cells associated with allergic immune response and the release of inflammatory cytokines, which negatively affect GI function (Konturek, Brzozowski, & Konturek, 2011). Following gastric bypass surgery people frequently develop immune-related arthritis, due to the production of antigens by the intestinal bacteria, which then move into the bloodstream. This likely explains why short fasting periods (Sundqvist et al., 1982) and even antibiotic therapies followed by restoration of healthy flora benefit people with rheumatoid arthritis who suffer from high rates of depression.

Also associated with excess permeability is SIBO, which occurs when large numbers of bacteria grow in the small intestine, and cause symptoms similar to inflammatory bowel syndrome. It can occur in response to chronic use of nonsteroidal anti-inflammatory drugs (NSAIDS) (Muraki et al., 2014) and proton pump inhibitors. Herbal medicines have proved to be as effective as antibiotics in treatment (Chedid et al., 2014). Among the most effective natural antibiotic is oil of oregano.

The Large Intestine, Rectum, and Anus

Once nutrients are absorbed through the small intestines into the bloodstream, what is left is undigested food. This becomes a waste product that moves into the large intestine (colon), where any remaining water and nutrients are absorbed. As water is extracted, the waste becomes solid in the form of stool, which then passes via more peristaltic waves toward the rectum, which holds the stool until it is pushed out through the anus.

Stress and nutritionally related digestive problems can also affect the end of the alimentary canal, at the rectum and anus. For example, if fecal matter does not have enough fluid or fiber, it can lead to constipation and hemorrhoids. There is a significant association in children and adults between lower bowel function problems like hemorrhoids, constipation, and diarrhea and a history of sexual and physical abuse (Imhoff, Liwanag, & Varma, 2012; Rajindrajith et al., 2014). The combination of trauma treatment alongside nutrition is essential for improvement. This may include increased fiber and improving digestion through stress reduction, mindful eating, and belly self-massage (Korn, 2013).

FIBER AND FERMENTED FOODS— YOUR "BEST FRIENDS FOREVER"

Fiber intake is essential to a healthy colon and to mental health. There are digestible and nondigestible forms of fiber. The fiber sources that are indigestible carbohydrates are found in natural plant foods such as leafy green vegetables, fruits, legumes, nuts, and grains. Fiber has no calories or food energy, and yet it is a crucial component of a healthy diet. It passes through the digestive tract undigested, but in the process it sweeps up the debris along the colon walls and adds content to the digested food. Each day, women and men should obtain at least 25 grams and 38 grams of fiber, respectively. Fiber also causes the microbes in the gut to release a waste product called acetate, a short-chain fatty acid (Frost et al., 2014). Acetate goes to the hypothalamus and sends signals to stop eating, which then suppresses the appetite.

There are two types of fiber: soluble and insoluble. Soluble fiber slows down digestion by absorbing water and forming a gel in the digestive tract. It increases the feeling of fullness, and it slows down the rate at which the stomach empties, which also slows down the absorption of glucose, making it essential in the diets of people with diabetes. Soluble fiber is found in foods like oat bran, nuts, beans, lentils, psyllium husk, peas, chia seeds, barley, and some fruits and vegetables. In contrast, insoluble fiber does not dissolve in water, but rather it absorbs water and puffs up like a sponge, passing through the digestive tract and helping to push materials through. In this way it helps prevent constipation by providing a laxative effect. Insoluble fiber is found in wheat bran, corn, whole grains, oat bran, seeds and nuts, brown rice, flaxseed, and the skins of many fruits and vegetables.

Traditional or Paleolithic diets provide 10 times more fiber than the SAD diet. Also known as prebiotics, the larger quantity of fiber provides "soil" for the microbiome garden" of the colon and allows healthy bacteria to grow.

Prebiotics

Prebiotics set the stage in the colonic "garden" so probiotics or microbiota can flourish and not allow the harmful bacteria to propagate, much like healthy soil allows seeds to develop into fruit and be resistant to the effects of "pests." Prebiotics are soluble indigestible dietary fibers that support the beneficial gut microbiota (bacteria) that live in the colon. Prebiotics include raw and cooked onions, garlic, Jerusalem artichokes, leeks, asparagus, wheat, beans, bananas, agave and dandelion, and chicory root, often found in coffee substitutes.

Chia is an example of an exceptional prebiotic as it has a mix of both soluble and insoluble fiber and has the added benefit of being rich in Omega-3 fatty acids. Traditional dietary practices include drinking a glass of water each morning in which chia or flax has been soaked, thus providing fatty acids and fiber. While juicing has many benefits, its main detraction if done to the exclusion of eating whole fruits and vegetables is that it removes most of the fiber from foods.

Fermented Foods and Probiotics

Probiotics are beneficial live microorganisms that colonize the intestines, maintaining a balance of the beneficial gut microbiota (bacteria). There are 400–500 different kinds of healthy microbiota that inhabit the gut. They promote a healthy digestive system; prevent infections, diarrhea, and inflammation; and improve immune health. They also produce nutrients, such as vitamin K, B vitamins, some short-chain fatty acids like lactic acid, and folate. Preliminary research on the oral administration of GABA derived from *Lactobacillus hilgardii* fermentation has been shown to reduce anxiety (Bested, Logan, & Selhub, 2013).

Probiotics are also called "psychobiotics," referring to "a live organism that, when ingested in adequate amounts, produces a health benefit in patients suffering from psychiatric illness" (Dinan, Stanton, & Cryan, 2013, p. 720). These bacteria produce both GABA and serotonin and have been shown to reduce stress and decrease anxiety. Maintaining healthy bacterial levels in the gut supports NT activity in brain health. Early-life stress sensitizes specific gut microbiota to later life stress exposure. One study showed that lactobacillus, found in the traditional Korean food kimchi, increased hippocampal brain-derived neurotrophic factor (BDNF), a protein in the brain involved with neuronal survival (Jung, Jung, Kim, Han, & Kim, 2012).

The lack of intestinal microbiota has been shown to negatively affect health. *Lactobacillus GG* is safe at an early age and helps to reduce food allergies and associated inflammation. One of the reasons that breast-fed babies are thought to have fewer allergies is because breast milk contains beneficial microbiota. Even coming through the birth canal and being washed with the mother's bacteria provides improved immune system health in contrast to Cesarean-section-born children.

Sources of probiotics include fermented foods like sauerkraut, kombucha, kimchi, miso, micro-algaes, brewer's yeast, as well as yogurt and cheeses with live cultures, and probiotic supplements. Yakult is a probiotic drink made in Japan that has been shown to reduce bladder infection recurrence. One should ingest probiotic foods (or supplements) daily.

Varieties of Probiotics

Lactobacillus acidophilus is a lactic acid bacteria found in yogurt and kefir containing live and active cultures, kimchi, kombucha, fermented soy products, and dietary supplements.

- *Lactobacillus casei* is a lactic acid bacteria found in yogurt and kefir containing live and active cultures, naturally aged cheeses that are not pasteurized, and milk.
- *Lactobacillus bulgaricus* converts lactose and other sugars into lactic acid. It is found in foods like Swiss cheese and yogurt containing live and active cultures, and other fermented food products.
- *Streptococcus thermophilus* is a lactic acid bacterium that makes growth-promoting nutrients. It is found in fermented milk and cheese products.
- *Bifidobacteria* makes short-chain fatty acids and lactic acid and prevents gastrointestinal disorders. It is found in yogurt, cheese, and fermented soy products.

Probiotic supplements are also available and should be taken with food, not on an empty stomach.

Food Combinations

If you are taking digestive enzymes and eating well, and yet still having digestive trouble, it is worth looking into simplifying how you are combining foods. Eating only one or two types of food that combine well together (foods that require similar acid- or alkaline-based enzymes) enhances digestion. For example: Are you combining large amounts of starch, like noodles, with protein foods like meat and then feeling digestive upset? Certain food combinations will not digest well because of the way digestion works. One way to think about food combining is to consider the mixing or combining of various paint colors; while you might mix any color together, if you mix several competing colors at once the results become muddied. While some colors work well together and enhance the overall palette, others do not. Food combining works in a similar way. Starches are digested in the mouth with the enzymes present in saliva, while protein is digested by stomach acid. If you ask the body to simultaneously produce both an acid environment (to digest protein) alongside alkalinizing enzymes in order to digest starches, it can delay digestion as the body figures out which food takes priority. This often leads to fermentation and gas.

Gas

Gas is a natural by-product of digestion of sugars and starches, and elimination via the oral route (belching) or anal route (flatulence) is normal. Excessive gas production can lead to discomfort or pain in the belly and even legs, and this signals poor digestion that will benefit from both digestive enzymes and the fine-tuning of food combinations. Beans are an example of a food containing a sugar called

TABLE 2.1
Food Combinations

Combine	With
Proteins	Nonstarchy/green vegetables
Fats and oils	Nonstarchy/green vegetables Vegetables Starches Proteins (use small amount of fat/oils)
Protein and fats	Nonstarchy/green vegetables Sour fruits
Grains and starches	Nonstarchy/green vegetables
Fermented dairy products	Nonstarchy/green vegetables Sour fruits Seeds and nuts
Beans and legumes	Nonstarchy/green vegetables Cultured vegetables
Fermented foods and drinks	Everything
Water and cold liquids	Nothing
Fruit	Nothing
Acid fruits	Subacid fruits
Subacid fruits	Acid or sweet fruits
Sweet fruits	Subacid fruits

oligosaccharide, which is not digestible and thus leads to gas. Yet its benefit is experienced when it serves as a prebiotic once it reaches the colon.

When you eat starches and protein together, the starches can absorb the stomach acid and delay the digestion of protein. Food combining often requires that we go against established social dietary norms; we like baked potatoes (starch) and steak (protein) for dinner, or tuna or turkey sandwiches for lunch, or a fruit cup before a heavy dinner. Exploring individual reactions to food can begin simply by limiting food types at a meal and then experimenting with each combination to observe digestive reactions.

One can also add spices and herbs (called carminatives) to food that decrease the development of gas or aid its release once formed. Providing a handful of fennel seeds and licorice after an Indian meal is a practice of serving carminative herbs just like the Mexican culinary tradition of adding the green herb *epazote* (wormseed) to cooked beans. Adding black pepper, dill, basil, ginger, cardamom, and parsley to cooked or raw food also reduces gas, as does drinking a cup of peppermint tea following a meal.

Mixing and matching food combinations for optimal digestion is described in Table 2.1

Basic Principles of Food Combining

1. Eat fruit separately from meals by at least 30 minutes, longer if eating after a meal.
2. Drink water and liquids, especially cold liquids, at least 30–60 minutes before a meal.
3. Avoid combining proteins with starchy vegetables and grains.
4. Combine nonstarchy vegetables with animal proteins.
5. Combine nonstarchy vegetables and fats with starches like grains, seeds, and starchy vegetables.

Nonstarchy vegetables include leafy greens, broccoli, asparagus, cauliflower, carrots, bok choy, cabbage, celery, lettuces, green beans, garlic, fennel, onions, chives, turnips, sprouts, red radish, yellow squash, zucchini, cucumber, and beets.

Nonstarchy vegetables and ocean vegetables can be combined with proteins, oils and butter, grains, starchy vegetables, lemons and limes, and soaked and sprouted nuts and seeds.

Starchy vegetables include acorn and butternut squash, lima beans, peas, corn, water chestnuts, artichokes, pumpkin, and potatoes.

Starches include cereals and grains, dried beans, pasta, breads, and peas.

Fats and oils combine with vegetables, grains, and protein. Avoid large amounts of fat with protein (like the mayonnaise in tuna salad) because it slows digestion. Instead, use a small amount of oil to cook and oil-free dressings.

Protein and fats include avocado, olives, seeds and nuts, cheese, and milk (except peanuts and chestnuts, which are starches). Combine these with nonstarchy vegetables and sour fruits.

Acid fruits include citrus fruits, pineapples, plums (sour), pomegranates, strawberries, and sour fruits.

Subacid fruits include apples, apricots, cherries, grapes, mangoes, papayas, pears, and nectarines.

Sweet fruits include bananas, dates, figs, prunes, raisins, and persimmons.

Avocado combines best with nonstarchy/green vegetables and acid or subacid fruits.

Tomatoes combine best with nonstarchy/green vegetables and protein.

Melons are best eaten without other foods as they will digest quickly and easily when eaten alone.

Essential Next Steps

I have explored the second brain and how digestion works throughout in order to communicate with the first brain. Many of the foods we eat nourish this complex network, and some poor-quality foods can interrupt the communication, leading to mental health problems. Creating change at almost any stage of this process or substituting a different food will bring improvement. It becomes a step-by-step process of change.

- Eat only when relaxed.
- Incorporate rituals of mindfulness before meals.
- Chew food until it is almost liquid.
- Eliminate trans fats from the diet.
- Ensure sufficient digestive enzymes.
- Identify each organ of digestion and ensure it is working well.
- Treat gut permeability.
- Eat a variety of prebiotic foods, including soluble and insoluble fibers.
- Eat a variety of probiotic "fermented" foods.
- Follow food combination principles for better digestion.

CHAPTER 3

Listening to Your Clients About Their Diet and Health: Assessment Techniques

Diet Essential: Symptoms tell a story of nutritional and emotional challenges.

We begin an integrative mental health nutrition assessment during the first meeting with a client. As mental health practitioners, we usually conduct psychologically oriented intakes and assessments; however, one of the most illuminating additions to mental health assessment is the inclusion of a comprehensive physical health and nutrition/dietary history.

Over time, as we learn to put together the pieces of someone's story, and the meaning it has for her health and well-being, so do we learn to see the patterns of their physical health history and the bidirectional effects of physical and mental influences on health.

The inclusion of a physical health history along with a nutritional history and current food and preparation patterns will help identify and prioritize the next steps, including underlying causes that can be corrected through dietary and nutritional interventions.

ASSESSMENT AS EDUCATION

The partnership model suggests that clinician and client work together as partners in finding the best approaches for the client. The clinician works to empower the client and walk with her step by step when necessary. It is not authoritarian; it is authoritative. The clinician supports the client to discover what works best for him or her in the context of best available knowledge. Most people are conditioned to being told what to do by health practitioners; the clinician finds opportunities to empower the client as her or his own agent of change.

When conducting a client assessment, I share with the client the metaphor of a jigsaw puzzle that we are co-constructing. Most of my clients have tried many approaches to restoring their health, often with limited success. This is in part because each clinician puts together a few pieces of the puzzle, but the client never has the opportunity to see how all the pieces fit together. In my experience this is the major challenge facing clients when they seek help. They see specialists for each type of symptom, whether mental or physical, but no one helps them to "put the pieces together" in order to tell a coherent story. I share with the client that we will identify and put together seemingly disparate pieces about one's whole health history and symptoms in order to understand how everything fits together, and from this we will create a new picture that provides insight into causative factors. These then will point us in the direction of the next steps to take.

People want to know why they feel the way they do, and they will more readily engage in making changes if they understand how these changes will help them. Symptoms tell a story of nutritional and emotional challenges. Our role is to listen to the story and, together with the client, make the story coherent and actionable.

The assessment process begins to . . .

1. Educate the client about the nutritional basis for her or his symptoms.
2. Connect mental health symptoms with physical symptoms or condition.
3. Bridge health experiences and symptoms of the past with those in the present.
4. Identify where food-related behaviors may be an effort to reestablish balance in the system.
5. Identify some alternatives to current behaviors that will bring positive, lasting results.
6. Provide hope for methods that can reduce any current side effects .
7. Identify three nutritional goals to begin the change process.

Avoid Shame During Assessment

Any illness or symptom can result in a sense of shame. This is especially so with alcohol/chemical dependency, obsessive-compulsive disorder (OCD) behaviors, body dysmorphic disorder (recall that this involves a person believing one's body is somehow defective), eating disorders including purging, and obesity. The client may not readily explore these elements of her or his history unless prompted. If I sense that a client would benefit from exploring these areas and she or he does not seem comfortable raising the topics or responding during the intake, I identify them as topics we can explore down the road. I may say: "I can appreciate that right now it may be difficult to talk about this. How about if we focus on (name a less triggering topic) right now and we can revisit this down the road?"

Because there is a high correlation between the experience of trauma in early life and substance use and eating disorders, I always educate the client about the role of affective dysregulation and the disruption of biochemistry by chronic stress—and the tools that exist to nourish the brain, mind, and body toward balance.

In response to a client who has bulimia and is a survivor, I might say, "We know from clinical experience that most people who experience bulimia have histories of sexual abuse. While we don't understand all of the interrelationships, we do understand that it is by and large an effort to reestablish balance. Let's explore what your behaviors are telling us about what your body-mind needs in order to establish balance and a sense of well-being, and then we can explore what options are out there that may more effectively support your health."

When discussing management and self-care behaviors, it is important to avoid language or attitudes that may inadvertently add to the feelings of shame. This requires a matter-of-fact approach; there are many explanatory systems about mental health illness rooted in cultural, religious, and popular belief systems.

Shame is closely related to self-criticism and blame arising from affect dysregulation. Building in compassion-based skills to address these issues early and as they arise will improve self-care and adherence behaviors and ultimately overall outcomes. Compassion therapy (Gilbert, 2009) applies a mindfulness approach and reinforces and stimulates feelings of safeness, warmth, and connectedness that lead to self-soothing. Because food and drugs and medications are often central to these efforts, understanding the role they play will be essential to avoid engaging in shaming dialogue. Women with eating disorders who reduced shame and increased self-compassion have better treatment outcomes for eating disorders (Kelly, Carter, & Borairi, 2014). This suggests that when someone "falls off the wagon" with a particular protocol or regimen, she or he is supported in a nonjudgmental way to identify what they need to return to their program. This will include reframing shame-based statements.

SAMPLE DIALOGUE 1: REFRAMING SHAME-BASED STATEMENTS

Client 1: I just have no willpower when it comes to donuts. If I see them at work on the break table, I just gobble them up. I have always been bad that way.

Therapist: Donuts are designed with so much sugar and flour that they act like drugs. No wonder you and many people find it hard to turn down donuts. It is not about willpower. Let's strategize some nutritional support that will help you.

Client 2: I went to my friend's birthday party and she offered me a platter, and I ate two pastries, and now I have ruined everything I was working toward.

Therapist: You have not ruined everything you are working toward. You have had a brief setback, but there's nothing keeping you from your goals. It's hard to say no at a birthday party. Did you feel you would "standout" or offend your host if you said "no thank you"?

Client 3: I have been depressed all my life and on meds since I was 11. I just think this is the way I am. There's just something wrong with me and that's how it is going to be.

Therapist: I can appreciate you feel despair at times. You have worked with great courage to restore your health and I am confident of your success. I am thinking about the time you shared with me that you grew up very poor, and often went hungry, and that when you did eat, it was mainly cereal. In many ways this set the stage for your body to crave alcohol and likely led to your body and brain not getting what you needed. You have come a long way in recovery. I know that we can work together to identify the foods and support you need to feel better, and we will work together to identify that and I will support you in achieving that (see Appendix B for the Client Intake Form).

INITIAL INTAKE FORM AND ANALYSIS

The following sections map the assessment (provided in handout printable format in the Appendix). In what follows, I provide an explanation of the meaning of the questions in the context of mental health nutrition and how answers may be understood and interpreted.

There are a number of sections to the assessment, and you may find that you will conduct it in several stages. The client can fill out the assessment and then review it in the office as a basis for discussion and amplification of answers. Like many assessments, it need not be reviewed in order but tailored to the presenting need and tolerance of your client. There will be some parts to the assessment that may feel overwhelming at times to your client, in which case you can proceed slowly, as needed. It is also possible that a client will leave parts blank, in which case you can review the content verbally.

Food-Mood Diary and Clinician Checklist

The Food-Mood diary provides a 3-day window into food habits and patterns and how the client links mood and energy to food quality, quantity, and timing of intake. It provides the clinician with a quick visual of client nutrition and helps to identify initial places to start the change process. I provide this handout after the first appointment so that I can explain it to my client. The client can take it home, and we can review it together at the second appointment. Then, together with a review of the complete intake and a review of this diary, we can begin to identify goals for change. The Food-Mood diary may also serve to initiate some quick changes that will bring about significant improvement in mood and energy and thus engage hope and positive attitude. Hence, one need not wait until the complete intake is finished to engage the change process.

As you sit with the client to review the Food-Mood diary, use the Clinician Checklist as a step-by-step approach to review each section of the Food-Mood diary. Use the interpretation and suggestions as initial steps/goals for the client toward well-being. When analyzing the Food-Mood diary, ask the client to follow along with a copy of the diary, which you will also have in hand. She or he can amplify anything. Some clients feel impatient filling out diaries and make notes only. In this case you can use these notes as prompts to clarify or deepen the answers provided.

In Boxes 3.1 and 3.2, I have provided examples of a Food-Mood diary and Clinician Checklist followed by a dialogue with review and analysis.

Box 3.1
Sample Food-Mood Diary

Food/Mood Diary
Name:_____(Joan Client)_____ Date: (dd/mm/yy)
Write down everything you eat and drink for three days, including all snacks, beverages, and water. Please include approximate amounts. Describe energy, mood, or digestive responses associated with a meal/snack and record it in the right-hand columns. Use an up arrow (↑) for an increase in energy/mood, down arrow (↓) for a decrease in energy/mood, and an equal sign (=) if energy/mood is unchanged.
Time of waking:_____6:30_____a.m./p.m.

Meal	Beverages	Energy Level (↑,↓, or =)	Mood (↑,↓, or =)	Digestive Response (gas, bloating, gurgling, elimination, etc.)
Breakfast (Time: 7:00 a.m.) No breakfast	Coffee, creamer, 2 Equal	Good	Energy low around 9:30 a.m., starting to feel stress of the day	Pain in stomach
Snacks (Time: 9:30 a.m.) Danish pastry	Coffee, creamer, 2 Equal	Was low but then got better	Stressed about work deadlines	
Lunch (Time: 1:00 p.m.) Salad bar, French dressing, wheat roll with butter, fruit cocktail	Diet coke Glass of water	Better during lunch, dreading afternoon	Good lunch with coworker	Gurgling and a little discomfort about an hour after lunch
Snacks (Time: 3:20 p.m.) 1 Reese's peanut butter cup	Coffee, creamer, Equal	Flagging, headache		
Dinner (Time: 7 p.m.) Lean Cuisine Pizza, Applesauce	Iced tea	Exhausted	Tired and irritable	
Snacks (Time: 8:30 p.m.) Reese's peanut butter cup				

Box 3.2
Clinician Checklist for the Food Diary

Joan's Checklist #1

Question	Fill in Answer/ Notes	Goals and Recommendations
1. How much time passed between when the client awakens and when the client eats breakfast? Is the client eating breakfast?	3 hr /not eating breakfast	One should always eat breakfast, containing at least 3–4 ounces of protein within 30 minutes of waking for proper energy and blood sugar balancing.
2. How much water/broth is the client drinking throughout the day?	3 coffees 2 diet cokes 1 ice tea 8 oz. water Joan =180 lb/50% Needs at least 60–90 oz/day	Water intake should be about 50% of body weight every day in ounces (example: if a person weighs 160 lb, she or he should be drinking 80 ounces of water daily).

3. How often is the client eating? How many hours between each meal or snack?	Is snacking but with sugary products not food per se; 6 hr between lunch and dinner	Food should be eaten every 3–4 hours to prevent mood swings, and the client should have at least 3 meals/day and 2 snacks.
4. How many servings of vegetables is the client eating per day?	1 salad	At least 3 servings of vegetables should be eaten every day. A serving equals from ½ to 1 cup.
5. Is the client eating raw vegetables and fruits?	1 salad/maybe 1 apple/applesauce	At least 1–3 servings of raw fruit or vegetables should be eaten every day.
6. Is the client eating enough protein? Note if lack of protein corresponds to drops in mood.	Very limited protein	Proteins help to stabilize energy and balance mood and should be emphasized during the daytime hours.
7. Is the client eating enough fats? Note if lack of fats corresponds to mood shifts.	Poor-quality fats	Fats help to stabilize energy and balance mood and should be emphasized during the daytime hours.
8. How many servings of starchy carbohydrates is the client eating and at what times of day?	Throughout day/ pastries, candy, roll/pizza	During the day carbohydrates are best when combined with protein, and carbohydrates should be emphasized in the evening for relaxation.
9. What is the quality of the food the client is eating (freshly prepared vs. canned or prepackaged foods)?	Poor-quality food	Recommend whole, fresh, organic foods over packaged and canned foods.
10. Is the client eating enough soluble fiber?	Some fiber: apples	Soluble fiber is found in foods like oat bran, nuts, beans, lentils, psyllium husk, peas, chia seeds, barley, and some fruits and vegetables. Men should be eating about 38 grams/day and women 25 grams/day.
11. Is the client eating enough insoluble fiber?	Some in grain sources	Insoluble fiber is found in wheat bran, corn, whole grains, oat bran, seeds and nuts, brown rice, flaxseed, and the skins of many fruits and vegetables.

During the review of the Food-Mood diary, you have the opportunity to identify basic dietary patterns and to ask additional questions. This initial review also allows an assessment of client willingness to make certain changes within the context of the overall stages of change (see Chapter 9). With the completion of the Food-Mood diary, there is enough information to begin goal setting (see Appendix C for printable versions of the Food-Mood Diary and Clinician Checklist).

SAMPLE DIALOGUE 2: FOOD-MOOD DIARY

Clinician: Hi Joan, thank you for filling out this Food-Mood diary. I'd like to review it with you, and we may be able to discover some ways to improve your sense of well-being. One of the first things I notice is that you don't actually eat breakfast. Is that because you're not hungry when you wake up?

Joan: Yeah, I just don't have any appetite.

Clinician: I see that you drink coffee, and I notice that you have some pain in your stomach in the morning. Can you tell me about that?

Joan: I wake up with it every morning, I don't know if it is just stress, but it is kind of pain and nausea.

Clinician: Does it get better or worse when you drink coffee?

Joan: It stays the same . . . maybe a little worse but I need the energy so I just put up with it and if it gets real bad I take an aspirin.

Clinician: Joan, I think that is a priority we can work on and help you feel better. Around 9:30 you had a pastry with another coffee. One of the things you said here is that your energy is a little low by 9:30. That is very common when we don't eat breakfast. Our energy drops and then we grab something to boost it. One of the things we'll talk about are the ways you can increase your energy by changing some of the foods that you're eating and the times you eat. How does that sound to you?

Joan: That sounds good.

Clinician: It looks like at lunchtime you had a salad. Is this something you do every day or was this unusual?

Joan: Yes, though sometimes I have a lunchmeat sandwich. And sometimes instead of a fruit cocktail, I might just have an apple, but I really like the sweet in the fruit cocktail. I feel like it gives me a little energy. I had been drinking regular coke but then decided to switch to diet coke, because I thought that was better for me.

Clinician: I can understand that. In general, sugary foods only give a short-term energy boost and from what I see in your mood and energy sections later in the day your energy drops again. Again, with a few simple changes I think you will have more sustained energy throughout the day. One of the things I notice is that you had a little bit of discomfort after lunch.

Joan: Yeah, I always end up having cramping, low down in my stomach.

Clinician: Do you mean your stomach, or lower down in your belly where your intestines are? (Note: Point to the different locations of the abdomen as people often call their intestines their stomach.)

Joan: Oh, I guess it is lower down than the stomach.

Clinician: Can you place your hands on your belly where you feel the pain?

[Joan places her hands on her descending colon.]

Clinician: Ok. We will talk about that in a bit.

Clinician: Could I clarify, this next area under mood is not filled in, but I noticed that by the middle of the afternoon your energy drops. What happens to your mood at that time?

Joan: I start to get depressed and bark at my office manager.

Clinician: Do you feel better after the coffee and the Reese's peanut butter cup?

Joan: Well, I think so, maybe for an hour, but then I feel a little nauseated and I still find it hard to get through the rest of the workday. I start to feel antsy.

Clinician: I notice that you eat dinner at about 7 p.m.—a Lean Cuisine pizza and applesauce—is this a normal type of dinner for you and regular time?

Joan: Yes, I try to get something healthy that I can just throw in the microwave. I think the applesauce is good for my constipation, though then sometimes I get too loose.

Clinician: I notice that by this time you're really feeling exhausted and tired and irritable. How are you feeling in your belly?

Joan: Well, one of the things I notice before I go to bed is that I have kind of a hot pain coming up into my throat, especially when I lie down. Sometimes it is so bad I take some Tums.

Clinician: Joan, I notice that in the middle of the evening you have another peanut butter cup. Is that because you're hungry or you want something sweet?

Joan: Well, I feel like it settles my stomach. I'll be watching TV and . . . I don't know . . . it just tastes good. I feel a little lonely since my divorce. I know I shouldn't, but . . .

Clinician: I can imagine you feel very lonely since your divorce and feeling crummy every day like you have described here doesn't help either. I feel confident that we can help you feel better physically, and this in turn will help you get back on your feet again. I have no doubt of it, Joan. Is there anything else you want to tell me about your food diary before I share? You can make some nutritional changes that will help the depression, fatigue, and stress and pain we have been discussing.

Joan: Well, the only thing is that I do like to cook, but I just don't seem to have the time or energy after a day of work. I know some of this probably isn't that great for me. I just feel so overwhelmed and stressed most of the time I just can't take on anymore.

Clinician: Yes, I can appreciate that. I am glad you like to cook. It is really important for you to do so and you also lead a busy professional life. I will have some suggestions for you so that you can do some more cooking. It will make a big difference in your energy and health, and I don't think it will take up too much of your time.

Dialogue Analysis and Recommendations

Clinician: I'd like to review some areas in this diet where we can find some initial improvement and they won't be too difficult to implement. And I think I have some answers as to why you feel the way you do. If you undertake some initial changes, you will experience very good improvement in your energy and depression pretty quickly. I know that we are working on your feelings about the divorce and John leaving you and your sadness. We have talked about how those feelings won't go away quickly, but let's focus on some areas you can control now and 'tease out" how your diet is affecting your mood and energy. Once we clear that up, then we will know a bit more about the best ways to focus on your sadness and depression. Shall we go through this together?

Joan: Yes.

Clinician: The first thing I notice is that when you wake up, you have some pain, but you also aren't very hungry and you drink coffee, but not until 9:30 do you put anything in your stomach. I'd like to work with you to eat something, even if it is small and simple, soon after you wake up. Is that doable for you?

Joan: Yes, I can try.

Clinician: Once you try it for a few weeks, I know you will get the results you want. Let's also focus on reducing the pain in your stomach; when you drink coffee on an empty stomach, it can create excess acid; I suspect you may have some acid problems because what you describe at night when you feel that hot pain is also a sign of that. Things like a lot of coffee and starches can cause the symptoms you describe. And, even though you take aspirin for the pain, the aspirin just makes it worse. So it is important never to drink coffee on an empty stomach. You might look into the low-acid coffees on the market, and once we get your energy boosted a bit, how would you feel about just having some coffee in the morning and passing on the afternoon cup? Would you think about that? Could you also tell me why you choose to use a creamer and Equal?

Joan: I thought a creamer was better than cream, and that Equal was better than sugar.

Clinician: Well, Joan, believe it or not, creamer and Equal can actually be worse for your health than cream and sugar. I'd like to recommend that you have some good organic cream, and instead of Equal or sugar, would you be willing to try a natural sweetener? Like honey or a few drops of stevia? There are a lot of additives in both of those products that can affect mood, and I want to rule out anything that can be affecting your mood. Since you drink coffee at work, maybe you could bring a little bit of organic cream and some stevia and keep it at the office with you.

Joan: Yes, I could do that.

Clinician: Wonderful. And from today onward I want you to consider this mantra: "Food is medicine." This means all the food that goes into your body should be used to help you in some way. If it has no health value, then chuck it. So begin with a good low-acid coffee and cream; and cream is better for you than milk. Focus on just two cups in the morning and don't drink unless your belly has some food in it.

Clinician: The next thing I notice is that when I review all of the liquids, you're not getting too much liquid, and when you are, it is not ideal for your health. We know that dehydration can actually contribute to headaches and fatigue, and I'd like to rule out the possibility that this might be affecting you. Would you be willing to drink more water or herb tea during the day?

Joan: Yes.

Clinician: You might purchase rhodiola herb tea. It will give you a boost similar to coffee but it won't make you wired or hurt your belly. I wouldn't drink it after 3 p.m., however. Let me know when I see you next week how you respond to it.

Clinician: I do notice that a lot of the liquids you're drinking are stimulants, and this can affect the difficulty with sleeping that you've been having, and I'd like us to work toward the goal of limiting the stimulants to earlier in the day; let's rely on foods and nutrients as we continue in our discussions to support your energy. Does that sound workable for you?

Joan: Well, I guess.

Clinician: We'll put that on the back burner for right now, but just know I think that's the direction we'll go in, and I promise you that you'll notice a big difference in how you feel. I'll work with you to find some good substitutions.

[Review goals and recommendations in the Clinician Checklist for question 2.]

Clinician: One of the things I notice in your Food-Mood diary is that there is a lot of time in between some meals. For example, between lunch and dinner is 5.5 hours or so, and the middle of the day is a challenging time for you. Your energy drops, your mood drops, you have a headache. I'm wondering whether instead of the Reese's peanut butter cup, why not get a jar of peanut butter or almond butter and some crackers or maybe an apple or a banana. I know you like chocolate also and why not bring some organic cocoa powder to work and you can make yourself a nice cup of hot cocoa, sweeten it with stevia and use some cream or almond milk and enjoy the nut butter. You will still have the foods you like, but now they are medicinal and nutritious rather than making things worse. Does that sound like something you can do? Would you try this for the next week and then tell me how you feel; we can review that again. Would that work for you?

Joan: Yeah, I have a stove at work and a fridge.

Clinician: Great. I have a few recipes for this I will give you before you leave today. I am excited for you making these changes, Joan.

[Review goals and recommendations for question 3.]

Clinician: I notice that you eat a salad almost daily, and that is great. Do you like vegetables?

Joan: Yes, but I just don't have time to cook or prepare them.

Clinician: I can appreciate that. Well, let's put on our to-do list to explore some recipes that you would enjoy, that would include some more vegetables that are quick to prepare. You might even try bringing some celery to work. Peanut butter goes really nicely with celery and celery is known to reduce anxiety.

[Review question number 4.]

Clinician: Joan, I notice that you're eating fruit cocktail and some applesauce, both of which are loaded with sugar. Apples are a perfect fruit for you. I'd like to encourage you to choose apples instead of the fruit cocktail and the applesauce because the sugar in both of those products is exacerbating your symptoms. Research shows that sugar can cause inflammation in our bodies, and this contributes to depression. Again, I want to reduce all these dietary causes of your depression, so we can focus on the life changes you want to make. Do you think that's feasible for you to do? Could you start that this week?

Joan: Yes, I could do that.

Clinician: I know we are going through a lot here and I am making a lot of suggestions. How are you feeling at this point? I don't want to overwhelm you, and we can stop here if you prefer.

Joan: No, this is great! It is giving me a lot of ideas. I didn't realize all of these things.

Clinician: Joan, I am convinced that you would feel better if you were eating more protein. Brain chemicals that help us feel happy rely on protein. What are the kinds of proteins that you like? For example: chicken, eggs, fish, beans, meat . . . .

Joan: Well, I like chicken, eggs, and tuna fish. Sometimes I eat a steak in a restaurant.

Clinician: Wonderful! We talked about you eating in the morning. How about if you begin with an egg? Perhaps a soft-boiled or hard-boiled egg . . . ? Really however you like it. Even a light scramble with some butter would be fine. Some of my clients who are very busy like you boil eggs the night before and then carry a few to work. This would be ideal for you also. Also, add some chicken or salmon to your salad at lunch everyday, and then also have a little chicken or tuna for dinner. Think of the protein as energy for you. If you eat a little of it throughout the day, I guarantee you that your energy will be much stronger. If you start doing this tomorrow, when you come in next week I think you will feel very differently. Can you commit to doing this?

Joan: Yes, I can. I am starting to feel excited about these changes.

Clinician: Joan, before we wrap up for today, I want to discuss fats because they are helpful for stabilizing your energy and mood. I notice that when you have salad, you have French dressing. Do they have olive oil at this restaurant? Do you like olive oil and vinegar, or olive oil and lemon? Maybe you could check and that would be a good change to make that would begin to get you the kinds of fats that are healthy for you.

Clinician: I'm looking at these last few items on my checklist. One of the things we're going to focus on as we move down the road is making sure you get food that's satisfying and better quality . . . the better quality the food, the better your energy and mood. Remember your mantra: Food is medicine. Since you like to cook, I have some healthy Crock-Pot recipes (see Appendix D) that require only 15 minutes, so they will fit your schedule. We can address that more next week, but just give that some thought. Right now, let's review some of the changes you're going to explore this week. I will follow up with you by sending you an e-mail later listing some of the changes we discussed. I am also going to include the names of two nutrients I'd like you to purchase that will help reduce and eliminate the pain in your belly. If you can at all avoid taking the aspirin, please do.

Do you have any questions for me before we end? Let's recap the changes you have agreed to make this week. We have identified some changes that will bring you the quickest and lasting results. I'm going to be eager when you come in next week to hear how your week went.

GOAL SETTING

The goal for the first and second assessment sessions is for the client to share her or his primary concerns and to elicit one or two goals. Additional goals may also emerge from the review of the Food-Mood diary, and the clinician can link the client's identified goals with the Food-Mood diary and overall assessment findings.

Clients will leave with at least one action (and possibly several) they have agreed to undertake until we meet again.

Week 1 Goals for Joan

- Eat an egg for breakfast.
- Substitute cream for creamer.
- Use healthy fat (olive oil) on salad.
- Add protein to lunch salad.
- Obtain low-acid coffee.
- Substitute apple instead of applesauce.
- Substitute peanut butter and chocolate and stevia for candy.
- Reduce aspirin use.

Week 2 Goals Revealed

- Reduce or eliminate soda pop.
- Increase the amount of water drinking.
- Buy a Crock-Pot to cook a chicken.

Essential Outcomes for Client Education During the Food-Mood Assessment

1. The client knows more about the connections between her or his food intake and mood and energy levels.
2. The client understands that a combination of protein, complex carbohydrates, and fats every few hours will sustain mood and energy.
3. The client understands that depression, pain, and anxiety result, in part, from inflammatory foods.
4. The client calculates a range of water/healthy fluid intake that is optimal for energy and well-being.
5. The client commits to one to three goals of nutritional behavior change than can be transformed during the first week.
6. The client has heard about some additional goals for the future weeks to consider.

INTAKE FORM INTERPRETATION (CONT.)

1. Current Health Information (Access Appendix B for the Client Intake Form)

Height/Weight Measures and Their Meaning

Some of the things that people worry about the most and that form the basis for nutritional or medical recommendations include what people weigh and the number for their body mass index (BMI) (this is a general measure of body fat based on height/weight ratio). This information can form a focus of obsessive-compulsive behavior or be useful for change. What matters is what it means to the individual, and it can often be a source of shame. While the BMI is commonly used, it is not particularly meaningful to health because where the excess weight is carried is more important. For example, I had a client who was an athlete who was 5 feet 8 inches and weighed 200 lbs. By BMI standards she would be considered obese. However, as an athlete, she carried 150 lb of lean body mass muscle and bone and was in top condition. Fortunately, our work together was not about weight loss but optimal athletic performance.

If clients are obsessive about weight and BMI, I encourage them to consider hip-waist ratio as a more effective tool *if* they require a measure. Moreover, I emphasize condition and well-being, focusing on active choices that improve overall well-being with less of a focus on weight per se. For these "always dieting" clients, educating them about the "Obesity paradox" is essential. The Obesity paradox suggests that being overweight or moderately obese may not be deleterious to health and that people who are ill and overweight have better mortality rates than people who are underweight. Like all epidemiological research, these findings have to be applied to the individual to be of value. However, these outcomes are relevant to our work because the "paradox" suggests that we deemphasize weight as a measure of health and instead focus on measures of health, including the reduction of systemic inflammation and oxidative stress, and improving aerobic and anaerobic conditioning and flexibility. If a client wants to measure and chart progress, a hip-waist ratio is a more accurate reading of *potential* health risk (see Box 3.3).

Box 3.3
Hip-Waist Ratio

To accurately measure the waist and hip ratio, follow these steps:
  Place a tape measure around your bare stomach just above the upper hipbone.

Make sure the measuring tape is parallel to the floor (slanting can falsely increase your measurement). Also ensure that the tape measure is snug to your body, but not so tight that it compresses the skin. Exhale while measuring and relax your abdomen—sucking in is not allowed!

Using a tape measure, measure the circumference of your hips.

First look in a mirror and identify the widest part of your buttocks. Then place the tape measure at this location and measure around the circumference of your hips and buttocks. Using your waist circumference measurement, calculate your waist-to-hip ratio by dividing your waist circumference by your hip measurement. Divide the waist measurement by the hip measurement; a result above 0.9 for men or 0.85 for women indicates abdominal obesity and an elevated health risk.

Treatment Received, Experience With Practitioners

Understanding previous treatment and results, attitudes and experiences, benefits, connections, and mistreatment all inform our work as clinicians. I want to understand whether my client has felt heard, understood, and taken seriously, especially when the client may have been told that her or his symptoms are "psychosomatic" since the physical and mental are mediated so completely via nutrition.

Daily Activities, Stress, Pain

Understanding current levels of activity will inform possible issues of energy and inflammation and pain that are linked to nutrition. It is also important to identify what people engage in and where they may enjoy activities and receive support to return to those activities.

2. Health History

One of the most important steps a clinician can integrate is a comprehensive health history. Mental health symptoms give clues to physical problems, and physical problems also reflect emotional or cognitive issues. To understand these relationships, a health history is required.

Surgeries give insight into a variety of factors. The removal of digestive organs can occur as a response to illness, or in turn it can lead to nutrient deficits. Appendicitis may reflect chronic intestinal problems; removal of the gallbladder leads to problems digesting fats. Bariatric surgeries create absorption problems and often-lifelong deficits that must be closely managed. Thyroid surgery is also common and affects metabolism and mood. Surgery for chronic pain conditions is always linked to the inflammatory process and often linked to a history of early-life trauma. It also often follows from or leads to prescription painkiller abuse, which in turn affects one's digestion and depression.

A history of elective surgeries may also illuminate body dysmorphia, addictions, and a history of complex traumatic stress. Elective surgeries such as liposuction or cosmetic surgeries are highly correlated with histories of trauma (Korn, 2013).

A thorough history of treatments tried, and whether or not they have been successful or failed, will also inform the choices people have made and what has worked or failed.

3. Lifestyle Factors—Physical Activity and Exercise

Physical activity and exercise is the third part of the triad of healing and recovery in mental health along with nutrition and counseling. Understanding the role of exercise in self-care practices includes the three main types of movement, including stretching, aerobic, and anaerobic (muscle strength exercises). Exercise also affects nutritional status, increasing needs, altering appetite and increasing brain NTs and hormones. Exercise is a vital part of eliminating medications and improving mood, and this is a good place to educate about that. Most people do better on their nutritional plans when they are exercising. The assessment may also provide information about obstacles or phobias about movement that can be addressed. People who are overexercising have special nutritional requirements, and chronic overexercise can be a sign of an eating disorder.

4. Family Medical History

For the purposes of a comprehensive assessment, I explore family history to identify and deconstruct belief systems about the hereditary or inevitability of a disease process. Reviewing family history gives insight into family belief systems and behaviors and can be incorporated into exploring faulty beliefs. While there are some hereditary diseases and genetic vulnerabilities (like celiac disease), few are inevitable. Generally, most illnesses, both mental and physical, are lifestyle related and stress related, and even genetic illnesses are epigenetic in nature. They are not necessarily inevitable, but many are "triggered" by environmental stressors that can be prevented or reduced in severity. Family medical history and treatment also sheds light on family beliefs related to use of medications, fear of medications, or other behaviors that will influence the client's choices.

5. Current Dietary Habits

Understanding current diets and the decisions and beliefs underlying those choices and behaviors is central to developing a nutritional plan. A client may be open to new options or ironclad in his commitment to his current diet. Often the client is following a diet that is not appropriate for the specific biochemical individual needs, and this provides an opportunity to educate about areas for change. I also ask about eating behaviors, including meal/snack patterns, eating style, eating with people or alone, and behavioral issues like dining out (e.g., what kinds of places?).

Food Allergies/Sensitivities—Known and Suspected

In Chapter 5, I review in depth the role of food allergies and sensitivities and their contribution to mental illness. Here is where you might explore if any testing has been done. People may know of allergies/sensitivities or may suspect them but have never been tested or conducted an elimination diet. The question about "foods that you could not give up" reveals potential obstacles to dietary change.

Current Food Preparation Methods

This section explores activities surrounding food gathering and preparation. Both past and present practices will illuminate strengths and obstacles. People who have cooked in the past will more easily start again, while people who have not enjoyed cooking or are afraid of cooking will pose different challenges than those who have never learned but would like to. The answers in this section will guide "cooking coaching" options outlined in Chapters 6.

6. Diet History

Early dietary experiences can set the stage for childhood and adult physical and mental illness. These experiences can influence the willingness as well as the knowledge base that will inform adherence and compliance. Understanding the types of foods an individual is used to eating, as well as what foods she grew up on, will reveal dietary habits that may be difficult to change.

For example, did the client's mother eat a diet rich in essential fatty acids? Was the client fed formula? Did she experience ear infections? How about the use of antibiotics? This history could expose the possibility of dairy sensitivity and microbiome imbalance.

Digestive Problems Currently, During Childhood, and During the Teen Years

Did the client complain of stomach pains during childhood? Acne can be associated with food sensitivities to dairy. When did the symptoms of eating disorders begin? Were they resolved, or are they current, and how have the symptoms changed?

History of Fasting, Purging, History of Binging/Purging (SAD or Triggers)

Fasting, purging, and binging provide insight into chronic or acute responses to stress and nutrient deficits. Understood in context, these practices reveal where healing should be focused. Someone who fasts for a day a week because he believes in the calorie restriction theory of longevity is assessed differently than a young woman who had decided to fast for 10 days on water to lose weight. Even purging, while not a commonly practiced behavior that we see outside of pathology, has a long history as part of religious and health rituals around the world. Thus, a client who discusses purging as part of her spiritual or consciousness practices must be understood in the context and outcomes of these practices. Overall while fasting, binging, and purging are often associated with eating disorders, like all behaviors they must be understood for their meaning and outcomes.

Where there is a history of chronic binging and purging in particular, nutritional status should be evaluated immediately and treatment initiated.

History of Meals, and Mealtime, Current and in the Past

This section will reveal potential strengths and obstacles to engaging in a program of self-nourishment. Was the client a "latch-key" kid? Did he cook for himself and brothers and sisters? Was there fighting at mealtime? Were foods prepared from packages or homemade, or were they special types of meals? What about low-fat substitute use? Is she a practicing vegetarian? Is her diet based on religious or spiritual beliefs?

7. Medications: Current and Past Use

In mental health intakes we collect information on psychotropic medicine use. However, in the integrative assessment we collect information on all the medications a client is using, as well as herbal preparations, vitamins, and minerals. It is essential that all use of medications, including prescription, self-prescribed, and recreational or abused medications, be identified. Why is this important? One, there can be complex drug-nutrient-herb interactions. For example, fish oil is a blood thinner; if a client is already taking a blood thinner, it is important to know. Knowing what the complete medication list contains may also prompt collaboration with the prescribing clinician. For example, you may feel that 3 g of fish oil is useful for your client's depression, but he may already be taking a blood thinner. Taking high-dose fish oil can help thin the blood and actually may even reduce the dosage required of a blood thinner; however, this kind of recommendation should be coordinated with the prescribing clinician.

A number of approaches to improving mood stability involve nutrients that can lower blood sugar; clients with diabetes who may be on blood sugar–lowering medications such as metformin or insulin will want to be advised of the potential effects of these helpful nutrients in order to prevent blood sugar from going too low. This subject is explored further in Chapter 8.

Past Use of Medications—Pharmaceuticals, Antibiotics
Address drug-nutrient-herb-food interactions.

8. Use of Nonpharmaceutical Substances

What and how people use medications or substances to self-medicate also gives insight into the options we will suggest. Some clients will begin by withdrawing from substances, others may have done so years before, and still others do not want to take any supplements. Some may present a list of 20 items they take and have significant beliefs and associations about their benefits. Still others have prescriptions from multiple clinicians. I call these "serial clients"; they will move from clinician to clinician without always following recommendations, or they have many at once and compare and contrast what each says. All of this will contribute to our understanding of how to coach clients and make recommendations.

With a list of all medications and substances, one can evaluate their interactions by using an online database and explore potential nutrition deficits or dangerous interactions. There are many excellent databases identified in Appendix Z.

9. Use of Nutritional Supplements and Herbs

The main purpose of this section is to identify whether someone is already taking nutritional supports and at what level. If the client is not taking any supplements, that is as informative as the individual who has a comprehensive plan underway. The source and quality of the nutrients are very important as poor-quality supplements have fillers, additives, sugar, and food colors, so often the place to start is improving the quality of the supplements. Who, if anyone, prescribed them? What are the dosages, and are they adequate or excessive? What is their potential for negative interactions with medication? Assess their efficacy relative to current goals.

10. Detoxification Section

Types of detoxification the client has undergone or tried, currently and previously.

This section provides insight into the spectrum ranging from self-care to self-harm. It is as important to know what people are doing as well as why they are doing it. Detox fads make the rounds just as do dietary and food fads. Elsewhere I have written extensively on detoxification and the scientific basis for its benefits (Korn 2013). There are significant benefits to detoxification when done correctly; however, some transient nutritional harm can result at times if done incorrectly or for long periods. I also want to understand if these behaviors are linked to mental health or undue concerns about feeling dirty or unclean, and integrate this understanding into our work toward health.

11. Pain and Discomfort

Pain levels can be assessed using the visual form and the visual analogue. Pain provides insight into inflammation levels; it often co-occurs in depression, either as a co-occurring or a secondary result of living with pain (a hallmark of fibromyalgia). The potential to reduce pain may motivate a client to change her diet. This is accomplished by eliminating inflamatory foods and increasing anti-inflamatory foods and nutrients. If pain is a primary concern, it can be the focus of initial dietary and supplement protocol.

12. Current and Previous Medical Conditions and Their Link to the Mental Health Nutritional Checklist

In this section people may again consider symptoms they experience.

Headaches

What types and how often, and what seems to trigger incidents? Gluten and food allergies are major triggers for headaches; use of medications for headaches can cause digestive problems.

Fatigue may signal nutrient deficiencies or signal chronic stress/hypoglycemia. Infections and sinus symptoms may signify food allergies, especially to dairy.

Skin Conditions

Chronic rashes and fungal infections may indicate high levels of sugar consumption or low essential fatty acid levels.

Allergies

Allergic reactions to scents, oils, lotions, and detergents may signal chemical sensitivity, which may reflect chronic stress response and adrenal fatigue. Clients should be encouraged to eliminate these exposures.

Muscles and Joints

Somatic signs of stress signify inflammatory levels and food allergies; pain may point to inflammation also underlying depression and other cognitive symptoms. Such symptoms may indicate the need for dietary anti-inflammatories.

Nervous System

Head injuries, concussions, dizziness, ringing in ears, loss of memory, confusion, numbness, tingling, sciatica, shooting pain, chronic pain, depression, and other similar responses.

There is a range of implications for cognitive function and inflammatory process in the body. History of head injuries can contribute to chronic headaches and be a risk factor for depression and cognitive decline.

Respiratory and Cardiovascular

These symptoms will likely necessitate a referral or collaboration with the prescribing practitioner. Thiamine may be used to increase blood pressure in people with low blood pressure. Supplemental fish oil can enhance circulation; sleep disorders such as sleep apnea are risk factors for cognitive decline. Hyperventilation may signal anxiety.

Digestion/Elimination

Identifying symptoms in this section will clarify digestion from "top to bottom." Symptoms can be prioritized and addressed with dietary and supplemental nutrients.

Endocrine System

Most answers in this area will alert to the need for collaboration or a referral.

Reproductive System

Reproductive organ symptoms are often associated with poor mental health either as cause or reaction. Significant improvements can be obtained with nutritional therapies. For example, vitamin D is associated with reduction of fibroids in perimenopausal women.

Cancer/Tumors

History of cancer or current cancer may signal the need to collaborate with other clinicians.

13. Meaning of Food

The meaning of food in the client's life may be revealed in a discussion of the food diary. Food means something to everyone and people have a variety of associations. Understanding these associations will aid change or present barriers. The meaning of food is especially important during the exploration of eating disorders or for a bariatric assessment. Food may be explored in the context of types of foods, and their positive or negative associations with how foods are used for energy, for self-medication, relaxation, and in the context of early or current family life.

Sometimes clients live alone and do not prepare food for themselves or do not have time to cook. Or, people may have a difficult time answering this question. At this stage, there may be an opening to understand food-related behaviors and discuss the role of mindfulness and eating.

This is also a good stage in the intake to take a break and teach your client the mindfulness exercise discussed in Chapter 2.

14. Motivation for Nutritional Change/Obstacles

This section explores areas and activities where the client has previously been most successful, what has not worked, and the challenges/obstacles. This will provide insight into special areas for focus.

Identify the differing needs within the current family, history of cooking, and so on.

What is currently working? What are the obstacles to change? (See nutritional change questionnaire at the end of the Client Intake Form.)

There can be a number of factors, including biochemical individuality. Not everyone in the family needs the same kinds of foods in the same amounts, but oftentimes one person will sublimate her or his needs to the other without realizing its detrimental health effects.

The information gathered here can be used further when we explore "putting it all together" for coaching in Chapter 9.

NEXT STEPS FOLLOWING THE INITIAL INTAKE AND ASSESSMENT

Once the intake is complete, the clinician will review it and analyze it in preparation for sharing results and ideas for prioritizing next steps. It is important to collect information about the financial resources a client has available to allocate to a nutritional program since food and nutritional supplements can add up to several hundred dollars a month. Understanding the client's own timeline for change is also useful as it helps to gauge the rate of change that will be established during goal setting. The development of a report and identifying change strategies are found in Chapter 9.

Before any assessment is complete, however, there are additional factors that must be integrated into the analysis. Assessment of mental health and nutritional status is not a linear process. It is an ongoing process of integrating the many factors affecting the way nutrition and dietary behaviors contribute to our individual client's wellbeing. Here we transition away from the particulars of the individual to incorporate factors that intersect with nutrition that are absolutely essential to understanding the underlying causes of mental illness. In Chapter 4 you will find I apply these factors to specific diagnoses, and in Chapter 7 I review treatment strategies.

Five Essential Mental Health Nutritional Factors to Assess in Everyone

Many similar damaging processes result in a variety of symptoms and different diagnoses. This requires that we assess five essential factors that underlie poor mental health and that are caused by poor nutrition and can be addressed by nutritional therapies. Next I describe these factors and in subsequent chapters I describe the range of interventions that treat these five essential factors.

People come into the world with various strengths and weaknesses that can be genetic and also result from in utero and perinatal exposures. Early-life patterns and life stressors can strengthen or exacerbate these genetic patterns. Not all "genetic propensities" are necessarily evident. Environmental toxins and, most important, nutrition can activate dormant genetic responses for good or for ill. This is called epigenetics.

Consider what happens when a brand-new car is exposed to salt on the road every winter for several years. The original fine sheen begins to rust; at first perhaps a small area on the fender, then the hood has a larger area, and then rust breaks through the metal floor and spreads. Your neighbor's car, however, is exposed to the same salt, but the rust doesn't seem so bad, or it starts near the hubcaps. Meanwhile the tires on your car are wearing thin a bit sooner than your neighbors, even though they have the same mileage. Step by step the systems required for the car to function suffer; this depends upon the year of the car, its original quality, and its history—maybe it was mishandled in an accident at the factory, or perhaps your neighbor's car was garaged while yours was not. It is these many variables combined with the care or neglect and the various types of exposures that will determine the unique ways in which the car begins to break down. The human mind and body are not so different.

All of these five essential factors directly influence mental health and must be assessed in the context of each individual's specific responses.

Five Essential Factors That Affect Mental Health

1. "Chrononutrition" imbalance
2. Blood sugar and functional hypoglycemia
3. Food sensitivities, especially gluten/casein sensitivity
4. Inflammation, including mitochondrial energy and oxidative stress
5. Methylation: conversion of folic acid (B-9) to l-methylfolate

Essential Step 1

Assess for chrononutrition imbalance. Chrononutrition refers to the dynamic relationship between the timing of food intake and nutrient deficits; the sum total of these effects on circadian rhythm underlies mental health. As with other conditions, diet supplementation and food behaviors can rebalance circadian rhythm and thus contribute to improved mental health.

Think of a major clock in the brain that is linked to the great "clock" of daytime and night time, of light and dark. This master clock then regulates other smaller clocks in the body that in turn regulate digestion, glucose handling, and hunger. Mood disorders occur when the "brain clock" is out of sync with the master clock of light and dark, and in turn this dysregulates the smaller clocks. Thus, to reset these clocks so they are all synched, we use being awake, sleep light and dark therapies, and nutritional therapies that help move the "hands" of the clock backward or forward.

Circadian rhythm significantly influences depression, anxiety, PTSD, chronic pain (fibromyalgia), menstrual problems, OCD, bipolar disorder, eating disorders, and insomnia. Medications, nutrients, and light exposure can all affect adversely or beneficially the sleep-wake cycle and mood. Early-morning wakening, morning depression, chronic sleeping in late, awakening with exhaustion, feeling wired at night, and using medication to sleep are all signs of circadian rhythm disruption.

Stress alters the circadian rhythm and cortisol levels, which affect sleep, wakefulness, and fatigue. Excess cortisol can reduce sleep quality and duration, and circadian rhythm governs the rise and fall of amyloid-beta production, which is implicated in the development of Alzheimer's disease. Sleep deprivation is a risk factor for the development of dementia (Kang et al., 2009). Night shift workers are more vulnerable to stress-related illnesses, including depression and anxiety (Bara & Arber, 2009) and cancer.

Assessment Essentials for Circadian Rhythm
Review sleep-wake cycle.

> *24-hour salivary cortisol test*: This at-home test measures cortisol at four data points. Cortisol follows circadian rhythm and provides insight into the relationship between stress, adrenal function, sugar handling function, and the sleep-wake cycle.

> *Automated Morningness-Eveningness Questionnaire (AutoMEQ)*: This 19-question assessment provides information about sleep habits and your circadian rhythm type (see Appendix Z: Resources).

Essential Step 2
Assess blood sugar handling and eliminate functional (reactive) hypoglycemia. The next most important function to assess is blood sugar handling, functional hypoglycemia, and hyperglycemia/diabetes. Most everyone with mood lability has poor glucose handling. Without evaluating blood sugar handling, we will not know truly what is causing mood lability. Hypoglycemia causes significant mood lability that can appear to be anxiety, bipolar disorder, irritability, ADHD, or affective dysregulation. Chronic stress gives rise to hypoglycemia, which in turn leads to these many symptoms. Blood sugar levels are also intimately related to circadian rhythm and adrenal function so that people with chronic stress often have reactive hypoglycemia, which can develop into type 2 diabetes. The role of blood glucose and its effect on mental function has been a focus over the last 30 years with the rise of type 2 diabetes and mood lability in children and adults alike. What occurs in the body occurs in the brain. The term "diabetes type 3" (de la Monte & Wands, 2008) was coined to reflect the new understanding that Alzheimer's disease is a type of diabetes of the brain associated with diets high in refined carbohydrates.

Assessment Essentials: Blood Sugar Handling and Hypoglycemia

1. Identify the daily use of refined carbohydrates and sugars, low protein intake, long periods between meals or using refined carbohydrates every few hours to sustain energy, and periods of sleepiness during the day. These are all signs of functional hypoglycemia.

2. Assess for functional or reactive hypoglycemia by conducting a review of the Food-Mood diary, especially questions 1, 3, 6, 8, and 10.

3. Review the following checklist of major symptoms of hypoglycemia and poor blood sugar handling:

   Dizziness

   Feeling shaky

   Confusion

   Hunger

   Agitation

   Crying

   Headache

   Irritability

   Rage

   Tired

   Inability to focus

   Pounding heart; racing pulse

4. Following the hypoglycemia diet (see Appendix A for General Guidelines for a Hypoglycemic Diet) for 1 week is also a "rule-out" method. People with functional symptoms will feel much better when following this diet.

Essential Step 3

Assess for gluten/casein/food sensitivity/allergy. Celiac disease, nonceliac gluten sensitivity, and casein sensitivity are all important causes of mental illness. Significant clinical evidence has established casein and gluten sensitivity in people with mood disorders, anxiety, major depression, and schizophrenia (Cascella et al., 2011; Samaroo et al., 2010). People with bipolar disorder (Dickerson et al., 2012), OCD, autism, ADHD, and eating disorders have been found by practitioners to react to gluten and casein.

Gluten is the protein found in certain grains (wheat, barley, and rye) that causes grains to "glue" together. Gliadins are proteins that are components of gluten. Celiac disease affects about 1 in 250 people and is an autoimmune disease that manifests in severe digestive and frequently neurological symptoms. Nonceliac gluten sensitivity is an immune response leading to both digestive and neurological problems (Jackson, Eaton, Cascella, Fasano, & Kelly, 2012) but may not manifest in digestive distress and thus may go undiagnosed.

Casein is the protein found in dairy milk products. Both gluten and casein contain proteins to which people may be either allergic or sensitive. About 50% of people who are sensitive to gluten are sensitive to casein. This is called "cross reactivity."

Assessment Essentials

There are two basic approaches to assessment: the elimination diet and blood and/or salivary tests. Testing for both celiac and the various antibodies to gliadin and other gluten protein or an elimination diet should be enacted as a first step.

There are different tests for nonceliac gluten sensitivity; one assesses blood and the other saliva. Comprehensive testing should include testing for antibody production to a variety of proteins, enzymes and peptides including Transglutaminase, Deamidated Gliadin, Glutenin, Gluteomorphins/Prodynorphin, Wheat Germ Agglutinin, and foods that are Cross- reactive to gluten.

Adherence to a gluten- and casein-free diet is challenging for many people, especially children. Thus, it is important to conduct highly specific testing. New tests are available for both urine and serum and extend immune system testing to include the testing of peptides, which act as undigested proteins contributing to gastrointestinal, neurological, and neurodevelopmental disorders. These neuropeptides called casomorphins and gliadorphins act like opiates in the brain; they affect cognitive function, speech, and auditory integration and decrease the ability to feel pain. For example, binging associated with bulimia is linked to gluten sensitivity, which releases opioid peptides, accounting for the binging/withdrawal response to grains, especially wheat. Cravings for wheat and grains are often associated with mood elevation upon eating these foods.

> *Celiac disease:* The standard test is called the tissue transglutaminase antibodies (tTG-IgA) blood test for antibodies to gluten.
> *Gluten/casein intolerance*: Some labs conduct highly specific tests that analyze up to 24 possible substances that affect digestive immunological and brain health, including gluten/casein intolerance.
> *Urinary/serum peptide tests*: The gluten/casein peptides test determines the effects

of sensitivities to the opiate-like peptides in response to gluten or casein, even if an individual has no IgE or IgG allergic reactions (see Appendix Z: Resources).

Assessment With the Elimination Diet

It is not always practical due to financial resources to undergo blood or salivary testing. I recommend these tests to clients while remaining aware that they may not always be affordable. In this case a diet that eliminates all exposure to gluten and casein can be used. Gluten is found in many foods, not just bread products, and the elimination diet must be exacting. I recommend eliminating gluten first. It takes at least 4–12 weeks to experience the effects (see Appendix E for a comprehensive list of gluten-containing foods). Following the gluten elimination diet, I recommend the casein (dairy) elimination diet since gluten and casein cross-react about 50% of the time.

Essential Step 4

Assess inflammation, oxidative stress, and mitochondrial energy. Oxidative stress occurs as a function of living, just like a car rusts and ages over time. One theory of aging is the rate at which one "rusts." Thus, we assume some oxidative stress and mitochondrial dysfunction based on aging and symptoms alike. Oxidative stress is similar to when your car becomes rusty. Over time, if the rust is not addressed, it affects the little engines that fire up the car (the mitochondria inside the cells); as a result, they in turn cannot convert nutrients into energy. Mitochondrial dysfunction is involved in depression, bipolar disorder (Stork & Renshaw, 2005), Alzheimer's disease, schizophrenia (Jou, Chiu, & Liu, 2009), chronic fatigue, and fibromyalgia. Chronic alcohol and drug use, and poor-quality diet leads to oxidative stress. Chronic stress damages mitochondrial function in response to chronically high glucose levels (Picard, Juster, & McEwen, 2014) that in turn lead to systemic inflammation to neuronal damage and cell death.

Assessment Essentials

In addition to the mental health symptoms I have discussed earlier, pain, heat or inflammation around joints, along with cataracts, and heart disease are signs of inflammation. Oxidative stress precedes neurological diseases and mitochondrial energy failure occurs in fibromyalgia and chronic fatigue.

Basic inflammatory markers in blood tests
Homocysteine

High-sensitivity C-reactive protein (CRP): norms, under 0.55 mg/L in men and under 1.0 mg/L in women

Fibrinogen: 200–300 mg/dL

(See Appendix Z: Resources)

Telomere testing: Telomeres are genetic material at the end of each chromosome. Their primary function is to prevent chromosomal "fraying." Think of the plastic tip at the end of a shoelace that keeps the shoelace from unraveling. It is normal for telomeres to shorten over time with age, leading to cell death. The oxidative stress hastens this death just like rock salt hastens the rust buildup on a car in New York City, in contrast to the same car with no salt garaged in Arizona. A variety of stressors appear to cause telomere damage, including overconsumption of sugar and chronic stress in early life (Mitchell et al., 2014). Telomere length appears to be influenced positively by intake of antioxidants that combat oxidative stress (Shen et al., 2009). Testing telomeres can reveal the effects of oxidative stress on DNA (see Appendix Z: Resources).

Essential Step 5

Assess methylation: conversion of folic acid (B-9) to I-methylfolate. A significant number of individuals lack the ability to convert folates (or its synthetic form folic acid [B-9]) to l-methylfolate, due to natural genetic mutations. The process of folate conversion requires an enzyme called MTHFR (5,10-methylenetetrahydrofolate reductase) to convert folic acid and food folate into 5-methylenetetrahydrofolate. This processing deficiency is quite common among patients with depression (Rush et al., 2006), and up to 70% of patients with depression test positive for the inability to convert folic acid into L-methylfolate. This renders folic acid in vitamin B supplements and enriched foods ineffective for this group of patients. This leads to problems in what is called the "methylation pathway." Defects in methylation conversion pathways set the stage for a variety of symptoms due to the body's inability to metabolize specific vitamins and NTs like dopamine, necessary for physical and mental health. One of the signs of folate (and vitamin B12) deficiency and a possible MTHRF mutation is elevated homocysteine levels—a risk factor for both depression and cognitive decline.

Methylation Pathway

Orthomolecular clinicians consider the role of either overmethylation or undermethylation processes in the contribution to psychiatric illness. Different nutrients increase or decrease methylation. Methylation pathway problems contribute to high homocysteine levels, which are a marker for both heart disease and depression. The methylation pathway is also responsible for the synthesis of CoQ10 in the body.

CoQ10 is required for mitochondrial energy production. Fibromyalgia and chronic fatigue are two signs of methylation dysfunction that benefit from B vitamins. The body must convert folates into a usable form. Folates are found in plant foods, such as spinach, or in the synthetic form called folic acid found in multivitamins, and in "enriched" flour or other processed foods. Folic acid or folate is routinely administered to pregnant women to prevent neural tube defect. There is a correlation between low levels of folate and poor response to SSRIs, which had led to folate/folic acid supplementation to improve the efficacy of SSRIs. Diets high in folates, such as the traditional Chinese diet, are linked with lower lifetime rates of depression (Korn, 2013).

Assessment Essentials

High homocysteine levels indicate that the methylation process is inadequate.

MTHFR mutation is a simple blood test that is widely available and generally covered by insurance (see Appendix Z: Resources).

Lab work: Completion of the history and specialized assessments will also lead to a discussion of further testing that may involve lab work. Some people want lab work right away, and others may not for reasons of affordability. A great deal of improvement can be achieved without specialized lab work, and thus its costs and benefits should be discussed with the client. I will suggest to a client that if results are not obtained following 3–6 months of dietary and nutrient changes we will explore laboratory testing.

DIAGNOSTIC AND SYMPTOM-SPECIFIC ASSESSMENTS

Following a review and analysis of the overall assessment, symptom-specific assessments may be incorporated. In the following section I address eating disorders and bariatric surgery because so many people seek help with eating issues and because eligibility for bariatric surgery requires a psychological assessment. In Chapter 4, I continue exploring nutrition and the contribution of nutrient deficits to specific diagnostic categories.

Eating Disorders

People come for counseling and nutritional therapies to talk about chronic or acute eating disorders. They may also want to be evaluated for bariatric surgery. Frequently a discussion of food behaviors surfaces during the treatment of depression, anxiety, or PTSD when self-care habits are associated with a sense of helplessness. To obtain bariatric surgery a client requires a psychological review. A clinician who understands mental health nutrition can be a vital resource to the client before, during, and after surgery.

Anorexia nervosa (AN), bulimia, and binge eating disorder (BED) affect all ethnicities in the United States. Latinos and African Americans tend to have higher rates of bulimia nervosa (BN). Bariatric surgery patients have a 27% lifetime prevalence of BED (Herrin & Larkin, 2013). There is a high rate of eating disorders among women and men who were victimized in childhood (Korn, 2013). There are elevated levels of anxiety and depression among bariatric surgery candidates and higher rates of mental disorders among the obese and then even higher rates of mental disorders in obese people who seek bariatric surgery (Mitchell & Zwaan, 2011). Bisexual and gay men have a higher risk for eating disorders with as many as 15% (Herrin & Larkin, 2013). Eating disorders are highly comorbid with obsessive-compulsive disorder, and the nutritional treatment is very similar. Balancing serotonin levels is central to the range of symptoms that occur along the eating disorders continuum.

Eating disorders reflect complex psychobiological stressors, efforts to regulate affect through food and food behaviors, and complex nutritional imbalances. Eating disorders often have a dissociative and obsessive-compulsive component. At a larger social level are the influences of pressure and advertisements on children and adults of what constitutes a perfect body and the ways that food or lack thereof may achieve that. Eating disorders often co-occur with orthorexia, which I explain in Chapter 5.

The eating disorders in general are linked to dissociation and alternate states of consciousness achieved through food types and binging/fasting/purging activities. Bulimia and purging are anxiolytic behaviors. For example, purging activates vagal response. If you have ever thrown up, you know that afterward you are exhausted and fall asleep. Indeed, there are many cultural practices throughout the world that actively engage purging and regurgitation as methods of altering states of consciousness. People generally use carbohydrates as their food of choice in bulimia, though they can choose fatty foods as well. These are mood altering by way of the serotonergic system, but they also lead to a sense of fullness.

People who often engage in fasting and or purging frequently engage in intensive exercise. Or, as regulation of food intake becomes more balanced, intensive exercise can increase. These behaviors alter consciousness by inducing endorphin response, which reduces anxiety, but it can also exacerbate dissociative symptoms. Foods themselves have psychoactive components, which are enhanced when there are allergies or sensitivities, for example, to the opiate-like chemistry of gluten and casein that affects many people with eating disorders.

Bulimia Nervosa

Bulimia nervosa (BN) tends to include impulsive and secretive behaviors, as well as mood lability (Herrin & Larkin, 2013). Higher rates of BN are found in those with a history of trauma. The difference between BN and BED is that bulimics will compensate for the binge by self-induced vomiting or other measures like exercising excessively, restricting their food intake, or excessive intake of diuretics and laxatives (Herrin & Larkin, 2013).

Purging Behaviors

AN and BN behaviors both may include purging and extreme use of laxatives, which upset the digestive process and also the health balance of intestinal flora. Chronic purging can be dangerous and lead to nutritional deficits, GERD, and even death. Most eating disorder treatment approaches have a goal of eliminating purging behaviors, including self-induced vomiting. However, not all purging behavior is harmful, and frequency and the meaning of the practice should be assessed with each individual. Historically and across cultures humans (and other animals) are known to engage in these ritualized behaviors. Thus, understanding the spectrum of these behaviors ranging from adaptive and healthy to maladaptive and leading to self-harm and, in particular, the cultural context, will be valuable.

Binge Eating Disorder

BED may include grazing patterns where people eat small amounts of food throughout the day. Compulsive eating is similar to grazing in that eating may continue for hours; there is a tendency to repeatedly reach for food and feel overfull and out of control, and to become preoccupied with eating. It is not uncommon that individuals with BED and BN have blood sugar imbalances related to excessive starchy carbohydrate intake and insulin resistance. These are especially associated with cravings for these kinds of foods. They can never be satisfied as long as they are fed with refined carbohydrates. Grazing patterns can be interrupted or reframed when applied to hypoglycemia, which should be ruled out.

Emotional Eating

Emotional eating occurs as an effort to regulate stress or boredom or other uncomfortable emotions. Comfort foods are part of emotional eating—often high carbohydrate or high fat because both increase relaxation.

Night Eating Syndrome

Night eating syndrome is distinguished from BN and BED by the timing of food intake and the fact that the food is eaten in small repeated snacks rather than true binges (O'Reardon, Peshek, & Allison, 2005). It also does not include purging behaviors.

Anorexia Nervosa

AN is a disorder of starvation that leads to malnutrition and often death. When addressing nutritional support for AN, it is important to distinguish between pre-AN deficits and the nutritional biochemistry arising out of long-term AN behaviors and nutrient losses. Thus, a history alongside testing will reveal current nutritional status. Common nutritional deficits are low levels of zinc and potassium. Hormonal disruption, amenorrhea, and osteoporosis are also major complications. Epling & Pierce (1996) suggest that the concept of "activity anorexia," which co-occurs at a high rate with AN, is characterized by an increase in exercise in response to a decrease in food intake that can lead to starvation and death. This suggests the need to include an exercise history alongside food history during the assessment process.

Avoidant/Restrictive Food Intake Disorder

Known also as selective eating disorder (SED), it is an eating disorder that prevents the consumption of certain foods.

Assessment Essentials

The night eating syndrome (NES) questionnaire is used to screen (with a score of 30) as the cutoff for bariatric surgery (Mitchell & Zwann, 2011, p. 44).

NES history and inventory are available from Allison et al. (2008).

Eating Attitudes Test 26: This test can be used for education and screening. A score of 20 or greater implies the need for further assessment (http://www.eat-26.com/)

Blood tests include the following:

Food sensitivities testing

Nutrient status tests

Salivary test

Zinc taste test: The zinc taste test is a simple way to test functional deficiency, which is common in eating disorders. Take a teaspoon full of liquid zinc (see Appendix Z: Resources) and you will find that you experience varying tastes based on your body's current needs. If you are deficient in zinc, the liquid will taste like water, while if you have adequate levels it will taste bitter.

24-hr cortisol test to evaluate HPA axis function

Amino acid levels testing (urinary and blood)

Tissue mineral analysis

The Bariatric Client

Bariatric gastric bypass surgery restricts food intake by making it difficult to ingest large amounts of food. Its efficacy, however, is based on altering the appetite to decrease hunger and increase satiety and not the food restriction itself. Predicting who will be successful in losing weight and maintaining weight loss in those who undergo this surgery is difficult, and recent research identifies genetically based variations affecting success (Hatoum et al., 2013).

Weight-loss surgical procedures are categorized into three groups: (1) the laparoscopic adjustable gastric band, (2) the Roux-enY gastric bypass, and (3) the sleeve gastrectomy (Mitchell & Zwaan, 2011). Malabsorption of macronutrients is more common in these combination procedures.

A client is required to undergo a psychological assessment prior to acceptance for bariatric surgery. Most people consider bariatric surgery after many years of attempted weight loss. Nevertheless, every effort should be made to combine a weight-loss program with exercise and adjunctive methods to improve well-being. Differentiation should be made between morbidly obese individuals (BMI over 40) who have life-threatening conditions associated with obesity and the population of people with a BMI of 30–35 who wish to undergo surgery.

From a mental health nutrition perspective, bariatric surgery should be the last resort; bariatric surgery frequently leads to complications, including impaired nutritional status due to malabsorption syndrome as well as psychological sequelae. However, there are clients for whom it represents a viable alternative to improving health. Thus, it is up to the clinician to use all the tools at her or his disposal to provide an integrative approach.

Clients who are both obese or morbidly obese (and who may or may not have type 2 diabetes) may be advised by a health professional to undergo bariatric surgery, or a client may raise the option of surgery with us during treatment. Over 100,000 bariatric surgeries are performed annually in the United States. There are many types of surgeries. They range from reversible to permanent procedures. The lap band reduces the size of the stomach by sectioning off a portion with an adjustable (and reversible) gastric band. Gastric bypass may be performed, which surgically reroutes food to the lower intestine.

There is a high rate of complications post surgery and during the years following surgery, requiring specialized and ongoing management. Furthermore, a range of studies demonstrate there is significant weight gain in 50% of individuals within 2–5 years following surgery. For some people the surgeries are very successful and lead to improvement or elimination of type 2 diabetes and sleep apnea, and for others they are less successful. While a number of studies have identified some of the psychological predictors of success, they are inconclusive. Substance abuse and psychosis are among the contraindications. A number of studies demonstrate significantly high rates of self-reported childhood maltreatment emotionally and sexually among male and female obese individuals seeking bariatric surgery. Noncompliance with postsurgical requirements is high. A number of studies have identified high rates of post–bariatric surgery psychiatric hospitalization and suicidality among childhood sexual abuse survivors (Clark et al., 2007).

Where people with BN or BED seek bariatric surgery, an assessment should include a history of exposure to complex trauma. There are high rates of traumatic stress and developmental trauma disorders leading to higher rates of somatic symptoms. Caution should be taken to ensure that bariatric surgery is not suggested as another in the list of surgeries in the attempt to "cut out" the trauma that is held in the body memory. Likewise, assessment for eating as a self-regulation, self-medication method should be addressed prior to bariatric surgery. Food, carbohydrate, and fat addiction, in particular, should be assessed as well.

People will come to bariatric surgery after trying other forms of surgery such as liposuction or cosmetic surgery. These clients can also have body dysmorphia or body image issues. Bariatric surgery will not solve any of the underlying issues that may contribute to BED; indeed, it can make them worse.

A comprehensive assessment can define whether an individual is a candidate from a mental health nutrition perspective. Because bariatric surgery is a business, a therapist must serve as an advocate for the client, and the nutritionally oriented therapist can provide alternatives to surgery that have not been considered previously.

While a client may be a candidate physically and in need of weight loss, not all clients will do well, especially people who are compulsive eaters, unless they can manage the day-to-day changes that will be required for a lifetime. Furthermore, food addiction often transforms into alcohol abuse or other addictive behaviors. Where compulsive eating and being overweight are associated with a history of childhood sexual abuse, weight loss can trigger memories and flashbacks and it is advisable to address childhood trauma prior to surgery. Many people show improvement in physical health and self-esteem due to weight loss, yet many continue to struggle psychologically (Kubik, Gill, Laffin, & Shahzeer, 2013). Bariatric surgery patients show higher suicide rates than the general population (Peterhänsel, Petroff, Klinitzke, Kersting, & Wagner, 2013).

A comprehensive assessment that results with recommendations for surgery should lead to an individualized treatment plan that is strengths based, improves resilience, and engages social supports, while exploring obstacles and strategies for postsurgery adaptation (Mitchell & Zwaan, 2011).

A qualitative interview should include comprehensive weight and diet history, general eating behaviors, history of past or present eating disorders (*DSM-V*), BED (which is the most common reason people come to bariatric surgery), purging or compensatory behaviors, night eating syndrome, emotional eating, exercise, substance abuse, trauma history, treatment history, stressors and coping skills, and social supports. The intake form provides sections for all of these areas. The assessment should include psychoeducation about the surgery and postsurgery nutrition and include expectations of surgical outcomes.

A comprehensive nutritional assessment should be undertaken prior to surgery including nutrient status. This can be done with laboratory workups with a registered dietician or other professional. While bariatric specific recommendations focus on thiamine, vitamin B12, folate, iron, calcium, zinc, and vitamin D, a more comprehensive nutritional analysis outlined in this book will benefit the client along with specialized food allergy/sensitivity testing, especially given the high rates of gluten sensitivity found in bulimic clients. Specialized blood tests are available that can measure vitamin mineral status prior to surgery (see Spectracell in Appendix Z: Resources), and a client can elect to optimize nutritional status. SIBO is common post bariatric surgery and attending to gut health in advance is essential.

Following a comprehensive evaluation, the clinician can provide a report to the bariatric medical team or make recommendations for mental health treatment required prior to surgery, for example, if there is a mood disorder. The client may also require further education about the lifestyle changes required post surgery. Suggestions to attend a post-bariatric surgery support group may also be beneficial.

Assessment Essentials

Weight and Lifestyle Inventory (WALI) (Wadden & Foster, 2006)

Boston Interview for Bariatric Surgery (Sogg & Mori, 2009)

Cleveland Clinical Behavioral Rating System (Heinberg, Ashton, & Windover, 2010)

Micronutrient tests (blood). These tests measure the function of 35 nutritional components, including vitamins, antioxidants, minerals, and amino acids within our white blood cells.

Inability to Gain Weight

Some clients want to discuss being underweight and problems with gaining weight. Being underweight can be a risk factor for poor mental health, yet contrary to popular belief there appears to be no association between poor mental health and poor body satisfaction or other body image issues in the non-eating-disordered underweight population. Underweight may result due to poverty, digestive problems, hyperthyroidism, genetics, or drug or alcohol use. A number of problems can underlie inability to gain weight; stimulants and thyroid problems can cause weight loss or prevent weight gain. They include malabsorption associated with gluten or other food allergies, Crohn's disease, and colitis. Elderly clients may experience sacopenia, which results in muscle loss and is a risk factor for falls and cognitive decline. It generally results from reduced levels of exercise and hormone changes.

Nutritional suggestions for weight gain include high-quality proteins and fats, root vegetables and whole grains, raw nuts, and supplemental smoothies with whey or pea protein added. Weight gain should concentrate on muscle (not fat) gain through amino acid supplementation.

As I have explored earlier, many different symptoms can derive from similar types of imbalances or combinations of complex nutritional deficits. One of the first steps I take following assessment is to provide clients with a handout of a delicious beverage (smoothie) recipe that can be modified according to their specific taste or nutrient needs. Whether they wish to lose or gain weight, decrease depression or anxiety, or improve their energy and cognitive function at any age, this first initial step starts the process of nutritional change (see Appendix F for the Pineapple Coconut Cognitive Smoothie recipe).

PRACTITIONERS WORKING IN THE FIELD OF NUTRITION

The following practitioners can serve as resources and referrals for collaboration and for prescribing nutritional programs. Following these descriptions, review the table in the appendix that includes the training and credentials for each profession (see Appendix G). This list may be reviewed with and provided to the client.

Nutritional Counselors/Therapists

These include certified clinical nutritionists, certified nutritional consultants, certified nutritionists, and board-certified physician nutrition specialists (medical professionals with specialized training in nutrition).

Nutritional counselors work with people to assess their nutritional needs and make recommendations for dietary changes to improve health and well-being. A nutritionist has specific nutritional training but is not a registered dietitian.

Registered Dietitians

Registered dieticians (RDs) can help to manage and prevent chronic illness, provide sports nutrition and culinary education, assist with presurgery and postsurgery nutrition, help with eating disorders, lead community efforts to improve food resources, provide guidance with prenatal and perinatal nutrition, and assist with healthy food and nutrition for the elderly. RDs administer medical nutrition therapy in which they review a person's eating habits, review her or his nutritional health, and create a nutritional treatment plan that is personalized for the individual. Often, though not always, the course of study promotes conventional nutritional guidelines rather than more progressive ones, and thus one should explore the approach taken by the dietician.

Naturopathic Physicians

Naturopathy is a holistic medical system that is guided by the major principle: The Healing Power of Nature (Vis Medicatrix Naturae). It is a blend of natural medicine and allopathic medicine. Naturopathic doctors (NDs) are licensed as primary care physicians in some states in the United States. Naturopathic practice includes the following diagnostic and therapeutic modalities: clinical and laboratory diagnostic testing, nutritional medicine, botanical medicine, physical medicine (including manipulative therapy), counseling, minor surgery, homeopathy, acupuncture, prescription medication, and obstetrics (natural childbirth).

Functional Medicine Practitioners

Functional medicine uses a systems-oriented and patient-centered approach, addressing the patient as a whole person. Practitioners of functional medicine take extensive patient histories and take time to understand an individual's unique health needs. They draw from Western and complementary/alternative medicine focusing on science-based prevention and treatments for body, mind, spirit, lifestyle, family, career, and the environment.

Integrative Medical Practitioners

Integrative medicine draws on both allopathic and complementary/alternative medical practices. It is often evidence based and takes into account the patient as a whole person and the relationship between the practitioner and the patient; it uses all available therapies that may help in the treatment of a client.

Health Coaches

A health coach educates and serves as a role model to motivate individuals, couples, families, and communities to explore and enact positive health choices. A variety of health coach training and certification programs exist, and training hours credentials can vary.

Osteopathic Doctors

Osteopathy is a comprehensive medical system that focuses on disease prevention while using the technology of modern medicine to diagnose and treat illness. It is holistic, looking at the patient as a whole person and not just treating isolated symptoms. Osteopathic physicians (DO) are fully trained physicians like MDs; they are able to perform surgery and work with prescription drugs. They also emphasize nutritional therapies and manipulative therapies such as cranial osteopathy.

Traditional Chinese Medicine and Acupuncturists

Traditional Chinese medical practitioners and acupuncturists prescribe individualized diets for the whole person. They take a comprehensive history and conduct a thorough assessment that includes pulse taking, tongue reading, and facial diagnosis. The Chinese nutritional approach is based on having a balance of the five tastes (spicy, sour, bitter, sweet, and salty) and six food groups (meats, dairy, fruit, vegetables, grains, and herbs and spices). Chinese medicine also incorporates the concepts of yin and yang to nutrition and recommends different foods for different times of year.

Traditional Medicine Healers/Practitioners

Traditional medicine involves ways of healing that are passed on from one generation to the next, among families and healers, and is based on indigenous, practical, and observational arts and science. Medicinal plants, animals, foods, the elements, rituals, spirit ways, and touch are all part of the earth's gifts that make up traditional medicine. Traditional medicine is the property of the communities and nations from which it originates; it emphasizes restoration of balance and prevention of causes and requires the vital preservation of the culture and natural resources of its origin.

Essential Next Steps

After the comprehensive physical and mental health intake, you then may discuss the following with the client:

- Further testing: discuss timeline, priorities, and costs
- Elimination diets
- Additional resources: handouts, reading
- Allow time for questions and concerns.
- Discuss a referral or consider a future referral; educate your client about the various clinicians who may be of assistance.
- Research practitioners working in the field to whom you might refer and collaborate.

CHAPTER 4

Common Diagnoses and Typical Nutritional Culprits

Diet Essential: Where there is mental illness, there is always a history of digestive problems.

Nutritional deficits occur in almost everyone; over 40% of the population has been found to have inadequate intakes of vitamin A, C, D, and E, calcium, and magnesium, and more so among obese individuals (Agarwal, Reider, Brooks, & Fulgoni, 2015). Understanding the role of nutrient deficits as contributing factors to mental illness has evolved over the last 75 years with the research of psychiatrists and biochemists, who explored the role of nutrition and brain function in people with psychotic disorders. It is now well established that nutrition intersects with individual biochemistry to play an essential role in mental health.

Nutrient deficits and imbalances contribute to the five essential factors that underlie mental illness:

- Chrononutrition imbalance
- Blood sugar handling and functional hypoglycemia
- Food allergies and sensitivities
- Inflammation, oxidative stress, and mitochondrial function
- Methylation: conversion of folates/folic acid (B-9) to l-methylfolate

CULPRITS, DEFICITS, AND DIAGNOSTICS

In this chapter, I investigate some major diagnostic categories and the nutrient culprits and deficits known to contribute to mental illness. I also provide recommendations on further tests and assessments that are available, and you will understand how to identify the contributory factors more closely. Knowing the tests that are available, whether you conduct them or you refer to another practitioner, will help you and the client to fill in the pieces to the "jigsaw" puzzle that is the client's health.

Mood Disorders

Depression is often an end-stage symptom of chronic stress. Depression is also a disease that arises from systemic inflammation. Chronic stress disables the body's capacity to successfully "quench the fires" to fight inflammation. Inflammation affects the first and the second brain as cells called cytokines block tryptophan conversion to serotonin. The stress-depression dyad also underlies ADHD, cognitive decline, the dementias, and traumatic brain injury. Deficits in Omega-3 fatty acids also contribute to mood disorders (Parker et al., 2006). Vitamin and mineral deficiencies are common among people who are depressed; in particular, deficiencies include B vitamins (biotin, folic acid, B6, B1, and B12), vitamin C, and calcium, copper, iron, magnesium, potassium, and zinc. Alternately, excessive levels of lead and copper (regularly obtained from drinking well water, for example) can also contribute to depression. Low levels of magnesium are frequently present, especially with anxious depression. Too much calcium is often found in depression, which is why biochemical individuality demands, for example, that we not just administer large amounts of calcium to older people with osteoporosis unless we know they absolutely require it. Vitamin D deficiency is an important factor in depression. Deficiency in pregnenolone—the "master hormone" that is synthesized in the brain and the precursor from which all other hormones are made—is also linked to depression (George et al., 1994). Celiac disease leads to low iron levels (and anemia) and results in depression. Serotonin requires iron during the conversion of the amino acid tryptophan from foods.

Nutrition and hormones interact throughout the life cycle and play an important role in depression, especially by the age of 40 in both men and women. Women are vulnerable to depression associated with perimenopause or menopause in part because hormonal changes lower neurotransmitter levels. As estrogen levels decrease, serotonin levels can decrease. Progesterone deficiency at this stage is common not only because of the stage of life but because stress depletes progesterone. Bioidentical progesterone can improve mood and aid sleep. One should recognize that testosterone levels also affect the health of both men and women. Low levels of vitamin D and zinc contribute to low testosterone, as do statins and environmental toxins like herbicides. By contrast, supplementation of testosterone is an antidepressant in men who experience low/borderline testosterone levels (Pope, Cohane, Kanayama, Siegel, & Hudson, 2003).

Assessment Essentials

24-hour salivary cortisol test: This can indicate biological depression due to chronic stress. This is common in PTSD and other chronic stress and anxiety disorders; it occurs when 24-hour cortisol measures show low waking cortisol and high nighttime cortisol—that is a sign of biological depression.

Vitamin D (25-OH vitamin D) test: A serum vitamin D (25-OH vitamin D) test should be performed annually, with the optimal range being from 40 to 65 ng/mL (100 to 160 nmol/L) (Vasquez et al., 2004).

MTHFR mutation: This simple blood test assesses the MTHFR gene, which is responsible for methylation; Mutations in the gene are common and affect homosysteine and NT synthesis and are associated with mental health disorders.

Salivary hormone tests for men and women

Gluten/casein and food sensitivity tests

Bipolar Disorder

All of the five essential health factors I presented earlier could underlie bipolar disorder. The pharmaceutical approach to treatment of bipolar disorder frequently involves the use of lithium carbonate. Researchers believe administering this compound both lengthens circadian rhythm and improves mitochondrial energy production (Maurer, Schippel, & Volz, 2009). This suggests that both of these functions are dysregulated in bipolar disorder. High homocysteine levels in people with bipolar disorder are common, suggesting the impaired ability to convert folates as a result of MTHFR mutation.

Researchers have identified a range of nutritional deficits in people diagnosed with bipolar disorder. Insufficiencies in particular include fatty acid deficits and impaired phospholipid metabolism (Stork & Renshaw, 2005). Phospholipids are a special type of fatty acid that supports cellular membranes and signaling between neurons. Pyrrole disorder occurs at higher rates among people with bipolar disorder. Observed evidence suggests that many people with bipolar disorder have food sensitivities such as gluten and casein. They exhibit reactivity to artificial sweeteners such as aspartame that increase mood lability and also negatively alter the microbiome. Finally, hypoglycemia aggravates mood lability.

Assessment Essentials

Functional hypoglycemia should be assessed as a contributing factor in mood lability. Insomnia is common in bipolar disorder, and affect dysregulation and mood cycling in response to complex trauma can also appear like bipolar disorder.

Homocysteine is a chemical in the blood that is produced when the amino acid methionine is broken down in the body. High levels occur in response to the MTHFR mutation and increase risk of mental health disorders, dementia, and heart disease.

Seasonal Affective Disorder

Seasonal affective disorder (SAD) is a form of major depressive disorder. It is also called "winter depression" associated with the onset of winter and the reduced environmental light. It generally improves when the sun returns in the spring and summer. It occurs more often in women and is associated with disruptions of the visual processing of light, changes in melatonin secretion, and lower levels of serotonin (Rosenthal, 2009). Symptoms of SAD include difficulty waking up in the morning, oversleep, fatigue, low mood, craving for carbohydrates, and weight gain.

The reduction of light exposure and its effects on neurotransmitter function is a central factor in SAD. Vitamin D and carbohydrates in their role in the tryptophan-serotonin-melatonin pathway is the focus of most research and treatment.

Assessment Essential

Seasonal Pattern Assessment Questionnaire (SPAQ): The SPAQ is a brief, self-administered screening tool for SAD (Rosenthal, Bradt, & Wehr, 1984).

Anxiety Disorders

People with anxiety commonly have disordered breathing and hyperventilation and somatic symptoms. They complain of headaches, neck pain, jaw pain, leg and body cramps, and tension in the shoulder muscles. Anxiety is also correlated with asthma in children and adults. Signs of chronic anxiety may be observed during history taking. These may include sighing, suspension of breathing (apnea), breath holding, erratic breathing, and intermittent long sighs or gasps.

Hyperventilation or disordered/overbreathing is exacerbated by a vegetarian diet when undertaken by people who are more suited biochemically to a carnivore diet. In anxiety with hyperventilation, CO_2 builds up in the blood and the diaphragm tends to fatigue. With increased fatigue and reduced oxygen, hypoxia can affect the brain, contributing to headaches and depression. Increased lactic acid in the musculature also can contribute to anxiety in a bidirectional manner. Shallow breathing changes blood gases that reinforce alkalosis, which leads to increased lactic acid and a loss of magnesium as the body tries to compensate for the alkalosis. Thus, magnesium is depleted by hyperventilation in chronic anxiety and panic response.

Low levels of magnesium are a marker for anxiety (Satori, Whittle, Hetzenauer, & Singewald, 2012). Anxiety is also associated with low levels of the neurotransmitter gamma-amino butyric acid (GABA). Caffeine use inhibits GABA in the brain. In individuals with lifelong anxiety or family anxiety, there may be a genetic disorder that affects the enzyme glutamic acid transaminase, which converts glutamic acid to GABA. Low levels of essential fatty acids (Omega-3) are associated with increased anxiety as are low levels of the vitamin B complex and vitamin D. People who experience panic attacks also have similar nutrient deficiencies. Diet pills, amphetamines, asthma medications, caffeine, antihistamines, and steroids all can increase anxiety and panic.

Tests

When a client complains of dizziness, faintness, or vertigo, assess for hyperventilation syndrome as a possible cause. The Nijmegen scale is a 16-item measure useful for identifying anxiety and hyperventilation associated with somatic symptoms (van Dixhoorn & Duivenvoorden, 1985).

Kharrazian (2013) suggests a simple challenge test to ascertain glutamic acid-GABA conversion disorder. Take 3,000–4,000 mg of alpha-ketoglutaric acid. If there is a genetic basis for this conversion problem, you will feel very nervous and anxious. If you don't have this problem, then you might feel a little energized, but it will not cause anxiety or irritability.

Obsessive-Compulsive Disorder

Obsessive-compulsive disorder (OCD) causes people to have obsessive thoughts and ideas, and/or the compulsive need to repeat specific behaviors or mental acts. OCD behaviors can be highly individualistic. People with OCD may also experience depression, eating disorders, ADHD, bipolar disorder, and social phobias. Obsessive–compulsive spectrum disorders (OCSDs) also include tic disorders, trichotillomania (TTM), hypochondriasis, body dysmorphic disorder (BDD), and body-focused repetitive behaviors (BFRB). Currently SSRIs are used for pharmacological treatment though usually only 40%–60% of OCD patients receive benefit from first-line SSRI treatments.

Levels of vitamin B12 are often low in people with OCD (Greenblatt, 2013). Melatonin is reduced in people with OCD (Monteleone, Catapano, Tortorella, Di Martino, & Maj, 1995). High levels of estrogen can also exacerbate symptoms in women with OCD (Rapkin, Mikacich, Moatakef-Imani, & Rasgon, 2002).

Trichotillomania

Trichotillomania (TTM) is defined as a self-induced and recurrent loss of hair. It is commonly considered part of the OCD spectrum but may also be considered a tic, habit, or addiction. There is often a dissociative element to the behavior itself. More recently it has been included among "body-focused repetitive behaviors."

TTM co-occurs at high rates in people with a history of trauma (Gershuny et al., 2006) and may be a self-soothing behavior. It is also associated with celiac disease and the effect of malabsorption of nutrients leading to problems with NT synthesis. Significant improvement of trichotillomania was observed after 9 weeks of treatment with N-acetylcysteine (TTM) (Grant, Odlaug, & Kim, 2009).

Trauma and Stressor-Related Disorders

Posttrauamatic Stress Disorder / Complex Trauma / Developmental Trauma

People who have been traumatized often experience depression, anxiety, insomnia, and dissociation along with intractable physical symptoms, including pain, digestive problems, heart, respiratory problems, and reproductive problems (Korn, 2013). Substance abuse, including eating disorders, and self-injury and traumatic brain injury are common among trauma victims. People with PTSD have increased levels of inflammatory markers, increased allergies, and are vulnerable to higher rates of autoimmune diseases, depressed immune function, and therefore increased risk of infections. PTSD is associated with disruption of cortisol levels and depletion of NTs.

The major nutritional factors affecting PTSD are similar to those in chronic depression and anxiety. Nutritional deficits also result from the poor dietary habits associated with impaired self-care and the side effects associated with the use of pharmaceuticals to treat functional pain symptoms of fibromyalgia, migraines, and irritable bowel syndrome and long-term effects of substance abuse. For example, tobacco and cannabis use is high in PTSD and opiate and benzodiazepine use is common.

Assessment Essential

24-hour salivary cortisol test

Chemical Dependency and Substance Abuse

Humans everywhere seek to alter their consciousness. Alcohol, drugs, plants, and foods all alter consciousness. Distinguishing between altering consciousness as a ritual for healing or for self-medication and addiction is essential to mental health recovery. Understanding what is being altered and why is essential in order to identify alternative nutritional strategies.

In my practice I have observed success with the nutritional treatment of the addictions by combining two models of mental health nutrition: the model of self-medication and the model of nutrient deficit. The concept of addiction-as-self-medication (Khantzian, 1997) suggests that people choose substances to self-regulate painful affective states. This leads to using substances—whether self-prescribed or clinician prescribed—that medicate what the brain/body cannot do for itself. This concept is applied also to addiction-as-nutrient-deficit disease with strong evidence provided by Williams (1998), Hoffer (1962), Pfeiffer (1988), and Enig (2000). During the assessment process if we follow the substances that are used, we can understand what states of consciousness and thus what deficits are being medicated. We then analyze the affective and biochemical effects on the body/mind. If one understands what one is self-medicating, one can identify the nutrients that may be missing; this will complement all the other addiction therapies.

Drugs and alcohol stimulate neurotransmitter release and create a sense of pleasure and reward in the brain. But over time these exogenous chemicals suppress the ability of the brain to produce its own chemistry. The brain says, "I don't have to do much of anything and look how I am getting all this drug action without doing much at all." For example, almost all addictive substances cause an increased production of dopamine, one of the neurotransmitters involved in feelings of reward and pleasure. But overstimulation of dopamine leads to depleted dopamine levels and, in turn, a lack of pleasure in life. This, in turn, drives the cycle of reaching for more dopamine-stimulating substances to get that pleasurable feeling. It is like hitting your thumb with a hammer; you feel it the first time, but if you keep hitting it, it becomes numb.

The use of alcohol and drugs can contribute to primary or secondary malnutrition. Primary malnutrition occurs due to lack of food intake. This may be due to lack of money and access to food, being homeless, co-occurring disorders, or expenditures of resources on drugs. Secondary malnutrition occurs as a result of the ways the specific substance impairs digestion and absorption of nutrients. Co-occurring disorders such as PTSD, depression, and eating disorders are common and alcohol and drug abuse commonly occurs as a form of self-medication in response to traumatic stress. While each type of substance has specific deficits that lead to or result from use, the status of essential fatty acids (Omega-3) is the first area requiring assessment and intervention.

Alcohol

Alcohol is an example of a substance that when abused leads to both primary and secondary malnutrition. It is well established that nutrient deficits make one vulnerable to alcohol use and that the ability to digest and absorb nutrients and fatty acids is impaired as a result of chronic alcohol use. Alcohol use inhibits fat absorption and thereby impairs absorption of the Omega fatty acids and vitamins A, E, and D that are normally absorbed along with dietary fats. Low levels of folate and vitamin B12 have been found in depressed patients who had a history of alcoholism. Chronic excessive alcohol consumption depletes brain levels of Omega-3 fatty acids. Binge drinking leads to insulin resistance, making individuals with a history of alcohol abuse more likely to develop type 2 diabetes and, later, possibly dementia. A severe thiamine (vitamin B-1) deficiency can occur in heavy alcohol users leading to brain damage, called Wernicke–Korsakoff syndrome.

Alcohol addiction is also a physiological addiction to sugar that needs to be managed during active and long-term recovery. As people withdraw from alcohol, they often replace alcohol with refined sugar and simple carbohydrates, and increase coffee intake as part of the withdrawal and maintenance process. This can serve as a short-term transitional approach to ease withdrawal; however, it is not a long-term benefit, as the sugar will exacerbate cravings.

Assessment Essentials
Liver function tests
Assess for ability to eat and digest nutrients for the recovery process
Assess for IV nutrient support (Myer's cocktail)

Cannabis

Like many substances, cannabis can be medicinal or it can be the object of abuse. Cannabis has not been shown to have a physiological basis for addiction. It is often used to self-medicate symptoms of PTSD and chronic pain. Medical cannabis and increasingly recreational cannabis are being legalized in the United

States. Like every substance used to alter consciousness, mood, and physical sensation, a comprehensive analysis of the role of cannabis and its mode of ingestion/absorption is required to understand the meaning and psychobiological effects on the individual.

Chronic smoking of cannabis can lead to lung irritation, and people will benefit from vitamins and glandulars that support lung recovery. Cannabis users will benefit from new technologies that do not cause lung irritation. It is common for cannabis smokers to also smoke tobacco. In these cases cessation of tobacco should be enacted first and then cannabis withdrawal. There is some evidence that cannabis use in children and adolescents has a negative effect on the brain. Cannabis use should be limited until full brain development has occurred.

Cannabis withdrawal syndrome is now included in the *DSM-5*; irritability, nervousness, sleep difficulties, appetite changes, restlessness, and depressed mood are among the symptoms described. Research in the United States suggests that 9% of those who use cannabis become dependent, especially among heavy users who start when they are young. However, these criteria have been criticized because the criteria for dependence have not been well defined in these studies and may range from use throughout the day to an occasional toke.

There is evidence that essential fatty acids positively affect the endocannabinoid system in the brain, reinforcing the idea of supplementation for people who wish to decrease or eliminate recreational cannabis use. Hemp oil is a good fat of choice, along with fish oil, borage oil, and butter. Pregnenolone appears to reduce several effects of THC, suggesting it may be useful for the treatment of cannabis withdrawal (Vallée et al., 2014).

Butane Hash Oil (Dabs)

Butane hash oil is increasingly used in the United States. It is a highly concentrated form of marijuana that looks like honey and contains a high percentage of THC, the drug's psychoactive ingredient. People who abuse butane hash oil usually smoke it, vaporize it, ingest it in food, or apply it to the skin. One report among users describes hash oil as inducing greater tolerance and withdrawal (Loflin & Earleywine, 2014). The practice of making the preparations at home is also filled with danger of unexpected fires.

Cocaine

Most nutrition research examining the effects of cocaine has been conducted on animals. In animal models cocaine increases oxidative stress, and low cholesterol has been found in people who have detoxified but relapsed to cocaine addiction (Buydens-Branchey & Branchey, 2003), suggesting the importance of fats for brain function in maintaining recovery. Cocaine depletes dopamine in the brain and can also damage delicate mucus membranes. It decreases apetite and can lead to primary malnutrition and also depletes vitamin B6, thiamin, and vitamin C.

Ecstasy/Molly

MDMA (3,4-methylenedioxymethamphetamine) is a common component in Ecstasy. MDMA releases a flood of serotonin and dopamine and increases blood levels of the hormones oxytocin and prolactin. MDMA is used both therapeutically, for example to treat PTSD, and also as a street drug that is often impure or mixed with other substances.

The street drug Ecstasy often includes methamphetamine and cocaine or caffeine. Acute adverse effects, such as jaw clenching, dry mouth, and lack or loss of appetite, are common, especially among women (Liechti & Vollenweider, 2001). Street-obtained Ecstasy initiates a cascade of oxidative stress depending upon the chemistry of the drugs used and the chronicity of use. Withdrawal needs include addressing depression and mood lability following use and the use of L-tyrosine or DL phenylalanine to increase dopamine levels.

Methamphetamine

Methamphetamine (meth) is a very dangerous drug for the brain and leads to oxidative stress and neuronal damage. It can damage proteins in the brain that protect and repair dopamine, resulting in Parkinson-like symptoms. It also appears to damage the blood-brain barrier. Malnutrition is common among meth users since it decreases appetite.

Opiates

There are a wide variety of opiates in use, both legal and illegal; OxyContin and Vicodin are commonly prescribed opiates to which people may become addicted, and heroin is a widely used addictive substance. Opiates impair digestive function, and prolonged use impairs the body's capacity to reduce pain. People addicted to opiates (or who are on methadone treatment) are at risk for increased sugar intake (Mysels & Sullivan, 2010), leading to obesity, hypoglycemia, and diabetes. Among the major opiates in use are morphine, codeine, and the semisynthetic derivatives, hydrocodone, oxycodone, and hydromorphone. Among the effects of these medications/drugs is reduction of glutathione and selenium.

Tobacco/Nicotine

Smoking tobacco is a form of self-medication, though in some societies, most notably American Indian, it is used in small quantities as a ritual plant. Tobacco is a euphoriant; it increases cognitive function, can appear to reduce anxiety, and possibly helps to extinguish traumatic memories. As a result, tobacco use is high among people with PTSD. Because nicotine is an antidepressant, cessation often triggers depression. Nicotine also speeds metabolism, and weight gain often follows withdrawal.

Considerable toxicity is associated with nicotine. Commercial additives and other toxins contribute to increased oxidative stress in the body. These affect nutrient status, and smokers are known to have lower levels of B-complex, vitamin C, and the antioxidants beta-carotene and vitamin E (Preston, 1991). Mineral levels of selenium and zinc, known as antioxidant minerals, are measured at lower levels in smokers. This is likely due to chronic inflammation. Exposure to secondhand smoke appears to lower nutrient levels as well.

Withdrawal from nicotine generally begins within 30 minutes of smoking the last cigarette; consequent physical symptoms peak within 3 days and last for at least 4 weeks. People are subject to low energy, depression, and depressed cognitive function during the withdrawal process, so planning in advance with diet, nutrients, and exercise can mitigate those effects.

Preparation for withdrawal begins with improving diet and balancing blood sugar and oral needs by eating a mixture of high-protein, carbohydrates, and fats in meals every 3 to 4 hours. Choline-rich foods such as eggs, liver, and fish are very helpful.

In my clinical experience many people withdraw successfully from tobacco by substituting cannabis during the withdrawal period. The combination of the cannabis constituents and the inhalation process both likely contribute to their efficacy. THC, the psychoactive constituent, is associated with a reduction of somatic symptoms of nicotine withdrawal, suggesting the anecdotal evidence of use of cannabis during the withdrawal process has merit (Balerio, Aso, Berrendero, Murtra, & Maldonado, 2004). Tyrosine precursors have been used to ameliorate the effects of nicotine withdrawal. There is some evidence that use of CBD, a nonpsychoactive constituent of cannabis, is useful for the withdrawal from tobacco (Morgan, Das, Joye, Curran, & Kamboj, 2013). Prousky (2005) suggests the use of niacin to treat nicotine addiction. Walking and/or climbing or swimming to the point of breathing heavily helps to manage anxiety, decrease dissociation, and satisfy the urge to inhale. Heavy breathing mimics the sensation of inhaling smoke. Sweating in a sauna, steam bath, or ritual group sweat can be useful. Place ice packs on the spine between the shoulders to reduce depression and increase lung function.

Autism Spectrum/Neurodevelopmental Disorders

Like the psychotic disorders, the autism spectrum disorders (ASDs) are where we see the confluence of nearly all the problems of nutrition that can occur both from the point of view of deficits that are causative and subsequent challenges in obtaining good nutrition.

The reasons for the exponential increase of the ASDs in the United States and other industrialized countries has not been definitively identified, yet significant research points to deficits in nutrition required for the developing brain and exposure to toxins, both pharmaceutical and environmental. Lemer (2014) refers to the concept of "total load," which, like allostatic load, suggests that the cumulative burdens of physical and emotional stressors, environmental toxins, vaccines, and food allergies tip the body/mind into the autism spectrum. Acetaminophen use in genetically vulnerable children may contribute to autism (Shaw, 2013a), and the mother's exposure to air pollution in late-stage pregnancy increases risk of ASD in the child (Roberts et al., 2014). High oxalate levels from foods and fungus have also been identified in ASD (Shaw, 2013b).

Among the nutrient deficits that have been identified are essential fatty acids, as well as an excess of Omega-6 over Omega-3 ratios (Vancassel et al., 2001; van Elst et al., 2014). Inadequate levels of choline and betaine have been found in children with ASD, suggesting poor methylation (Hamlin et al., 2013). These children also show evidence of impaired methylation, increased oxidative stress (James et al., 2004), and dysbiosis (van De Sande, van Buul, & Brouns, 2014).

Essential fatty acid and phospholipid availability and processing, respectively, are central to behavioral well-being in ASD. Phospholipids play an important role in ASD like most psychiatric disorders. Phospholipids are found in foods like fish oils, eggs, and lecithin. Antiphospholipid antibodies have been found in children with ASD, suggesting an autoimmune response (Careaga, Hansen, Hertz-Piccotto, Van de Water, & Ashwood, 2013) may influence their behavior. These antibodies likely also represent inflammatory processes and impair the ability to utilize fats at the neuronal level. Whether this may be part of a larger ongoing autoimmune dysfunction associated with food-mediated allergens is yet unknown, but it does reinforce the idea of reduction of hyperreactivity of immune response at all levels. The phospholipase 2 (PLA2) enzyme destroys essential fatty acids and has been identified as being high in ASD. Therefore, PLA2 stimulants, such as refined foods that raise insulin (Bell et al., 2004), should be avoided. These clients will benefit from a diet with low carbohydrates and rich in EPA from fish oil, evening primrose oil, and phosphatidylcholine.

ASD children often have very challenging food eating patterns and are highly selective about foods, with a preference for carbohydrates and sugars, which may also reflect allergic cravings. Food selectivity also exacerbates nutritional deficits and leads to low levels of calcium and protein (Sharp et al., 2013). Gimpl and Fahrenholz (2002) suggest that a low level of oxytocin (the love hormone that supports prosocial behavior) is common in people along the autism spectrum. Oxytocin is strongly dependent on good cholesterol levels, suggesting the use of foods with saturated fats like whole cream, eggs, and liver may be important in the diet. Aggressive behaviors and self-injury have improved with cholesterol supplementation (Aneja & Tierney, 2008). Where there are food allergies or dislike of cholesterol-rich foods, there is a cholesterol supplement available in powder form that may be added to juices.

Assessment Essentials
Gluten/casein sensitivity test

MTHFR mutation test

Organic acids test: Oxalates and intestinal bacteria test (urine) examines oxalate levels along with intestinal levels bacteria and yeast.

Cognitive Function and the Dementias

There are many nutritional problems that contribute to memory loss and cognitive decline. Once cognitive decline becomes symptomatic it reflects a well-established process of oxidative stress and inflammation. DNA and lipids in the brain are damaged by oxidation as we age, causing neuronal death contributing to Alzheimer's and cognitive impairment. Just as the intestines can become hyperpermeable in response to inflammation, so can the brain. In contrast to commonly held opinion, mild memory loss is not a normal part of aging and likely constitutes early stages of dementia (Wilson et al., 2010).

Health risk factors include history of brain injury, chronic depression, PTSD, and poor-quality sleep/untreated sleep apnea, diabetes, smoking, and chronic depression. There is a growing body of evidence that implicates the herpes simplex type 1 virus in the development of Alzheimer's dementia (Rubey, 2010). People with elevated homocysteine levels have a greater risk of cognitive decline since high levels of homocysteine cause memory impairment, reduce brain circulation, and brain volume. Aluminum is a known neurotoxin, and occupational exposure to aluminum has been implicated in neurological disease, including Alzheimer's disease (Exley, 2014). There is significant evidence that exposure to environmental toxins affects cognition negatively and increases the risk of the dementias. These toxins include the range of pesticides, herbicides, and fungicides (Baldi et al., 2001); cumulative exposure to lead (Bakulski, Rozek, Dolinoy, Paulson, & Hu, 2012); and work exposure to low-frequency electromagnetic fields and exposure to cell phones and electronics.

Dietary risk factors include foods that increase inflammation and insulin levels such as simple carbohydrates, sugars, and trans fats; a relative deficiency in dietary fats and cholesterol contributes to the development of Alzheimer's disease (Seneff, Wainwright, & Mascitelliemail, 2011). Numerous studies have demonstrated that there is no significant relationship between cholesterol intake and heart disease (McNamara, 2014) but rather that people with cholesterol below 200 consistently show lower cognitive functional capacity (Elias et al., 2005). Low levels of the carotenoids xanthophylls, lutein, and zeaxanthin are associated with cognitive decline (Johnson, 2012), and vitamin D deficiency accelerates age-related cognitive decline.

Cognitive decline is also attributed to the aging process where the neurons' ability to manage intracellular calcium levels via calcium-binding proteins decreases. The buildup of calcium in the brain is a major contributor to age-related cognitive decline (Oliveira & Bading, 2011). A decline in calcium-binding proteins is a key factor in calcium accumulation and appears to affect both Alzheimer's type and vascular dementia (Nimmrich & Eckert, 2013).

One of the major theories of Alzheimer's is that amyloid beta peptide builds up plaque in the brain. Bredesen (2014), however, asserts that the amyloid beta peptide has a normal function in the brain, and rather the problem lies with an imbalance in nerve cell signaling. This has led to his design of a comprehensive approach to improving brain signaling using intensive nutrient supplementation, which has demonstrated reversal of cognitive decline in small clinical trials of Alzheimer's patients.

All of the NTs are essential for the maintenance of cognitive health. One of the most important for cognitive function is acetylcholine, which is required for sleep, memory, and neuromuscular function. Acetylcholine declines with age, and this contributes to decline in neurological function. Dietary choline is one of the nutritional precursors of acetylcholine and is often deficient in the diets of vegetarians and vegans as well as people on low-fat and low-cholesterol diets, or those who abuse alcohol. Consumption of low levels of folate and vitamin B12 are also risk factors for the development of dementia (Wang et al., 2001), suggesting that vegetarians who are at risk for B12 deficits may be at higher risk.

Assessment Essentials

Neuropsychological testing to establish baseline function is important in people expressing concerns about cognitive decline.

Sensitive C-reactive protein (sCRP). This is a marker of inflammation associated with heart disease and with systemic inflammation. Dietary change and the use of suggested nutrients below should show changes in this marker overtime.

24-hour cortisol test

Blood test that assesses for sex hormones

Serum testosterone

Homocysteine (blood)

Fasting insulin

Traumatic Brain Injury/Concussion Syndrome

Traumatic brain injury may be acute or chronic. The causes range from violence, abuse, accidents (car/motorcycle), athletic injuries, and exposures during war. Secondary to the initial event is a cascade of secondary damage as a result of inflammation, oxidative stress from free radicals, chemical imbalances (cytotoxicity and calcium influx into neurons), loss of circulation, and insufficient oxygenation, all of which lead to tissue and neuron damage. Traumatic brain injury is diagnosed based on the level of injury from mild to severe and location of the injury in the brain.

Nutritional treatment is an important adjunct to controlling secondary effects in the acute stage. Head injury patients are at risk of zinc deficiency, and zinc loss is ongoing following acute injury and is proportional to injury severity. Up to 12 mg a day of zinc may improve physical status and survival (Cope, Morris, & Levenson, 2012).

Attention-Deficit/Hyperactivity Disorder

The diagnostic category of ADHD is fraught with controversy, including overdiagnosis and misdiagnosis. Some clinicians question its existence and express concern over the significant side effects of stimulants on the developing brain (Baughman, 2006). Problems maintaining attention are multifocal. Poverty, environmental stress, violence, household stress, and developmental trauma lead to learning and attention problems (Burke, Hellman, Scott, Weems, & Carrion, 2011) and may be mistaken for ADHD. Many children with a diagnosis of ADHD may be hungry, may not eat breakfast, or if they do, it may be a highly refined carbohydrate-rich breakfast. Their behaviors may reflect functional hypoglycemia and deficits of essential fatty acids. The reduction and elimination of physical exercise programs in schools and the mandatory requirement to sit for long hours, along with limits of learning style and teaching methods, all contribute to behavior problems. Medications such as Adderall and Ritalin, the commonly prescribed medications, can lead to problems sleeping, weight loss, and irritability. These medications also create functional changes in the brain, which are then further medicated.

Children with ADHD often have low levels of zinc and iron, both of which are required for neurotransmitter synthesis. Dopamine levels may be low in ADHD, and essential fatty acid and phospholipid metabolism is likely impaired. Food sensitivities, a highly refined carbohydrate diet, food coloring, microbiome imbalance, and toxic exposures such as heavy metals and environmental toxins are also common (Kidd, 2000). Some children and adults are also sensitive to foods containing salicylates.

Assessment Essential
MTHFR mutation

Sleep/Wake Disorders

Insomnia
Insomnia affects a high percentage of people and is associated with major depression, anxiety disorder, and alcohol and drug abuse. Insomnia commonly occurs with bipolar disorder during both depressive and manic episodes. People require individualized treatment approaches to insomnia.

Sleep/wakefulness is governed by the HPA axis, which controls cortisol production on a 24-hour circadian rhythm. Hyperarousal prevents sleep and is often associated with high levels of evening cortisol. While small doses of caffeine improve mood and the ability to focus, higher doses interfere with the delta waves of deep, restorative sleep (Landolt, Dijk, Gaus, & Borbely, 1995).

Transient insomnia lasts for less than a week and can be caused by an illness, changes in the sleep environment, the timing of sleep, severe depression, or by stress. Acute insomnia is the inability to consistently stay asleep for a period of less than a month and can include difficulty falling asleep, staying asleep, or restless sleep. Chronic insomnia lasts for longer than a month. It can be caused by a medical or psychiatric disorder, or it can be a primary disorder. Chronic insomnia is a risk factor for the use of sleep medications, including benzodiazepines, which further decrease REM and restorative sleep.

Insomnia can lead to drug and alcohol use, but substance abuse can also increase the likelihood of insomnia. Chronic and acute pain affects sleep. Exploring pretrauma functioning can identify reasonable goals for improved sleep. Early-childhood trauma survivors may have never had a satisfactory sleep rhythm; these individuals may require more time to be treated effectively. High allostatic load (AL) is associated with sleep disturbances. African Americans and Hispanic populations have higher levels of AL (Chen, Redline, Shields, Williams, & Williams, 2014), suggesting the role of chronic stress and minority status and its impact on restful sleep. High levels of glucose and insulin resistance, diabetes, and sleep apnea are also associated with insomnia, and insomnia increases insulin resistance and weight gain. The role of (hidden) caffeine in insomnia is described in Janet's story in Box 4.1

Box 4.1
Janet's Story

Janet was a 20-year-old college student who came to the office complaining of insomnia and nervousness. She said that while she was under some stress at school, she had always handled it well and that she did not think that anything had changed in her life. During our intake, she reached into her bag and pulled out an energy drink that contained 160 mg of caffeine and taurine, an energizing amino acid. Janet told me that she drank three cans a day. I explained to Janet that she was drinking the equivalent of 4–5 cups of coffee a day and that we would want to explore her slowly stopping the use of these drinks. I added that we would find alternatives that would still help her to focus and keep her energy strong but that would not affect her sleep or cause anxiety.

Assessment Essential

Evaluation of the type of insomnia (sleep-onset insomnia or sleep-maintaining insomnia) is required for effective treatment.

The Pittsburgh Sleep Quality Index (PSQI) is available in 56 languages. It is a self-rating scale that assesses sleep quality and disturbances (Buysse, Reynolds, Monk, Berman, & Kupfer, 1989).

Evaluate evening functional hypoglycemia when people describe that they can fall asleep but awaken 2–4 hours later. They may fulfill criteria for sleep-maintaining insomnia. When blood sugar drops, the body awakens in an alarm state. These individuals benefit from eating a few ounces of protein and carbohydrate just before bed. If they awaken in the night, they can also eat a little food to stabilize blood sugar levels.

Psychosis/Schizophrenia

Schizophrenia is associated with low levels of essential fatty acids and poor phospholipid metabolism. Early theories of the cause of schizophrenia focused on phospholipid function but left mainstream thought in favor of the NT theory of illness, especially the dopamine theory. While NTs are crucial to healthy cognitive and affective function, the direct treatment of NTs via pharmaceuticals has generally failed to achieve the hoped-for results. Recently the phospholipid concepts have been reexamined, especially in the light of the decline in dietary phospholipids and essential fatty acids to support brain function.

There is evidence that people with the diagnosis of schizophrenia and psychotic disorders are especially sensitive to gluten and other food allergens. As early as World War II, clinicians observed that countries that limited bread and cereal consumption led to a significant decrease in hospitalizations for schizophrenia (Dohan, 1966). The overgrowth of the gastrointestinal tract by multiple *Clostridia* species and yeast/fungal species and its effects on a variety of physical and mental health disorders has been well documented (Shaw, 2011). Shaw (2011) found that intestinal infection with *C. difficle* species produced a dysbiosis in people with schizophrenia and autism, and led to disruption of dopamine function. Healing gut dysfunction (dysbiosis) in psychotic disorders may require medications like antibiotics or antifungals initially to eradicate dangerous levels of bacteria.

Approximately 80% of people with schizophrenia do not "flush" in response to the administration of 200 mg of niacin, which is suggestive of phospholipid signaling dysfunction (Lake, 2006). Deficiencies in folate, vitamin C, and niacin appear to worsen the symptoms of schizophrenia (Hoffer, 2008).

Assessment Essential

Niacin challenge test: The niacin challenge test may be used to distinguish symptoms of schizophrenia from other severe symptoms (Lake, 2006). Use (approximately) 200 mg of niacin to observe a "flush." People with phospholipid-impaired schizophrenia do not "flush" in response to administration of oral or topical niacin. The dose required may vary according to genetics.

MEDICAL PROBLEMS THAT INTERSECT WITH NUTRITION

Adrenal Fatigue

Adrenal fatigue occurs in response to chronic stress. Adrenal fatigue underlies depression, anxiety, chronic pain, insomnia, and PTSD. Adrenal hormones follow a circadian cycle. They are like your body's engine, ready to pump out hormones in response to stressors in your environment. Imagine trying to drive a car with your foot on the accelerator while the car is in neutral. Eventually this will cause the engine to burn out. When the adrenal glands are repeatedly overstimulated, for example in response to prolonged stress, poor diet, and excess caffeine, they become overworked.

Under normal conditions cortisol levels are high in the morning and decrease during the day and are lowest in the evening before sleep. But in adrenal fatigue the opposite occurs; this is biological depression. Without the assessment and nutritional treatment of adrenal fatigue, the treatment of illness often fails.

Assessment Essential

24-hour cortisol test

Obesity and Bariatric Surgery

Research shows that in general people lose weight undertaking a range of programs; what matters is persistence and what people feel is a good "fit" for them. This also reflects nutritional and biochemical individuality discussed in Chapter 1. Some people will do better on an Atkins-type carnivore diet, others will do better on a Weight Watchers approach, and others will do better on a vegetarian-style diet. The needs of the obese client who has a history of trauma are more specialized because trauma disrupts metabolic function, alters NT function, and increases inflammation, depression, and anxiety. SSRIs also cause weight gain. Obesity occurs in response to diminished sleep and an altered microbiome. People may binge on grain-based and sugary carbohydrates (and poor-quality fats) and have resulting insulin resistance. Addressing these issues first is an alternative to surgery. Exploring in depth the postsurgical requirements to adhere to a restrictive diet program and intensive nutritional supplementation is also essential.

One of the areas where people lack compliance post surgery is in exercise. This may also occur among people who are obese. CBT and coaching activities can encourage people to exercise, which helps decrease dissociation. Exercise and movement may also trigger flashbacks as people experience their body sensations. Titrating these experiences may also include touch therapies (Korn, 2013) and other body-oriented activities like yoga, or receiving spa services as other methods for decreasing dissociation.

Intensive nutrient supplementation prior to surgery and improvement of HPA and amino acid/fatty acid levels is essential. While there are many protein powder mixes and supplements for the bariatric client, they most often have added corn syrup, sugars, corn oils, and preservatives, all of which should be avoided.

Diet After Bariatric Surgery

Following bariatric surgery, intensive nutritional care is required. Special formulae containing easily absorbed vitamins and minerals along with healthy protein and fats can be used along with nutrients that boost immunity and support the healing of tissues. The nutritional imbalances that existed prior to surgery continue after surgery and worsen. Food and eating habits will need to be addressed after surgery, including the use of food as a coping mechanism or to stave off boredom, and emotional and social issues related to food, as well as eating disorders.

Complications and digestive problems are common after bariatric surgery; the most common is "dumping syndrome" in which the stomach empties into the small intestine at an increased rate. Dumping syndrome is exacerbated by the consumption of sugar and high-glycemic carbohydrates. Eating low-glycemic foods and complex carbohydrates is important in addition to proteins and healthy fats. Alcohol and other drug abuse commonly increases following surgery with 60% of people reporting no previous drinking problems (Ross, 2012). Immune-related arthritis can also develop following bariatric surgery (Bland, 2004).

Major nutritional complications of bariatric surgery continue over more than 20 years after surgery. Decreased intestinal absorption of iron (Bal, Finelli, & Koch, 2011), vitamin B12, folate, thiamin, calcium, vitamins A, D, E, and K, protein, zinc, magnesium, copper, and selenium are common. Deficiencies related to red blood cell production and bone metabolism are especially common. Despite the suggested use of routine vitamin and mineral supplements after surgery, micronutrient deficiencies are significant in postoperative gastric bypass patients due to impaired ability of the intestines to absorb nutrients.

Candidiasis

Candidiasis is also known as Candida-related complex (CRC); it is a common fungal (yeast) infection (*Candida albicans*). Yeast overgrowth is associated with cognitive and affective dysfunction, chronic fatigue, depression, fibromyalgia, and pain.

Candida-related complex can develop as a result of antibiotic use that leads to yeast overgrowth in the colon and other parts of the body. *Candida albicans* is naturally present in the body, but it can also proliferate in people who are immune compromised such as people with HIV-AIDS, or also in response to a sugar-rich diet. Other risk factors include hypothyroidism, oral contraceptives, pregnancy, post surgery, stress, zinc and iron deficiency, and copper excess. Bread and other yeast-based products aggravate candidiasis. Yeast ferments sugar into alcohol, and endogenous alcohol production is elevated after eating foods rich in carbohydrates. Yeast converts the alcohol (ethanol) into acetaldehyde, thus changing the levels of gut flora and leading to chronic candidiasis. The acetaldehyde toxins can also cause leaky gut (permeability).

The yeast may also spread to other parts of the body, passing through a permeable gut into the blood, as well as spreading from the anus to the genital area, causing vaginal yeast infections in women. Symptoms include fatigue, vaginal discharge and infections, anal itching, mental fatigue, prostatitis, bloating, indigestion, halitosis, mucus in the stools, low immunity or frequent colds, athlete's foot, cravings for sugar and carbohydrates and yeast, and allergies to foods.

Chronic Fatigue Syndrome

Chronic fatigue syndrome is a complex condition characterized by profound fatigue that persists for more than 6 months. It is marked by cognitive difficulties, pain, depression, headaches, sore throat, and disrupted sleep. It is more common in women and co-occurs with fibromyalgia. It is associated with a history of viral infections like Epstein Barr, adrenal fatigue, a history of trauma and chronic stress, and exposure to chemicals and environmental toxins. It may represent a multiorgan systemic breakdown, including HPA axis, mitochondrial energy production, and phase 2 detoxification in the liver. Disruption of the microbiome and a high ratio of unhealthy bacteria to beneficial bacteria has been found along with low levels of CoQ10 (Lakhan & Kirchgessner, 2010).

Diabetes Mellitus Type 2

Diabetes is a chronic life-threatening condition that requires daily self-care and can co-occur with depression. Deficiencies of biotin, vitamin E, protein, zinc, B12, and B6 are often found in diabetes. These deficits interfere with the enzyme delta-6 desaturase, which is required for essential fatty acid metabolism. Metformin use reduces levels of B12, which can lead to impaired cognitive function.

Early Puberty

Early puberty is a growing mental health problem associated with environmental and nutritional changes in the diets of girls. It occurs when physical changes of puberty occur in girls as young as 7 and 8 years old. It is associated with psychological and medical health problems such as an increased risk of depression and suicidality, physical distress associated with mind-body interactions, headaches, stomachaches, insomnia, bulimia, poor academic achievement, substance abuse, and sexual activity. Early puberty increases the frequency of date rape and poor social adjustment with peers (Mendle, Turkheimer, & Emery, 2007). African American and Hispanic girls experience early puberty at higher rates.

Among the suspected causes are obesity, which is associated with hormonal changes and inflammation; exposure to environmental toxins, especially endocrine gland disruptors that mimic estrogen; antibiotic use; and exposure to hormones in nonorganic animal proteins. Stress, especially early-life adversity, also contributes to early maturation.

Nutrition can make an important contribution to slowing down puberty in young girls (and boys). Starting in pregnancy and during development, the basic principles of health nutrition apply: eating organic foods, washing all foods to reduce pesticides, avoiding plastic bottles, and refraining from reheating plastics.

Hypochlorhydria and Gastroesophageal Reflux Disease

Gastroesophageal reflux disease (GERD) is a common occurrence and is generally associated with excess stomach acid production. However, in contrast, integrative medicine practitioners believe that it is in fact a result of insufficient stomach acid production called hypochlorhydria. Hypochlorhydria reduces the tone of the lower esophageal sphincter, which then allows the contents of the stomach to be refluxed. Major factors in GERD are excessive (refined) carbohydrate use, smoking, and alcohol.

Among the causes of reduced acid output are age, heartburn medications or those used for gastric reflux and stomach ulcers, antacids and proton pump inhibitors, chronic *Helicobacter pylori* infections, pernicious anemia, small intestinal bacteria overgrowth, stress, and anxiety.

Hypertension (High Blood Pressure)

Hypertension is commonly associated with stress and PTSD. Nutrient deficits that may contribute are vitamin B, vitamin C, and zinc; the amino acids arginine and lysine; and the minerals magnesium, calcium, potassium, and coenzyme Q10. Blood pressure medications can worsen nutrient deficiencies.

Pain/Fibromyalgia

Chronic pain commonly co-occurs with PTSD, depression, anxiety, and substance abuse and contributes to insomnia. Fibromyalgia is a sleep/pain syndrome that co-occurs at high rates with a history of interpersonal trauma, suggesting that the chronic disruption of the HPA axis and overall oxidative stress and mitochondrial dysfunction is impaired. Low levels of EFAs make one vulnerable to pain. Where pain is acute, treatment is fairly straightforward and swift. However, chronic pain initiates a cycle of helplessness and depression rooted in systemic inflammation. Fibromyalgia co-occurs at high rates with a history of adverse childhood events and circadian rhythm disruption.

Nutritional approaches are essential to reduce inflammation systemically and locally and thus increase physical mobility and decrease depression and pain.

Assessment Essential

A serum vitamin D (25-OH Vitamin D) test should be performed annually, with the optimal range being from 40 to 65 ng/mL (100 to 160 nmol/L).

Skin Disorders

There are numerous skin disorders associated with poor mental health. Many skin disorders result from food allergies and sensitivities. For example, people with disfiguring skin problems like acne, eczema/dermatitis, and psoriasis are at risk for anxiety, depression, and suicidality (Gupta & Gupta, 1998) with those with psoriasis having the highest risk next to acne. Among those with psoriasis, those who had antibodies to gliadins showed significant improvement in psoriatic symptoms when they eliminated gluten. Acne also shows important connections between the skin symptoms and mental health and nutritional status. It is widely observed that many people with acne are also angry and are at risk for depression and anxiety. Similarly, nutritional deficits have been found to contribute to acne (and anger and depression), particularly zinc, folic acid, selenium, chromium, and Omega-3 fatty acids, and an altered microbiome (Katzman & Logan, 2007). In eczema the intensity of itching is linked to depression, and eczema is associated with casein allergy and sometimes gluten sensitivity. It has been observed for over 100 years that sugar and carbohydrate metabolism may contribute to eczema. Severe eczema correlates with intake of fast foods by children.

Thyroid Disorders

The Thyroid and Mental Health

Clients who are depressed, sluggish, fatigued, have a difficult time awakening and getting active in the morning, and who always feel cold, especially cold hands and feet, should be assessed for thyroid function. Poor thyroid function is an important cause or contributing factor in depression. Fatigue, depression, and chronic pain can be mistaken for mood disorders, and hypothyroidism should be ruled out or treated; blood tests of TSH are not always adequate for a diagnosis. Subclinical symptoms may not show up on blood tests. Some foods called goitrogenic can decrease thyroid activity when eaten in large quantities by blocking the conversion of T4 to T3. These include soy along with cruciferous vegetables like kale, white turnips, brussels sprouts, broccoli, horseradish, and cabbage, which exacerbate hypothyroid. To inactivate this effect, these vegetables require cooking. Fluoridation and chlorinated water also decrease thyroid function.

Some drugs like Cordarone, Colsalide, Prozac, interferon-alfa, lithium, methimazole, potassium iodide, propylthiouracil, and corticosteroids cause hypothyroidism as an adverse reaction.

Assessment Essential

Blood tests are the conventional methods for diagnosing hypothyroidism. However, many clinicians believe there is a subclinical hypothyroidism that may not show up on blood tests but can be assessed based on low basal body temperature and clinical symptoms (see Appendix H).

A blood test is used to diagnose Hashimoto's thyroiditis, an autoimmune disorder that can be associated with food allergies.

Hyperthyroidism: The Overactive Thyroid

When the thyroid is overactive and produces too much of the thyroid hormone thyroxine, it is referred to as hyperthyroidism. This condition speeds up metabolism and can cause nervousness, weight loss, increased heart rate, irritability, and sweating. There are many causes of hyperthyroidism, among which may be the overconsumption of iodine-rich foods like seaweed or iodine supplements. Hyperthyroidism is less common, but it should also be assessed as a medical issue in clients with symptoms of nervousness, palpitations, tremors, and excessive perspiration.

Essential Next Steps

- Consider the role of nutritional deficits and how they may contribute to client symptoms.
- Link a client's signs and symptoms obtained during the assessment to what is known about nutritional deficits in those disorders.
- Counsel the client about how nutritional deficits can influence mental well-being.
- Consider what additional tests may be used to address the needs of clients and make appropriate referrals.
- Identify the relationships between mental and physical health symptoms and their concomitant nutritional factors.

CHAPTER 5

Food Allergies, Sensitivities, and Special Diets

Diet Essential: Mental illness is affected significantly by diet and exposure to food toxins and allergies.

People make food choices based on family experience, religious and cultural belief systems, and the conditioning of their sense of taste and satisfaction. Spiritual and religious faith also influences dietary choices, such as beliefs that prohibit eating of pork (Judaism and Islam), that include the drinking of human and bovine urine (Jainism, Buddhism), or that call for periodic fasting (Islam and Christianity).

People may also make choices or feel driven to eat certain foods due to allergies and sensitivities. What people choose to eat can be a response to cravings and the effects of food chemicals on the brain/mind. People are frequently unaware of their allergies or sensitivities even as their body reacts to various foods they consume, because the effects may not be immediate but delayed for hours or days. Indeed, someone who is allergic to shellfish may break out in hives in a matter of moments, whereas the signs of gluten sensitivity build over months.

Mental and physical reactions to foods and to food additives can go undetected for many years. Some people experience minor or major reactions while others do not experience any reaction. Eliminating certain foods and additives greatly reduces sensitivities. Symptoms can improve and frequently the adverse reactions resolve.

The saying "If your food can go bad, it is good for you. If your food can't go bad, leave it alone" refers to the detrimental effects of preservatives in foods that prevent spoilage.

In this chapter, I first show what is known about how food allergies and sensitivities affect mental health and then review some dietary concepts that are beneficial (or detrimental) for mental health. Diets provide a roadmap for clients to follow.

TABLE 5.1

Nutritional Types and Best Foods

Type	Metabolism	Blood pH	Best Foods
Fast metabolizer	Burns carbohydrates fast	Acidic	Carnivore and purines, fats, low carbohydrates
Slow metabolizer	Burns carbohydrates more slowly	Alkaline	Vegetarian, carbohydrate rich (lacto-ovo and lean animal products)
Mixed metabolizer	Burns balanced	Balanced	Mixed animal and plant proteins/carbs

Some people like a map laid out for them, while others prefer to use their inner "homing device," their gut. As a mental health clinician, you need not be a nutritional expert on all diets to help and advise your client. Knowing the types of diets clients are using or what diets are available as a roadmap for their health will enable you to have a dialogue about their choices, free of bias, and thus enhance your partnership model of care. Review Table 5.1 to match the optimal food ratios for each nutritional type.

The first step to identifying an appropriate diet is to further explore the client's nutritional type (Carnivore, Mixed, Lacto/Ovo Vegetarian, Pesca-Vegetarian) and the ideal range of food types and ratios that will benefit her or him. The next step is to discover whether the client has food sensitivities or allergies and, if so, their effect on the client's mental health. Sometimes eliminating certain foods may be the easier first step for certain clients. Identifying allergies and sensitivities may be painstaking. Some may do well eating larger amounts of protein but may also experience milk sensitivities. As a basic first step, I encourage clients to eliminate all the packaged foods with additives and preservatives, regardless of whether they are sensitive to them, while advising them to choose fresh whole foods.

Another common challenge to dietary changes may involve working with a vegan or vegetarian who eats a lot of grains. Such clients may indeed be sensitive or allergic to grains containing glutens, or she or he may be a biological carnivore or mixed oxidizer and is resistant to incorporating animal proteins. This individual may then be willing to try a gluten-free diet as a pathway to improved well-being before she is willing to incorporate more animal proteins. Using diets to explain desired outcomes can be helpful, but understanding personality needs and the stage of change that I discuss in Chapter 9 is crucial to success.

FOOD ALLERGIES AND SENSITIVITIES

Food allergies and sensitivities are common in people who experience poor mental health. Inflammatory reactions caused by diet fall into three categories: Food Allergy, Food-Induced Autoimmune Disease, and Food Sensitivities. Some of the more common food allergies that affect mental health are glutinous grains and dairy products, but they are not limited to these major categories of food.

Food Allergies: Definitions

Food allergies involve reactivity of the immune system. Allergies are often genetic and hereditary. Allergies can be present in childhood through adulthood and are more likely if a parent has an allergy. They can also develop in response to foods that are eaten often. Allergies can also develop in adulthood and may be linked to chronic stress disrupting immune function. Allergies can also develop as a result of chronic infections, eating poor quality or pro-inflammatory foods, toxic exposure, nutritional deficits, and chronic stress.

Food allergies are serious, sometimes life-threatening reactions of the body and immune system to certain foods. An allergic reaction occurs when the immune system overreacts, attacking a normally harmless food protein. This is why food allergies are sometimes referred to as "body paranoia." The body may be overreacting to a threat that normally should not be threatening. Food allergies occur when the body produces large amounts of the antibody immunoglobin E (IgE) to neutralize the offending food protein. IgE then stimulates the immune system to release histamine and other chemicals, resulting in an allergic reaction.

Symptoms of food allergy can occur immediately after ingesting the food or up to several hours later. Symptoms may be mild or severe. Mild symptoms of food allergy include itching in the nose, mouth, eyes, and throat; hives; or gastrointestinal problems like vomiting and diarrhea. More severe reactions include angioedema or anaphylaxis.

Common Allergens

While common allergens include milk, eggs, wheat, soy, tree nuts, peanuts, fish, strawberries, and shellfish, nearly any food can cause an allergic reaction.

Pollen-food allergy syndrome occurs when certain vegetables, fruits, nuts, or other foods cause an allergic reaction in people who have hay fever due to a similarity in the proteins in the pollens and the foods. For example, a ragweed allergy can cause a food allergy to bananas, tomatoes, or melons. Cooking food usually prevents this cross-reactivity from occurring.

Testing and Treatment

Food allergies can be tested by a skin prick test, blood test, oral food challenge, the pulse test, or elimination diets. The best approach to treatment is elimination of the allergen.

Box 5.1
The Pulse Test

One way to begin to test for food allergy or sensitivity is the pulse test, a simple, do-it-yourself method for determining negative reactions to foods. It is not recommended in cases of severe allergic reactions like anaphylaxis.

Pulse Test Directions

1. Begin the day by taking your pulse before you get out of bed. Count your pulse beats for 1 minute and record them.
2. Take your pulse 1 minute before each meal.
3. Take your pulse 30 minutes after each meal, then again in another 30 minutes, and a third time 30 minutes after that.
4. Take your pulse just before going to bed.
5. Record each pulse that you take along with the foods eaten at each meal.
6. Continue the pulse taking and recording of meals eaten for 2–3 days.
7. Take note of meals that caused pulse increases of more than 6 to 8 beats per minute, and identify foods within those meals that could be the cause.
8. Foods that are suspected of causing pulse increases can then be tested individually. Take your pulse before eating the suspected food item and again 30 minutes afterward.
9. Eliminate foods that cause pulse increases of more than 6 to 8 beats per minute from your diet.

Food Sensitivities/Intolerance

Food sensitivities are the most common type of diet-induced inflammatory reaction. These sensitivities contribute to poor mental health and yet may be disguised in their presentation. Thus, it may take many years to realize that food sensitivities can be a cause or contributing factor to any diagnosis or symptom.

Definitions

Food and food-chemical sensitivities or intolerances, also called nonallergic (non-IgE) food hypersensitivities or nonceliac inflammatory reactions, differ from food allergies. Food and food-chemical sensitivities play a role in the inflammation and symptoms of many chronic conditions. It can be very difficult to identify trigger foods because the symptoms may not manifest directly after consuming the offending food, and the amount of food eaten can greatly affect the presentation of symptoms.

Symptoms of food intolerances vary widely and can manifest quickly after eating the food or may require up to several days to appear. Sometimes the skin shows signs of food intolerance, like eczema, acne dermatitis, rashes, or hives. The digestive system can be affected with symptoms such as gas, bloating, cramping, diarrhea, constipation, irritable bowel syndrome, nausea, and ulcers in the mouth. The respiratory tract can also be affected.

There are many mental health and physical conditions that may be related to food and food-chemical sensitivities, such as fibromyalgia, GERD, inflammatory bowel syndrome, obesity, migraines, ADHD, autism spectrum disorders, depression, insomnia, and chronic fatigue syndrome (Oxford Biomedical Technologies, 2013). Food intolerances and sensitivities can also have a psychological component when foods are associated with traumatizing events in state-dependent learning memory and behavior. This occurs when an offending food is associated with a negative event in one's life and the body associates the pain of the event and the symptoms with the food or even the time of year the event occurred. This can make teasing out cause and effect very challenging. Then the symptoms can become conditioned and no longer require the food or environmental trigger; they just continue. Juana's experience, which is described in Box 5.2, reflects how allergic reactions and sensitivities can combine with state-dependent memory and learning and behavior.

Box 5.2
Juana's Story

Juana came for treatment for depression and anxiety due to disability associated with unremitting hives and life-threatening angioedema. She experienced ongoing swelling around her neck and shoulders and around her clavicle. Her breathing was also affected, and she was on several medications, including antihistamines and sedatives. She was emotionally and physically hyperreactive. Together we worked on her diet for several months. She closely followed her overall health program and made some improvements.

Still she suffered terribly with the angioedema. I explored during her assessment her history of the events leading up to the start of her symptoms. When she was on her way home from shopping, she picked up some take-out food and then sustained a car accident. During the accident the seat belt caused bruising across her neck and upper body, and the air bag had activated while her arms were crossed, forcing her hands against her neck and injuring her. She developed PTSD from the accident, and her body/mind memory associated the grocery bags in the car at the time of the accident—which went flying throughout the car—with fear and the bruising and swelling across her upper body. Years later, as she sat in my office, what remained was the state-dependent memory of fear and swelling associated with food. We then integrated a series of hypnotherapeutic sessions to decondition this state-dependent memory as an adjunct to the dietary improvements she was making. Together with her dietary changes, she experienced improvement over time.

Common Foods That Cause Allergies and Sensitivities

Lactose

Lactose is a sugar that is present in dairy products. Lactose intolerance is an impaired ability of the body to digest lactose due to lactase deficiency—an enzyme needed to break down lactose. Lactose intolerance is different than a milk allergy, in which the immune system reacts to protein(s) in milk. Milk allergies are more common in infancy, whereas lactose intolerance is more common in adulthood.

Lactose intolerance is commonly undiagnosed. Humans lose the ability to synthesize lactase by about age 5, and by adulthood 70% of people in the world are lactose intolerant. They do not produce sufficient quantities of this enzyme. Lactose intolerance is genetically based and occurs at high rates among people genetically associated with cultures where dairy animals are not native to the environment. Lactose intolerance varies among ethnicities. African natives and peoples from Asia have the highest rates (80%–100%), followed by African Americans and Mexican natives (70%–80%), Mediterraneans and those of Jewish descent (60%–90%), and Northern Europeans (1%–5%). However, in keeping with our understanding of culture and biochemical individuality, understanding the genetic influences is what counts. For example, the Maasai of northeastern Africa are herding peoples and indeed drink raw milk mixed with bovine blood. This is in contrast to peoples of the west coast of Africa who do not drink milk. Hence, the origins of one's ancestors, coupled with the admixtures with Europeans, African Americans, and other peoples, will ultimately determine these types of food allergies and intolerances. This will be true with everyone.

Some people are able to handle small amounts of lactose without triggering a reaction. Some people with lactose intolerance may be able to tolerate dairy products that have a higher fat content, such as pure cream or butter, since the lactose content is lower in these products. Yogurt and other fermented dairy with live cultures can generally be consumed due to bacteria converting lactose to lactic acid. However, note that most commercially available fermented products are not truly fermented nor have live cultures.

Many processed foods contain lactose (see Appendix I for a list of Foods Containing Lactose). It is important to read food labels and check for milk, lactose, whey, curds, dry milk solids, nonfat dry milk powder, and milk by-products. As a rule, I discourage all children and adults from drinking cow's milk or eating cow's cheese. There are better options for their health.

Casein

Casein is a protein found in milk and milk products. Products with higher protein content, such as yogurt, cheese, kefir, milk, and ice cream, tend to be higher in casein. Butter and cream contain only small amounts of casein. Casein is often added to nondairy cheeses to give them the melting quality of real cheese (see Appendix J for a list of Foods Containing Casein and Dairy Alternatives).

Casein has been implicated in schizophrenia, depression, and the autism spectrum disorders. Casein is the major ingredient in the anxiolytics that have the generic term Lactium or brand name De-Stress. However, this is a specially prepared peptide derived from casein and does not appear to contribute to allergic or sensitive reactions.

Gluten

Gluten (think "glue") is comprised of the proteins gliadin (a prolamin protein) and glutenin that can cause immune system reactions. Approximately 50% of those who are sensitive to dairy are also gluten intolerant. Gluten reactions occur along a spectrum; type 1 is celiac disease, an autoimmune reaction, and type 2 is non-celiac gluten sensitivity (GS). Celiac disease is a genetic autoimmune reaction to gluten that causes damage to the small intestines, preventing the absorption of important nutrients. I have been examining throughout this book the contribution of gluten and its various proteins to poor mental health and suggesting its elimination from the diet as a priority.

GS is more common than celiac disease. In GS, gluten does not always cause intestinal damage, and it does not trigger tissue transglutaminase antibodies. Undiagnosed GS should be suspected and ruled out in depression, dementia, ADHD, skin disorders, joint pain, headaches, schizophrenia, and autism spectrum.

Many foods cross-react with gluten. This means that the proteins in these foods are similar enough to cause a reaction. Among these are casein, yeast, oats, sesame, and instant coffee (Kharrazian, 2013).

GLUTEN-FREE DIET

The easiest way to withdraw from gluten is to follow a 7-day high-protein diet. Generally the physiological craving for gluten and carbohydrates has diminished significantly after 7 days, but the diet can be continued longer if necessary. A modification of this diet involves incorporating root vegetables such as sweet potatoes, yucca (manioc or cassava), parsnips, carrots, and squash. These foods satisfy the need for fiber and for something sweet. Unlike other sweets, they raise the blood sugar level slowly and they contain nourishing vitamins and minerals. Sometimes people who are addicted to carbohydrates like the sensation of fullness that these foods bring. This can be produced with root vegetables or by taking some fiber in a drink—for example, a gluten-free source such as psyllium.

There are many gluten-free carbohydrate substitutes such as milled flours: rice, potato, coconut, almond, buckwheat, sorghum, sweet potato, bean/cassava/rice mixtures, and tapioca. Gluten sensitivity may also be tied to glucose dysregulation and thus mood lability. It is very effective to eat a hypoglycemic type of diet (see Appendix A for Guidelines for a Hypoglycemic Diet), ensuring the intake of proteins every 3 to 4 hours. This will generally stabilize mood. It is very helpful during this time, once the client is through the first initial 3 days of withdrawal, to keep a food diary. It takes 3 months, in general, for the intestinal inflammation associated with gluten sensitivity to heal. However, changes in mood, a reduction in joint stiffness, and the lifting of depression will be apparent sooner. In severe cases of sensitivity, it is always wise to eliminate all gluten products. In mild cases of carbohydrate addiction, it is possible to reintegrate the use of carbohydrates with gluten on some special occasions without adverse effects. However, as in the case of alcohol addiction, some people do better than others with total abstinence. Total abstinence is better for some, and others appear to manage limited quantities.

Since glutinous carbohydrates are considered comfort foods, applying the principle of substituting a less addictive substance for another could be used here—for example, making a non-sugar-based cup of hot cocoa or chocolate to which a natural sweetener such as stevia has been added can help one through tough times and will raise energy levels and endorphins.

Gluten/gliadins are found in wheat, wheat germ, wheat grass, bulgur, couscous, farina, graham flour, kamut, matzo, seitan, semolina, triticale, barley, rye, buckwheat, pearl barley, oats (unless they specify gluten-free), oat bran, oat fiber, and spelt. Some people who are gluten intolerant are able to handle small amounts of gluten (see Appendix E for a list of Foods That Often Contain Gluten).

The digestive enzyme called dipeptidyl peptidase-IV (DPP-IV) helps to break down gluten protein fragments (Kharrazian, 2013). While this enzyme should not be used as a supplement in order to eat gluten, it can assist in the case of accidental exposure to gluten. DPP-IV also helps to break down the allergenic protein casein found in dairy products. Both gluten and casein contain proline. The intestines normally produce DPP-IV to break down proline. Researchers commonly hold the view that these prolyl peptides act like opiates in the brain and may cause a worsening of symptoms in depression, schizophrenia, and autism spectrum disorders. Simply removing gluten, along with reducing carbohydrates and increasing healthy fats in the diet may improve conditions such as ADHD, depression, and dementia (Perlmutter, 2014). There are many satisfying options for gluten-free foods, as shown in Box 5.3.

Box 5.3

Gluten-Free and Casein-Free Pancakes Topped With Fruit Sauce

Children and adults alike love pancakes, but ordinarily they contain poor-quality flours and sugars. However, these pancakes are ideal for everyone. They are light and fluffy, sweet and satisfying, and make a wonderful Sunday morning meal. Place one or two poached eggs on the side with some organic bacon or sausage for an antihypoglycemic meal.

Dry Ingredients

1¾ cups rice flour

¼ cup buckwheat flour

¼ cup almond flour

1 tablespoon chia seeds (for fiber)

1½ teaspoons baking powder

¼ cup tapioca flour

pinch of sea salt

Wet Ingredients

1 cup almond milk or coconut milk

1 cup water (or as needed)

1 tablespoon vinegar

2 eggs, beaten

4 tablespoons coconut oil, melted

4 drops of liquid stevia

1 teaspoon vanilla extract

Sauce Ingredients

1 cup defrosted organic berries or other fruits like mango or pineapple chopped

1 tablespoon organic Butter

1–4 drops stevia liquid, to taste

Serving Suggestions

Top pancakes with butter, fresh berries, almond butter, yogurt, and/or nuts.

Directions

1. Whisk together the dry ingredients in a large mixing bowl. In a separate bowl, whisk together the wet ingredients. Add the wet ingredients to the dry ingredients and mix until almost smooth. The consistency should be pourable; if it is too thick, add a little more water or milk. Let sit for about 10 minutes to blend and hydrate the chia seeds. It should show signs of little gas bubbles due to the vinegar/baking powder reaction.

2. Lightly grease your pan or griddle with coconut oil and heat over medium-high heat.

3. When the pan is hot, use a ladle to pour the pancake batter into the pan. (Turn heat down a bit if the first cakes are a bit scorched.)

4. Wait until you see bubbles forming in the pancake and the edges look cooked, then flip the pancake with a spatula. Cook for another minute or two until firm, then serve. Repeat with the rest of the batter.

Making the Sauce

1. Defrost frozen berries or other fruits like mango and pineapple and lightly heat in a pan with added butter and stevia. Bring to a near boil, simmer for a few minutes, and decant into a syrup bowl with a spoon.

2. Pour over the top of the pancakes.

Tip: Pancakes are best when eaten immediately, but if you need to keep the pancakes warm, use a large, shallow serving bowl and place a towel inside of it. Wrap the pancakes in the towel. This will keep them warm and prevent them from drying out.

Always Read the Label

The key to understanding the gluten-free diet and the additive-free diet is to become a good ingredient label reader. Gluten is everywhere now and even used as an additive, so there is a lot of hidden gluten in prepared and packages foods. Just because it is not listed does not mean it is not there. There are many gluten-free foods and bread/grain substitutes. Choose from many fresh, healthy foods like fruits, vegetables, beans, dairy, nuts and nut flours, sweet potatoes, buckwheat, amaranth, potato flour, and gluten-free grains like sorghum, quinoa, or rice. Millet along with quinoa is highly nutritious, versatile, and easy to prepare (see Appendix K for a recipe for Curried Quinoa). It is rich in iron, B vitamins, and calcium, and it can be used as a breakfast cereal with butter and sweet juice added, mixed with cheese, or used with vegetables or animal proteins as desired (see Appendix K for instructions on how to cook millet). The best options are the natural flours made with nuts and seeds and flours made from coconut, almond, and rice, potato, and tapioca.

Gluten and Alcohols

Beer is made from grains and thereby contains gluten. Most other alcohols such as scotch, rye, and vodkas, while made from grains that are glutinous, are distilled, which removes the gluten, thereby making them safe to consume. Do keep in mind that alcohol, when mixed with gluten in food, magnifies the reaction in sensitive individuals and therefore should be avoided. Further, many patients who have celiac disease or who are gluten sensitive have a poor reaction to alcohol. All commercial oats are contaminated with gluten. To be sure about the quality of the oats, obtain certified gluten-free oats.

Corn

Corn is one of the more difficult food allergies to have inasmuch as corn is so prevalent in foods produced in the United States. From cornstarch and corn syrup to ingredients like dextrose, it is very difficult to find packaged foods that do not contain some form of corn (see Appendix L for a list of Foods That Commonly Contain

Corn). While not considered one of the top eight food allergens, corn allergy is becoming more common in the United States and corn-producing countries in Asia and Africa. Perhaps due to how ever-present corn is in our diets, allergic reactions to corn are increasing. The symptoms of corn allergy are similar to other food allergies and can range from mild to severe.

Another aspect of what makes corn an allergen is that most corn in the United States is now genetically modified. Genetically modified organisms (GMOs) are plants or animals that have been genetically engineered with DNA from bacteria, viruses, or other plants and animals. More than 60 countries, including those of the European Union, have placed restrictions or bans on the production and sale of GMO foods. GMO foods should be avoided.

Histamine

Histamine is a neurotransmitter released from mast cells. While necessary for our immune system function, at high levels histamine causes allergic reaction and influences mood and psychosis. For example, the treatment of schizophrenia with high-dose antihistamines has shown some success (Meskanen et al., 2013). High levels of systemic histamine are also associated with OCD, oppositional defiant disorder, and seasonal affective disorder. People who are histamine sensitive may experience anxiety, headaches, migraines, mood lability, itchiness, and have hives and asthma. Histamine is found especially in fermented foods like red wine, aged cheese, and sauerkraut (see Appendix M for a list of Foods Containing Histamines). A low-histamine diet may lead to improvement. This means eating only fresh food, not leftovers, and avoiding the following foods: fruits and vegetables that are overripe; additives and fermented foods (probiotic powders should be used instead); cultured, processed, smoked, and fermented meats; eggs in large amounts; citrus fruits; tea; chocolate; and alcohol.

Salicylates

Symptoms of salicylate intolerance are associated with anxiety and depression, and they are found in people who experience multiple-chemical sensitivity. Sensitivity to foods containing salicylates has been shown to contribute to ADHD in some children (Stevens, Kuczek, Burgess, Hurt, & Arnold, 2010).

Salicylates Derive from Salicylic Acid
Many plants like willow bark naturally contain salicylates, which act as an immune hormone and preservative that protects the plants from harmful bacteria, fungi,

insects, and diseases. There are also synthetic salicylates found in medications (like aspirin), perfumes, and preservatives (see Appendix N for Foods and Products That Are High in Salicylates). Most people can handle moderate amounts of salicylates in food; some people are intolerant of even small amounts of salicylates and experience adverse reactions. This is called "salicylate sensitivity" or "salicylate intolerance." Adverse effects may be seen when a certain amount of salicylates are consumed, or if salicylates accumulate in the body over time. Both the natural and the synthetic forms of salicylates are harmful to everyone in large amounts. Symptoms of salicylate sensitivity may include depression and anxiety; asthma and breathing problems; headaches; nasal congestion; itching, skin rash, or hives; swelling of the hands, feet, and face; and stomach pain.

Sulfites

Sulfites, or sulfur dioxide (SO2), are chemicals used as a preservative and food additive. Sulfites are commonly added to wine to stop the fermentation process and to preserve the wine. Organic wines tend to have a lower content of sulfites. Generally, white wines and sweeter wines contain more sulfites. Sulfites are added to dried fruits as a preservative. They may be a hidden ingredient added to frozen shrimp and also in some beverages and medications.

Sensitivity to sulfites may cause symptoms such as mood lability, headaches, sneezing, asthma, throat swelling, and hives. People with asthma tend to be more at risk of having sulfite sensitivity.

Reading food labels is important when trying to avoid sulfites. Things to look for include sulfur dioxide, potassium bisulfite or potassium metabisulfite, sodium bisulfite, sodium metabisulfite, or sodium sulfite (see Appendix O for Foods Containing Sulfites).

Nightshades

Nightshade foods are an important factor in mental health. They can cause intestinal permeability and inflammation, leading to the use of pain medications and antacids. Consuming these medications causes nutritional deficits and adversely affects gut function.

Members of the large plant family known as Solanaceae, nightshades comprise a wide variety of plants and foods, including tomatoes, potatoes (excluding sweet potatoes and yams), eggplant, and peppers (excluding black pepper). Peppers include all peppers, both spicy and mild, from habanero and jalapeno chilies to cayenne and paprika. Additionally, ashwagandha, goji berries, cape gooseberries, ground cherries, and garden huckleberries are in the nightshade family. Symptoms of nightshade sensitivity include muscle pain and tightness, arthritis, sensitivity to weather changes, morning stiffness, slow healing, gallbladder problems, heartburn, and GERD.

Test for Nightshade Sensitivity

Begin by conducting a self-inventory of pain and swelling of joints. Rate how you feel on a scale of 1 to 10 with 10 being in terrible joint pain with stiffness. Eliminate all nightshade foods during 4 weeks, and at the end of the period conduct another self-inventory. If you are sensitive to nightshades, you will feel better after 4 weeks without them. You can test this by returning to the use of nightshades for 1–2 weeks and observe that the pain and stiffness will return. Some people can sharply reduce their intake of nightshades and still tolerate them on occasion. If you enjoy barbecue sauce, look for a nightshade-free recipe called Papaya Barbecue Sauce in Appendix P.

General Treatment of Food Intolerances

- Reduce exposure to one food one at a time to test reactivity.
- Identify healthy substitutes where possible.
- Increase supplemental digestive enzymes.
- Address linkages to traumatic events and use hypnotherapy to decondition reactivity.

Assessment Essentials and Elimination Diets

Tests

The Mediator Release Test (MRT) is a blood test that identifies up to 150 foods and chemicals, which provoke the release of immune mediators that cause pain and inflammation (Pasula, 2014).

Conduct Specific Food Elimination Diet

The elimination diet is an effective and safe way to assess and treat food intolerances. Eliminating a food or food group for 3 or 4 weeks while monitoring symptoms allows sufficient time to observe symptom changes. If symptoms improve during this time, the food is reintroduced to see if it causes the symptoms to worsen. If symptoms improve when the food is eliminated and return when the food is reintroduced, the food should be excluded from the diet for at least 6 months. Strict adherence to the diet is necessary for accuracy. Allow sufficient time for inflammation caused by the food to heal. Once an offending food is identified, it may be possible to eat it once in a while without symptoms, but only on special occasions, and this must be assessed individually (see Appendix Q for a Guide to Foods on the Elimination Diet).

After 3 weeks on the elimination diet, one food at a time is reintroduced for 1 day. For example, if you decide to end the elimination diet by reintroducing corn, you would add corn or a corn product to a couple of meals for 1 day. Then for the next 2 days you would not eat corn, but you would monitor to see if any reactions occur. If not, you can continue to eat corn, and after those 2 days you can add another food back into your diet and follow the same process of 1 day with the new food and 2 days without while monitoring for symptoms. The elimination diet and reintroduction phase should take about 5–6 weeks total.

Among the first foods to start eliminating are grains containing gluten (wheat, bulgur, barley, rye, couscous, kamut, semolina, spelt, triticale, and oats), cow's milk (milk and cheese products), and soy, but any food or food group (salicylates, nightshades, additives) that can cause reactions can be eliminated.

Modified Elimination Diet

1. Begin by eliminating dairy products like milk, cheese, butter, ice cream, and so on. It may be okay to continue eating small amounts of plain, unsweetened yogurt with probiotics.
2. Eliminate gluten and other grains that may cause reactions.
3. Drink a minimum of 2 quarts of water daily.
4. Avoid alcohol and products containing alcohol, as well as all caffeinated drinks, decaffeinated coffee, and herbal coffee (see Appendix Q for a Guide to Foods on the Modified Elimination Diet).

CHEMICAL SENSITIVITIES

Multiple-Chemical Sensitivity

Multiple-chemical sensitivity (MCS) is also known as "environmental illness" or "multiple allergy" and environmental intolerance. It refers to a range of severe symptoms that are related to chemical, biologic, or physical irritants, or pollutants.

Understanding MCS is important to mental health treatment because people with unexplained symptoms can suffer from debilitating symptoms and as a result have significant mental health problems. Because there is no widespread or agreed-upon consensus about this syndrome, people are commonly misdiagnosed with somatic symptom disorder and illness anxiety disorder. While they may indeed benefit from psychological treatment, these individuals are often difficult to diagnose. The causes of their symptoms are wide ranging and invisible. There are several theories as to how MCS is possible, including (1) enzyme depletion, (2) immune system disorder including systemic inflammation, (3) nervous system sensitization, (4) HPA axis dysregulation, and (5) challenges in phase 2 liver detoxification.

In my own practice, every person suffering from MCS has experienced many years of chronic stress prior to diagnosis. Early-life events and high allostatic load affect the ability of their adrenal and immune systems to withstand significant environmental exposures. MCS sufferers are the proverbial canary in the coal mine for all of us. Many people are exposed to significant toxins at work and at war that cause multisystem health reactions. Symptoms include fatigue, dizziness, headaches, chest pain, skin rashes, nausea, sleep problems, digestive problems, sore throat, coughing, wheezing, muscle pain and stiffness, itching, heartbeat irregularities, difficulty concentrating, memory problems, bloating, confusion, and mood lability.

Some of the common triggers reported in MCS include solvents, exhaust, volatile organic compounds (VOCs), chlorine, perfume, tobacco smoke, insecticide, new carpet, paint, pollen, pet fur, and dust mites.

Neurotoxins

Neurotoxins and excitotoxins are substances added to foods that prevent nerves from functioning normally by interfering with their electrical activities. They are found in most packaged foods and include ingredients like dough conditioners; seasonings; yeast extract; carrageenan; maltodextrin; hydrolyzed vegetable protein; sodium fluoride; sodium caseinate; calcium caseinate; chicken, pork, or beef flavoring; disodium anything; smoke flavoring and anything called autolyzed; whey protein concentrate; natural flavors or spices; and additives such as glutamate and aspartate. Researchers and clinicians associate neurotoxins with the development of Alzheimer's and Parkinson's disease. Neurotoxic food additives are mostly derived from proteins in the form of free glutamic acids. Next I list the most prevalent neurotoxins to be avoided.

Monosodium Glutamate

Monosodium glutamate (MSG) is a flavor enhancer added to many processed foods, especially of Asian origin. It is a natural sodium salt of glutamic acid. It is usually made from fermented corn, rice, or potatoes. Animal studies repeatedly show that refined MSG causes depression and anxiety (Quinesa, et.al., 2014). Individually and together with aspartame, MSG disrupts cognitive function and increases oxidative stress in animals (Abu-Taweela, Zyadah, Ajarem, & Ahmad, 2014). Magnesium (Bland, 2004) and vitamins C and E are protective against the oxidative stress effects of MSG (Tawfik & Al-Badr, 2012).

Natural Flavors

While natural flavors are derived from natural foods like fruits and vegetables, they are also isolates of those foods and can become toxic. When consumed as part of the whole fruit or vegetable, the other compounds present balance them. In addition to "natural flavors," which sounds harmless, many companies use the term "spices" to refer to ingredients that are actually neurotoxic substances. Foods with natural flavors added are to be avoided.

Soda Pop

Sodas with sugar and diet sodas are one of the first substances to eliminate from the diet. Diet sodas have excitotoxins like aspartame. Ironically they have been shown to cause weight gain and diabetes. Artificial sweeteners (saccharin, sucralose, or aspartame) disrupt intestinal gut microbiota and alter metabolism of glucose (Suez et al., 2014). Caffeine-rich sodas contribute to anxiety and insomnia, and there is some evidence that regular consumption of sugar-sweetened soda alters DNA and shortens life span (Leung et al., 2014). Withdrawal involves withdrawal from sugar (or artificial sweeteners) and often caffeine. Soda drinking is a common habit, linked to work.

Beverage Sweetener Alternatives

I encourage people to make their own sodas by purchasing mineral water and flavoring with frozen fruit and stevia. See the recipe in Box 5.4 for a Raspberry Lime Rickey.

Box 5.4
Raspberry Lime Rickey

Ingredients

Crushed ice

Juice from 1 lime

½ cup frozen raspberries

1 glass of sparkling mineral water

1 to 5 drops liquid stevia, to taste

Directions

Fill glass with ice. Add lime juice, raspberries, sparkling water, and stevia; stir to combine.

Aspartame®

Manufactured by a Japanese company called Ajinomoto, Aspartame has many other names, including Equal®, NutraSweet®, Benevia®, Spoonful®, and more recently AminoSweet®. Aspartame is an artificial sweetener used in sugar-free products like gum and drinks. It is most often made from the feces of genetically modified bacteria. Aspartame breaks down into methanol, which is then converted into formaldehyde. At low levels with long-term exposure, formaldehyde damages the nervous system and immune system, and causes irreversible genetic damage. Research links aspartame to serious illnesses, including depression and irritability (Lindseth, Coolahan, Petros, & Lindseth, 2014), migraines, oxidative stress, diabetes, seizures, blindness, obesity, and neurological disorders, (Soffritti et al., 2014). A significant body of research has shown that aspartame, along with other food additives, causes neurological, psychiatric, and behavioral disorders and is associated with headaches and panic. People with a history of depression, pregnant women and lactating mothers, and young children appear to be especially vulnerable. Individuals with mood disorders are particularly sensitive to aspartame, and aspartame makes depression worse (Walton, Hudak, & Green-Waite, 1993). The use of artificial sweeteners is associated with higher rates of depression in the elderly (Guo et al. 2014).

Sucralose®

Sucralose, or Splenda®, is an artificial sweetener used in sugar-free products. Sucralose is a chlorinated compound that is a cousin to the chemical DDT. The body breaks down chlorinated compounds like sucralose and toxic chemicals are released.

Hydrolyzed Vegetable Protein

Found in junk foods, hydrolyzed vegetable protein is high in glutamate and aspartate, which overstimulates nerve cells and leads to cell death.

ELIMINATION OF DIETARY FOOD ADDITIVES

The Feingold Diet

The Feingold diet was developed especially for ADHD and behavioral disorders by Dr. Ben F. Feingold, who was a pediatric physician specializing in allergies. This is a food elimination program designed to identify food additives in the diet that may be causing symptoms like hyperactivity. Foods containing artificial dyes, preservatives, and flavors are eliminated permanently from the diet, while some fruits and vegetables are eliminated but later reintroduced based on tolerance. Food dyes are petroleum based and are contaminated with mercury, lead, and arsenic. Food additives include dyes (Red 3, Red 40, Blue 1, Blue 2, Green 3, etc.) and artificial flavors, artificial sweeteners (Equal®/aspartame, Splenda®/sucralose), and preservatives (BHA, BHT, TBHQ). Salicylates are eliminated. The Feingold program provides lists of foods that are to be eliminated.

Benefits

The Feingold diet benefits children and adults with symptoms of hyperactivity, impulsiveness, compulsive behaviors, and mood lability; learning problems, such as short attention span, neuromuscular problems, and cognitive and perceptual problems; and health problems, like asthma, bedwetting, ear infections, eczema, hives, seizures, and sleep problems.

Cautions/Deficiencies

There are no problems incorporating this approach alongside other diets. Elimination of all these additives is beneficial for everyone.

The Leap Diet

The Leap diet is also called "ImmunoCalm Nutrition" designed for people with food sensitivities and allergies. It emphasizes foods that are beneficial for the individual, rather than focusing on what the individual is sensitive to. Water is essential to flushing out toxins. In Box 5.5 learn how to calculate your specific needs for water.

Box 5.5
Calculate Your Requirements for Water

We are made up of water. Think of a big balloon filled with water and a big fat globule called the brain at the top. That's our body. Dehydration contributes to fatigue, depression, and toxicity. I suggest to my clients to fill water glasses and place them in every room they visit during the day so they will drink their requisite daily fluid. (Coffee and black teas do not count toward the total, but herbal tea and broths do.) As a general rule, we need to drink 30%–50% of our body weight in ounces of water daily. Calculate your body weight and divide it in half. These are the number of ounces of water to drink daily. For example, 150 pounds equals 50–75 ounces of water daily.

HEAVY METALS

Heavy metals are well-established causes of mental illness, in particular learning disorders (lead, molybdenum) and cognitive decline (arsenic, mercury, aluminum, lead). With the use of mercury in dental amalgam and ongoing increases in air pollution and the widespread use of chemicals in the food supply, it is impossible to avoid exposure. One hopes to reduce exposure and eat foods that aid the body to eliminate what has been stored.

Aluminum

Exposure to aluminum occurs at higher rates than any other known metal neurotoxin. Aluminum exposure and high levels in brain tissue are correlated with cognitive decline and Alzheimer's disease (Bhattacharjee, Zhao, Hill, Percy, & Lukiw, 2014), in large part because of the inflammation and oxidation it causes. It is found throughout the environment—in the air, water, and soil; in medicines; and in foods. Aluminum is naturally found in all foods; however, additives like coloring agents, preservatives, and leavening agents contribute a much larger amount of aluminum compounds. Aluminum is also found in larger amounts in processed cheeses, spices, pickles, and baked goods. It is also commonly present in drinking water, antacid medications, and vaccines, the latter of which contributes to the majority of aluminum toxicity cases since frequently it is injected into the body. Maintaining higher levels of magnesium can be protective against aluminum absorption. Percy, Kruck, Pogue, and Lukiw (2011) describe the use of the intramuscular antioxidant agent desferrioxamine to reduce levels of aluminum and iron in the brains of Alzheimer's patients and to slow down the disease process.

Methods to Avoid Aluminum Exposure
- Do not take antacids that contain aluminum hydroxide.
- Avoid using aluminum cookware
- Do not use aluminum foil.
- Do not use antiperspirant spray, especially if it contains aluminum chlorohydrate.

Mercury

Mercury is a toxic metal that easily destroys brain tissue and can cause memory loss, ataxia, fatigue, depression, and neurological disturbance. Most mercury in the diet is obtained through seafood and fish products, which tend to contain high concentrations of mercury. Other sources of mercury in the body can derive from bleaching skin creams, calomel laxatives, some cosmetics, hemorrhoid suppositories, photographic supplies, some vaccines, and contact lens solution containing thimerosal.

Elimination of Heavy Metals With Nutrition

When protein is deficient in the diet, then toxic metals like cadmium, lead, and mercury are more easily absorbed and retained. The sulfur compounds in proteins protect the cells from heavy metal toxicity. Sulfur is necessary for the methylation process of detoxification. Sulfur is rich in animal proteins, fish, and garlic and onions. Supplemental niacin also works to detoxify the liver. The cruciferous vegetables—like cabbage, broccoli, and brussels sprouts—enhance detoxification enzymes, and sulfur-containing onions and garlic, both raw and cooked, are most beneficial when used daily (see Appendix R for a selection of recipes using raw, cooked, and fermented cruciferous vegetables). Seaweeds are a significant detoxifying food source (particularly kelp with its natural sodium alginate compound built in). Sea plants with sodium alginate bind toxins in the intestinal tract, drawing them from the body's cells. Adding seaweed to soups or bean dishes or as a snack is healthy for the thyroid. Alginates from the brown seaweeds bind toxic metals to the digestive tract (Eliaz, Weil, & Wilk, 2007); capsules combining sodium alginate from brown seaweeds and modified citrus pectin can be used every 3 months to reduce heavy metals. Coriander is also known as cilantro or Chinese parsley. It is a powerful antioxidant that has been demonstrated to remove heavy metals from the body. Incorporate cilantro in your recipes like the one shown in Box 5.6.

Box 5.6
Cilantro/Parsley Pesto Heavy Metal Detox

This is a healthy and delicious pesto that can be used on gluten-free pasta or rice, or as a dipping sauce for vegetables. The added benefit is that it chelates (removes) heavy metals from the body. Double the recipe and freeze it in small containers so it can be pulled out for a quick healthy meal.

Ingredients

2 cups of firmly packed organic cilantro leaves and stems

2 cups of firmly packed organic Italian, flat leaf parsley leaves and stems

½ cup of chopped organic walnuts

½ cup of organic olive oil

1 teaspoon of kelp powder

¼ teaspoon of sea salt

2 garlic cloves

Directions

Using a food processor or blender, mix all ingredients together until smooth.

ELIMINATING TOXINS IN THE HOME

Environmental toxins are linked to a variety of mental health problems. Exposure is especially dangerous in pregnant women and during the first years of life, but exposure at any stage is harmful. Although we cannot eliminate all exposures, we can reduce risk where we have control. This starts in the home with cleaning products and outside the home with pesticides or fertilizers, as well as detoxifying fruits and vegetables prior to consumption. To eliminate pesticides and fertilizers from produce, fill a sink with water and add ½ cup of either hydrogen peroxide or bleach. Let the vegetables and fruits soak for 5 minutes, then wash, rinse, and dry thoroughly. Look underneath your sink and in your garage for toxic cleaning supplies, as well as drain and oven cleaners. If you have bought cleaning supplies in the store, they will be toxic. Throw out any toxic cleaning supplies. Replace them with a mixture of white or apple cider vinegar and water. Vinegar is a powerful antibacterial, antimold, and antifungal cleanser and it is less expensive than cleaners. If you like, add a little essential oil with your favorite fragrance. This mixture can be used to clean dishes, counters, floors, toilets, and tubs. If you need to scrub, just add some baking soda and salt. Also avoid dry cleaning.

FOOD ADDICTIONS, CRAVINGS, AND ORTHOREXIA

When people are addicted to fast foods, such as those containing high levels of sugar and salt, they become inured to taste and lose the ability to taste foods in their natural state. Our work is to educate clients that they are in a process of learning to perceive these tastes. Processed food tastes are much more potent, so they blunt the capacity to taste and appreciate the authentic flavors of foods. People may be unaware of this, which leads them to say they do not like certain foods or simple foods "don't taste like much." Someone who salts heavily with table salt may not be able to taste the saltiness of sodium in celery and may feel the need to salt celery and other foods. This is an example of how people have overwhelmed and excited their own taste buds and inner chemistry. Part of the whole process of changing food and dietary patterns and addictive processes is to slowly eliminate these high-stress excitotoxins as they are replaced with their natural counterparts.

There are several factors that contribute to food cravings:

- Nutrient deficits may cause people to crave food with nutrients they need. This is "cravings as self-medication."
- Specific foods are formulated to be addictive and lead to cravings, especially processed foods. This is "cravings as addiction."
- Foods that people are allergic to can cause cravings for those foods; this is "cravings as allergy/sensitivity."

Cravings

Mood affects food cravings, and food cravings also affect mood. Cravings are complex and may derive from several causes. Understanding the foods, the time of day, the food-as-self-medication factor, food allergies, and mood prior to cravings is essential and can be reviewed during the assessment process. Hormones contribute to cravings. Ghrelin is the hormone that cues hunger and responds to chrononutrition. Sleep and ghrelin interact; the less one sleeps, the more one is hungry, and this also leads to obesity. Gastric bypass decreases ghrelin levels, though over time they rise again. Cholecystokinin and peptide YY cue satiety by slowing the emptying of food by the stomach and peptide YY signals satiety in response to protein, supporting the idea that protein provides more satiety than carbohydrates. People have different levels of each hormone, which can account for the ranges in appetite and cravings. Certain foods dysregulate these hormones, and boredom and anxiety can precede food cravings. People who are tense and distressed may crave sweet carbohydrates and then feel more relaxed after eating, while protein craving is often related to anxiety and hunger and then followed by more energy.

Nutritional deficiencies also contribute to food cravings as part of the self-medication response. Women tend to crave carbohydrates and sweet goods during the luteal phase (around midway through the menstrual cycle), which is suggestive of the need to increase dietary tryptophan and serotonin.

The elaborated intrusion theory of desires (May, Andrade, Kavanagh, & Hetherington, 2012) is a cognitive-emotional approach to understanding the role of imagery and intrusive thoughts on cravings, positing that alternative visual/spatial tasks such as mindfulness meditation, the computer game Tetris, and exercises that engage working memory can compete successfully for attention for cravings.

Decreasing the negative effects of cravings on health requires a multifaceted approach to understanding the types of foods being craved and how they alter mood, and identifying nutritional substitutes along with cognitive-behavioral management methods that decrease craving behaviors.

Nutritional and Behavioral Tips for Dealing With Food Cravings

- Reduce stress to help avoid the tendency to reach for addictive substances as a coping mechanism.
- Keeping addictive foods out of sight can help keep them off of your mind.
- Identify foods that precede or trigger your cravings and avoid them.
- Engage in alternative strategies for attention such as computer games, relaxation, and exercise.
- Drink water throughout the day.
- When a craving is for a comfort food not in alignment with your diet goals, substitute something healthy instead.
- Just rinsing the mouth with starchy carbohydrates triggers brain response and increases energy.

- Plan "snacks ahead" so if you grab something, it is healthier but satisfying.
- Allow some compassion with your cravings, but in small portions; for example allow craving responses twice a week and not every night.

Nutrient Supplementation for Reducing Cravings

- Vitamin B complex is useful in raising serotonin levels, improving mood and the body's ability to metabolize carbohydrates.
- Chromium and L-glutamine both help to regulate blood sugar levels and can reduce cravings for carbohydrates and sugars.
- Fish oil helps to reduce cravings for sugar by enhancing insulin sensitivity.
- L-tyrosine supports the production of dopamine that contributes to improving mood.
- Magnesium is useful in reducing stress, balancing blood sugar, and improving sleep.
- DL-phenylalanine increases endorphin levels, and tryptophan raises serotonin levels and reduces cravings for carbohydrates.

Orthorexia Nervosa

Orthorexia, from the Greek *orthos*, meaning "correct or right," and *orexis*, meaning "appetite," refers to a fixation on a way of eating that is characterized by an unhealthy obsession with what is considered healthy. There may be a feeling of superiority over others with less healthy eating habits, and there is an obsession with how much to eat, what types of food, the quality and purity of the food, as well as a tendency toward self-punishment if the diet is not strictly followed. A sense of self-righteousness is common. Social isolation may result from orthorexic tendencies, or people with similar dietary inclinations and philosophy may form together in communities. It may include self-abnegation and take the form of increased dietary restrictions, fasting, and exercise. Health may suffer if orthorexia becomes severe and as foods become so restricted that calories and the variety of nutrients are reduced.

Orthorexia can be related to a need for control, a fear of poor health, a desire to be thin, spiritual purity or other spiritual reasons, asserting identity through food choices, and self-esteem. There are some similarities between the symptoms of orthorexia nervosa and obsessive-compulsive disorder (Donini, Marsili, Graziani, Imbriale, & Cannella, 2004). Assessing whether or not healthy eating choices have become obsessive is the role of the practitioner.

One might also mistake orthorexia for rigid dietary practices that are required as a process to regain health. This can occur if clinicians are not familiar with the role of diet and supplementation in mental health. It may be misdiagnosed in people who have chronic illnesses such as gluten sensitivities, multiple chemical sensitivities, or specific needs that appear obsessive. Any of these may lead others to assess that they are being neurotic or obsessive. Thus, the overall picture requires assessment. In my own practice I have observed orthorexia, especially in addiction recovery clients, in persons practicing veganism, raw food diets, and vegetarian diets. Young people can also show symptoms as a result of group bonding, and others who are survivors of various cults may also show symptoms. These diet choices often reflect stage-of-life developmental processes associated with identity development and often change over time. In Box 5.7, I review an example of this process with the case of Suzanne.

Box 5.7
Suzanne's Story

Suzanne came to see me at the age of 24 complaining of depression, fatigue, low energy, and lots of bloating that caused discomfort. Suzanne had been a vegan for 7 years. She was in a relationship with a partner who introduced her to veganism. It became clear after a series of tests that while she was a vegan for spiritual and environmental reasons, her body and mind were suffering from this diet. First, we did some testing. We discovered that she had gluten and soy intolerances (two foods that had made up the majority of protein and calories in her diet). This was important for Suzanne to know. She was an intellectual, and it provided her with some answers to things she had wondered about. She made slow, consistent changes to her diet, beginning with the addition of certain foods and the exclusion of others. She began by reducing soy and gluten, and she began to eat eggs as her first animal protein. Almost immediately Suzanne noticed an increase in her energy. Exercise that normally left her feeling fatigued became easier and more enjoyable. After a couple months of including eggs in her diet, she also began to incorporate fish. She continued on this diet for a while but still experienced symptoms of low mood and fatigue. I encouraged her to try some other animal proteins, but Suzanne said, "I feel uncomfortable chewing flesh. Also, Brad, my boyfriend, is upset with me about making these changes." We spent a few sessions discussing her relationship. She invited Brad in for a meeting with us to explore these issues.

Suzanne felt better with the changes she had made, but her improvements stalled. It took several months to make this next shift, but when she did she noticed improvements in her overall energy and mood, and she began to feel more efficient in her life. We worked together over many years to make these changes. Like many spiritually minded vegetarians,

Suzanne had the belief that it was impure to eat animal flesh, and this sense of maintaining strict control over what went into her body reflected the need for her to stay sober after an adolescence of heavy drug and alcohol abuse. It was also a reaction to gain control over what had been a chaotic early-life experience with her family. This is not uncommon in people experiencing orthorexia and reflects a stage in their recovery.

I continued to work with Suzanne off and on for several years as she sought support. I focused on helping her pay attention to how her nutritional behaviors made her feel physically and emotionally as I suggested refinements in her dietary practices.

If I were to become too "heavy handed," then I would be repeating the patterns she had been in with other people who were often "making decisions" for her. Thus, my approach was to appeal to her intellectual understanding of dietary needs and then ask her to follow her intuition and what her "gut" told her that she needed.

DIETS AND THEIR VALUE FOR MENTAL HEALTH

There are nearly as many different diets as there are people. And there are as many diets as there are psychotherapies. Our clients frequently say to us that they follow certain dietary practices. Diet names come and go. But the basics of all diets are the same—the ratios of proteins, fats, and carbohydrates and the effects they purport to achieve. We know from our own experiences that a diet that does miraculous things for our neighbor or even a client may not have that effect at all in someone else. Thus, we return to the concept of biochemical individuality. If I suggested that my client who is an Inuit from Greenland become a vegetarian, I would be challenging her innate biochemistry; to return to our car analogy, I would be suggesting the car (her body/mind) could run on 89 octane when in fact it could run only on diesel. My client would likely become ill. Thus, the balance we seek for our clients is to help them identify what diets, or maps, might serve them, and like maps, there are several ways to get to the intended location, though some may be faster and others easier. In many ways the best approach for following a food system is to find one that feels "right" in the gut. Dietary needs shift over the life cycle as well. For example, orthorexia is common in young people who join groups based on belief systems, but they evolve out of the groups and beliefs or modify them, as I explored in the story of Suzanne.

Understanding the benefits and deficits of particular diets enables us to provide counsel for our clients. Let's remember our essential principle: There is no one right diet for everyone. The question we should ask: Is this diet right for my client?

People go through stages when it comes to making dietary changes. We reviewed during our assessment all the vagaries that affect one's dietary and food preparation choices. People's ability to taste subtle flavors improves as they explore new foods preparation methods and textures. It is unrealistic to think that most people will go from a SAD, fast food diet to a Paleo diet in a few months, though some are able to. More often, people make incremental changes. We often think that our clients will jump at the chance to feel better, faster, and some will, but many who have felt badly for a while need time to learn how to tolerate feeling good.

Identify which dietary changes are essential:

- Prioritize nutritional requirements.
- List health goals and link them to the dietary changes required.
- Identify where the fastest improvements will be experienced.
- Clarify which changes the client is willing to make and in what order.
- Identify appropriate substitutions for substances to be relinquished or reduced.

Next I describe some effective diets that provide a spectrum of approaches that address biochemical individuality; they range from carnivore to mixed types to vegetarian. I have organized them according to what I believe are best adapted for mental health and then additional specialty diets for health problems that intersect with mental wellness.

I previously suggested that one goal during the assessment process is to help clients consciously communicate between their second brain and their first brain, to identify how they feel when they eat certain foods and food combinations. When discussing dietary approaches with clients, I always ask them to pay attention to how the changes make them feel and to not to rely on what "the experts" say.

Gut and Psychology Syndrome Diet

Dr. Natasha Campbell-McBride, the neurologist and nutritionist, developed the Gut and Psychology Syndrome (GAPS) diet. The diet was developed to treat children (and adults) with the autism spectrum disorders, ADD/ADHD, dyspraxia, dyslexia, and schizophrenia in particular, but it may be beneficial for everyone who is reactive to dairy and gluten. It focuses on reducing inflammation of gut walls to reduce permeability and entry of toxins into the bloodstream. There are three main principles of the GAPS diet: (1) healing the gut, (2) restoring beneficial bacteria to the gut, and (3) detoxification.

The GAPS diet is undertaken in a series of stages beginning with a very restrictive introduction phase, which includes only easily digestible vegetables and homemade broths, fats, boiled meats, and fermented vegetable juices. All grains, starches, and sugars are eliminated from the diet. As digestive symptoms subside, more foods can be slowly added to the diet, such as raw vegetables, eggs, fruits, juices, and nuts. The diet emphasizes a range of whole foods in their natural and fermented states; especially healthy fat-rich butter, fermented foods, and eggs.

As emotional and mental health improves, one incorporates the full GAPS diet, which allows many whole foods but excludes grains, starchy root vegetables, sugars, and (unfermented) milk products. Some individuals can incorporate grains and dairy again, but others who are sensitive or allergic will not.

Benefits
The GAPS diet will help detoxify the body and repopulate the gut with healthy bacteria. It may reduce inflammation in the body and also improve mental health and overall well-being.

Cautions/Deficiencies
This diet is safe and effective for mental health disorders.

Carnivore Diets

Carnivore diets emphasize eating animal proteins, in particular raw or cooked meat and flesh. They vary by the amount of other food categories that are included. Cultures as diverse as those indigenous to the Arctic as well as East Africa are primarily flesh eating cultures. The Atkins and the Paleo diets represent two valuable approaches to a meat/flesh emphasis.

Atkin's Diet (Carnivore)
The Atkins diet is a low-carbohydrate diet often used for weight loss. This diet is very effective to eliminate carbohydrate cravings. By lowering carbohydrate consumption, the body switches from using glucose for energy to using stored body fat in a process called ketosis. Proteins and healthy fats are increased in the diet. Carbohydrates, like fruits, starchy vegetables, grains, breakfast cereals, flour, and sugars, are restricted. The diet can then be used as a healthy weight management diet for life if your metabolism requires heavy proteins and low carbohydrates. It does not work for people who require more carbohydrates. It is possible to become deficient in vitamins B5, C, D, E, and K. Fiber, selenium, potassium, magnesium, and B-complex vitamins and minerals should be supplemented.

Benefits

People who are eliminating carbohydrate addiction can be successful with this diet: carnivore/high protein metabolism weight loss.

Paleolithic (Paleo) Diet

The Paleo diet, also called the primal diet or cave person diet, is based on foods similar to the food groups eaten by hunter-gatherers in the preagricultural Paleolithic era. The diet is based on the belief that our Paleolithic ancestors did not have the current array of chronic diseases. The diet includes grass-fed meats, fish and seafood, nuts and seeds, vegetables, fruits, roots, eggs, and healthy oils, while excluding dairy, carbohydrates like potatoes and refined flour and sugar, grains, legumes, refined salt, and refined vegetable oils. It is higher in protein and fat while reducing the intake of carbohydrates.

Benefits

It is high in protein, fat, fiber, and nutrients, and low in carbohydrates and sodium. The diet is a superior diet for hypoglycemia and diabetes and is a beneficial diet for mental illness, including depression and anxiety and psychotic disorders.

Cautions/Deficiencies

It is important to ensure sufficient fiber in vegetables and fruits, and calcium and vitamin D sources.

Modified Carnivore

This diet is similar to the Paleo diet, but it allows dairy for people who are not sensitive to lactose or casein. This diet is also recommended for withdrawing from alcohol and sugar addiction.

Benefits

The diet is an excellent transitional diet off of fast food, allowing for animal proteins and fats that are satisfying. I recommend this diet to individuals who have a fast food and poor-quality protein and fat diet, and I ask them to substitute the fast food meats and fats for free-range steak, hamburger, eggs, and good-quality cheeses in lettuce wraps as they detoxify from fast foods.

Cautions/Deficiencies

People with kidney disease and women who are pregnant or breastfeeding should check with their health care practitioner before undertaking this diet. Low fiber intake can lead to constipation.

The Perfect Health Diet

P. Jaminet and S-C. Jaminet (2013) provide a valuable refinement of the Paleo diet. The diet consists of 20%–30% carbohydrates from starches like potatoes, sweet potatoes, and rice, beets, carrots, fruits, and berries; 15% animal protein, including some organ meat, derived mostly from beef, lamb, goat, wild bird and duck meat, and shellfish or freshwater fish; 55%–65% healthy fats like butter, sour cream, duck fat, beef tallow, coconut milk and oil, palm oil, avocado oil, macadamia nut butter, almond butter, cashew butter, and olive oil. Fats should ideally be combined with acids such as vinegar, lemon juice, or fermented vegetables. The diet also emphasizes the use of bone broths and soups, and it recommends small amounts of desserts from "pleasure foods" like chocolate, fruits and nuts, alcohol, cream, and fructose-free sweeteners like dextrose or rice syrup. Other foods are emphasized for their micronutrient content, such as egg yolks, liver, kidney, shellfish, seaweed, and fermented vegetables.

Certain foods are not consumed such as cereal grains (wheat, barley, oats, and corn) and products made from cereal grains (bread, pasta, cereal, oatmeal). White rice and white rice products (rice noodles, crackers, etc.), as well as gluten-free products made from rice flour and potato or tapioca starch, are considered "safe starches." Beans, soy, and peanuts are not recommended. Foods with added sugar or high-fructose corn syrup are not consumed on the diet, and sugary drinks are eliminated, while water, tea, and coffee are allowed.

Polyunsaturated fats (vegetable oils) should only be about 4% of the diet, so it is recommended to eliminate the consumption of soybean oil, corn oil, safflower oil, and canola oil. The basic principles of this approach are excellent and small increases in proteins and fewer fats may suit some clients better.

Ketogenic Diet

Primarily used to treat epilepsy in children, a ketogenic diet is high in fat and moderate protein, and low in carbohydrates. Between 50% and 80% of the calories on this diet come from fat, mostly high-quality butter, heavy cream, coconut oil, eggs, avocado, and raw nuts, with carbohydrates and protein making up the remaining 20%–50% of the calories. The diet is used to reduce the frequency of epileptic seizures by inducing ketosis in which ketone bodies are elevated in the blood. The ketones enter the brain as an energy source replacing glucose, normally obtained from carbohydrates. When glucose is eliminated in the diet, the body is forced to burn fat for energy instead. High-carbohydrate foods are avoided on this diet, such as starchy foods, sugar, and grains.

Benefits
The ketogenic diet can be an effective therapy for reducing seizures in epileptic children and youth, and it has also shown some benefit for adults with epilepsy.

Cautions/Deficiencies
Constipation, dehydration, and kidney stones or gallstones are the most common side effects of the ketogenic diet, and they may only affect some children. Drinking plenty of water and incorporating fiber into the diet are important to minimize these side effects. Qualified nutritionists, dieticians, or medical doctors and nurses should oversee administration of the diet.

Recommendations/Supplementation
Supplementation is necessary on this diet, as several important vitamins and minerals are deficient, including carnitine, calcium, magnesium, iron, and vitamins B, C, and D.

Diets That Focus on Reducing Inflammation

Anti-Inflammatory Diet (Mixed/Balanced Metabolism and Lacto Ovo Pescatarian)
The anti-inflammatory diet is designed to reduce the intake of inflammatory foods. It emphasizes eating a variety of fresh fruits and vegetables while eliminating the intake of processed and fast foods. The diet consists of 40%–50% carbohydrates, 30% fat, and 20%–30% protein. Carbohydrates are low-glycemic such as brown rice and bulgur wheat, beans, sweet potatoes, and winter squash. Animal proteins from fish and natural cheese and yogurt are emphasized, as well as vegetable protein.

Other aspects of the diet include drinking tea instead of coffee, drinking red wine in favor of other alcohols, and eating dark (sugarless) chocolate in moderation.

Benefits
This diet is an excellent first step approach for people in the process of changing their diets. It should be used for 2–4 weeks at a time. It is helpful for people with pain and depression. If it feels too restrictive, some of the inflammatory foods can be eliminated one at a time as beneficial foods are added. The diet is higher in carbohydrates than some people need so that people can still gain benefits by eliminat-

ing the inflammatory foods such as wheat, corn, soy, dairy, nightshade vegetables, sugar, margarine, partially hydrogenated oils, alcohol, and peanuts.

Cautions/Deficiencies

Over time people will need to add in saturated fats and people who are more naturally carnivore will benefit from adding in more animal-based proteins.

Recommendations/Supplementation

Can be done short term and periodically if eliminating all animal proteins and fats. This diet mistakenly suggests that saturated fats and animal proteins (meats) cause inflammation. Nevertheless, this is a cleansing diet that can be beneficial for almost anyone for short periods.

Dr. Sears Zone Diet

The Zone diet is a low-glycemic-index diet developed by Dr. Barry Sears as a way to reduce excess cellular inflammation, thereby leading to a balanced hormonal state, supporting a healthy inflammatory response. It comprises 30% lean protein, 40% carbohydrates (such as fruit and vegetables), and 30% "good" fats, including supplements with Omega-3 fatty acids from fish oil and purified polyphenol extracts.

Balanced/Mixed Diets

Mediterranean Diet

The Mediterranean diet is based on the traditional foods of the Mediterranean region. The diet emphasizes lots of plant-based foods and whole grains, healthy fats like olive oil, fish and poultry 2–3 times a week, red wine in moderation, and fresh fruit. Salt and red meat are reduced in the diet. Nuts are also an important part of the diet as they are high in healthy fats. Butter, saturated fats, and hydrogenated or trans fats are discouraged in favor of monounsaturated fats (found in olive oil) and fatty fish, which are rich in Omega-3 fatty acids. Exercise and eating with family and friends are other components of the diet. Herbs and spices are used to flavor food and to help reduce the need for salt and fat. Low-fat dairy products are also encouraged over the full-fat varieties.

Benefits

The Mediterranean diet is best for the mixed-oxidizer and vegetarian-type diet. It has been shown to reduce the risk of Parkinson's disease, Alzheimer's disease, cognitive decline, and diabetes.

Cautions/Deficiencies

The diet is very general in its requirements, which may make it easy or difficult, depending upon the personality of the client.

Raw Diet

A raw foods diet consists of fresh, uncooked, and unprocessed foods that can range from raw vegan and vegetarian diets to raw omnivorous diets. A raw foods diet may include raw fruits and vegetables, nuts, seeds, and sprouted legumes and grains, and sometimes raw eggs, meat, fish, dairy products, and fermented foods. Foods may be either completely unheated or heated only at very low temperatures (below 104 or 118 degrees Fahrenheit or 40–42 degrees Centigrade) or prepared using a dehydrator. Other raw food preparation techniques include sprouting, blending, pickling, fermenting, and juicing. A common reason for consuming a raw diet is that raw foods contain beneficial enzymes that are necessary for digestion, and cooking foods destroys these enzymes. Raw foods also contain beneficial bacteria and microorganisms that improve digestion and immunity and neurotransmitter production.

Benefits

Most people will benefit from the inclusion of raw foods in the diet, but few require or will benefit from a totally raw foods diet. Most people will benefit from including a range of raw food ranging from 25% to 50% of total daily intake. Another way to work with raw food is to undertake brief cleansing diets of raw foods that range from 3 to 10 days. Proponents of a raw foods diet believe that it increases energy, decreases the risk of disease, and promotes weight loss. Raw vegan and raw vegetarian diets are lower in saturated fats and cholesterol, and high in fiber, vitamins, minerals, and antioxidants. They are typically low in processed foods, and hence low in trans fats, sodium, and sugar.

Cautions/Deficiencies

A raw foods diet is not right for everyone, and I do not recommend a totally raw diet for clients with mental health challenges. People who are underweight, suffer from diabetes or hypoglycemia, or who have a history of eating disorders may not be candidates for a raw foods diet. The consumption of fruit juices can intensify hypoglycemia and diabetes. Low calorie intake can be a problem as well for people with difficulty gaining weight or who are prone to eating disorders. The rigorous nature of a raw foods diet can trigger an obsession for eating healthy foods. For some people a totally raw foods diet can lead to dissociated states. A raw foods diet requires a lot of preparation time, especially when a diversity of foods and menus is necessary to alleviate "food boredom."

Raw diets that do not include animal proteins are deficient in B12, vitamin D, Omega-3 fatty acids, zinc, and calories. Nutritional supplementation is recommended if undertaking a raw foods diet. When eating raw foods like meat, dairy and eggs, they should be organic and from a local, non-industrial farming source to ensure cleanliness. Even organic foods grown in large commercial operations are more subject to pathenogenic bacteria. Meat and fish can also be frozen for two weeks and then thawed prior to consumption.

Vegetarian Diets

While there is a wide range of vegetarian diets, from vegan to lacto-ovo vegetarian, the basic vegetarian diet excludes meat of any kind, including seafood, poultry, and red meat. One of the primary reasons people choose a vegetarian diet is generally due to the belief that it is unethical to kill animals for food. This diet is also chosen for health, religious, economic, environmental, political, or personal reasons. Frances Moore Lappé's book, *Diet for a Small Planet*, was one of the first books to describe the environmental and social impacts of large-scale meat production, and ongoing research confirms the inhumanity and toxicity of mass-produced animal foods. Lacto-ovo vegetarians eat eggs and dairy, ovo vegetarians eat eggs but not dairy, and lacto vegetarians eat dairy but not eggs.

Semivegetarian diets are primarily vegetarian but may include some animal flesh, such as pescatarianism in which seafood is the only meat consumed or a pollotarian diet in which poultry is allowed. Macrobiotic diets include whole grains and legumes, and they may also include some seafood. Semivegetarian diets are sometimes used when transitioning into or out of a completely vegetarian diet, or for other reasons such as a dislike for certain types of meat or to simply reduce meat consumption.

Benefits
Vegetarian diets are high in fiber, vitamins, minerals, antioxidants, and carbohydrates.

Cautions/Deficiencies
Animal protein is low in a vegetarian diet, but lacto-ovo vegetarians who consume animal by-products, such as cheese, milk, and eggs, are usually able to consume enough protein and the necessary amino acids. A vegetarian diet can provide adequate protein, but it is important to eat a wide variety of foods and proteins to ensure

proper nutrition. B12 deficiency is a risk for vegetarians, as this vitamin comes primarily from meat. Vegetarians can obtain some B12 from dairy and eggs, and other fortified packaged foods.

A deficiency of dietary sulfur can occur in those following a strict vegetarian or vegan diet, as they are not consuming the dietary protein that provides the sulfur-containing amino acids. A recent study shows that strict vegetarians may be susceptible to subclinical protein malnutrition that can lead to hyperhomocysteinemia and an increased risk of cardiovascular diseases (Ingenbleek & McCully, 2012). This protein deficiency also causes a concurrent sulfur deficiency, leading to problems with protein and enzyme activity in the body, as well as problems with bones, joints, metabolism, and connective tissues. Sulfur is important for the proper functioning of insulin, detoxification, carbohydrate metabolism, electron transport, and the synthesis of metabolic intermediates like glutathione.

Ayurvedic Diet—Vegetarian

Ayurveda is an ancient Indian system of medicine that is thousands of years old. The diet derived from this system is based on the principle of body types and a person's predominant constitution, referred to as "doshas." There are three doshas, Vata, Pitta, and Kapha, corresponding to the elements of air, fire, water and earth.

Ayurvedic diets vary based on one's constitution, but they are all vegetarian with an emphasis on wholesome, freshly cooked, or raw foods that are in season. Additionally, the diets incorporate a lot of spices, such as turmeric, ginger, coriander, fenugreek, and cumin. Meat may be prescribed as a medicine in cases of blood sugar issues or protein deficiency. Foods are divided into six tastes: sweet, sour, salty, bitter, pungent, and astringent, and each of these should ideally be present at every meal.

Benefits

The Ayurvedic diet aims to bring balance to specific constitutional types, so it is very personalized. It can increase energy levels, improve immunity, resolve digestive disorders, improve sleeping patterns, reduce toxicity, and improve overall health.

Cautions/Deficiencies

Using Ayurvedic dietary prescriptions and herbs could be problematic if not properly understood. Undertaking an Ayurvedic diet should be done under the care of a qualified Ayurvedic practitioner. Since this diet is mostly vegetarian, it may be deficient in vitamin B12 and it may be low in protein.

Five-Element Diet

The five-element diet comes from traditional Chinese medicine and is based on the five elements of water, wood, fire, earth, and metal, which correspond to the internal organs of the kidneys, liver, heart, stomach, and lungs. This diet incorporates fresh, local, plant-based foods and minimizes the use of animal proteins. The elements are also divided according to five tastes: salty, sour, bitter, sweet, and savory or pungent. Foods are chosen depending on the seasons, which correspond to the elements as well: Winter is water, spring is wood, early summer is fire, late summer is earth, and fall is metal. Light cooking techniques such as steaming and poaching are emphasized.

Benefits

A Chinese medicine practitioner familiar with the constitutional needs of the client may prescribe this diet. It is especially useful when a client is in recovery from illness and digestion is weak. It will be important to ensure adequate intake of fats and fat-soluble vitamins when on this diet.

Macrobiotic Diet

The macrobiotic diet is high in whole grains (40%–60%), fresh and cooked vegetables (20%–30%), beans, sprouts, nuts and seeds, seaweed, and small amounts of fish and seafood (5%–10%). High-quality, fresh, local foods are emphasized, whereas processed and packaged foods, dairy, eggs, meat, coffee, stimulants, and sugar are avoided. Nightshades are also avoided in this diet due to their tendency to cause inflammation in the body. Foods eaten vary based on the time of year, with lighter foods in spring and summer and heavier, denser foods in the winter. The macrobiotic diet differs from a vegetarian diet in that it includes fish and seafood, as well as other naturally raised meats, according to individual needs. The macrobiotic diet also dictates the role of food preparation—food is prepared in a peaceful environment, using pots and dishware made from glass, ceramics, stainless steel, and wood. Food is thoroughly chewed until it is a liquid to aid in digestion.

Benefits

The macrobiotic diet is both a way of eating and a way of life. Foods are eaten to balance yin and yang. The diet is also low in fat and high in fiber. The behavioral aspects of macrobiotics can be useful, such as food preparation and good food-chewing practice.

Cautions/Deficiencies

Not recommended for children, pregnant women, or nursing women; because it is low in dietary fats, supplemental fats would be necessary. Deficiencies could develop if one undertakes a strict vegetarian or vegan macrobiotic diet. Poor nutrition could result from a macrobiotic diet if it is not properly planned.

Vegan Diet

A vegan diet is a category of vegetarian diet. It is strictly plant based without the use of any animal products or by-products. This means that vegans do not eat anything that has been derived from an animal, including meat, fish, poultry, eggs, dairy, honey, or even gelatin. Vegans also believe that all sentient creatures have rights, and it is unethical to exploit animals as though they were commodities. Some people who follow a vegan diet also follow a vegan lifestyle, which eschews all clothing and personal products made from animals (leather, fur, wool, some cosmetics).

There are many reasons that people choose to adopt a vegan diet. Some approach it from an ethical standpoint and as a statement for animal rights. Vegans are against killing animals, and they also believe it is unethical to raise animals for their milk and eggs and keep them in cages. Many vegans are also concerned about the environmental effects of pollution from factory farms, large-scale deforestation for grazing land, and the use of fossil fuels in the meat industry. People also believe that being vegan is healthier and a more natural diet for human beings, claiming that cultures consuming a primarily plant-based diet live longer and have healthier lives. However, while there is good evidence for the health benefits of a diet rich in plants, there is no evidence of any indigenous culture or Paleolithic culture practicing veganism, suggesting that veganism is a relatively recent innovation in dietary practices among humans.

Benefits

Vegan diets are rich in carbohydrates, Omega-6 fatty acids, dietary fiber, carotenoids, folic acid, vitamin C, vitamin E, and magnesium.

Cautions/Deficiencies

It is common for people who are not well suited to veganism (or vegetarianism) to become depressed, anxious, and fatigued due to low protein levels, as well as develop neurological and mental health problems associated with vitamin B12 deficiencies. Veganism is especially dangerous for pregnant women and their fetuses due to the high amounts of essential fatty acids required for brain and nervous system development, available only from grass-fed animals. Omega-3s and the fat-soluble vitamins are required especially for neurological development and the brain. A vegan diet has low cholesterol and is low in saturated fats. The major drawback of a vegan diet is that it requires care and attention to ensure that essential nutrients are being included in the diet, as it is easy to become deficient in vitamins and nutrients essential to health. Protein in a vegan diet is limited to plant proteins, found in foods like legumes, nuts, seeds, and whole grains; however, only a few contain complete proteins. This results in deficits in obtaining all the essential amino acids, which are required for proper health. Vegan diets often include large amounts of soy and soy protein isolates, which can have negative effects on thyroid hormones and digestive enzymes. Other vitamins that are commonly missing, or very low in a vegan diet, are vitamin D, vitamin B12, calcium, and iron. The fat-soluble vitamins, A, E, D, and K, require saturated fats for absorption. Eating products fortified with these vitamins and minerals, and making sure that one's diet includes complete proteins as well as varied protein sources, is essential to maintaining a healthy vegan diet. However, it is questionable whether this type of diet is a match to human physiology.

Vegans are especially susceptible to vitamin B12 deficiency, a condition that, if left untreated, can cause serious health problems like depression, dementia, and Alzheimer's disease. Vitamin B12 is mainly found in animal products, and while it is found in some plant foods, such as spirulina algae, tempeh, and sea vegetables, the B12 found in these foods is an analog of B12 that actually blocks the absorption of vitamin B12. In effect, eating these foods can cause an increase in the body's B12 requirement. This deficiency can also cause the artery-damaging hormone, homocysteine, to increase. Even though the body's intestinal bacteria produces vitamin B12, it is not in a form that is readily absorbed and used by the body (Lam, Schneider, Zhao, & Corley, 2013).

Healthy nonmeat sources of B12 include organic free-range eggs, raw milk, and wild-caught Alaskan salmon. In terms of B12 supplements, the sublingual sprays are superior to other forms of consumption (Lam et al., 2013). Inasmuch as the diet is low in protein, saturated fat, Omega-3 fatty acids, retinol, vitamin B12, and zinc, vegans may have particularly low intakes of vitamin B12 and low intakes of calcium.

Recommendations/Supplementation

People who wish to adhere to a vegan diet should be encouraged to do so for very short periods of time. Because veganism is frequently linked to a strong belief system, it is important to inquire about the meaning of veganism: Is it about animals, the environment, and/or spiritual beliefs? In my practice with vegans, I discuss whether there are ways to balance out personal concerns for animal well-being with the need of the animal-human body for animal-based protein by ritually giving thanks to the animal who has shared its flesh.

Fasting and Detoxification Diets

Fasting is the voluntary act of abstaining from food and/or liquid for a given amount of time for health-related, spiritual, or political reasons. Fasts may include the consumption of only liquids. Mono diets may be used for elimination purposes.

Water fasts eliminate all food and liquids other than water from the diet. They are generally ill advised for mental or physical health, and people should be discouraged from water fasting. Many benefits can be obtained from juice or vegetable fasts, which include only fruit and vegetable juices and water but no other foods. Juice or vegetable fasts provide more nutrients and can be used for short periods of 1–3 days for detoxification.

Fruit and vegetable fasts restrict all foods except for fruits and vegetables, which are high in nutrients and allow digestion to rest and detoxification to occur. Mono diets are fasts in which only one food is consumed for a given period of time to give the digestive system a rest while supplying necessary nutrition, such as a rice fast or a diet of only one type of vegetable. For example, Khichadi (also *Khichari* or *Khichdi*) is an Indian dish made from split mung beans and rice, and sometimes other spices and vegetables; it is eaten as an Ayurvedic cleansing mono diet. This dish is easily digested and can be used after a period of intemperance or to eliminate allergens from the diet. It can also be used to transition into and out of other more extreme liquid fasts, as a recovery diet after surgery or other illnesses, or during times of emotional stress when digestion is taxed.

Fasts and detoxifications, like diets, follow "fad" periods. This does not necessarily mean they are without merit, just that they are promoted at the social level, often considered the latest "cure," and attract people via social contagion and may or may not be beneficial for individual mental health. When discussing fasts during the assessment, understanding the value of the fast and the duration along with its effect on mental health will be important.

One example is The Master Cleanse, a juice fast that was popular in the 1970s and returned to popularity recently. It is a 1- to 40-day fast in which the only liquid consumed is a mixture of freshly squeezed lemon juice, maple syrup, and cayenne pepper, which is added to pure water. It provides a sufficient amount of calories and nutrients (for a few days) while allowing the body to cleanse itself of toxins. The cleanse is undertaken in three phases, beginning with a 3-day period of slowly elimi-nating processed foods, then 10 days on the lemon juice mixture, and 3 days of slowly reincorporating solid foods back into the diet. The "cleanse" may include the use of nightly laxatives and a morning salt-water flush. The fast is very alkalizing, which might benefit people who are natural vegetarians/high carbohydrate/slow oxidizer metabolism types. But for carnivores it would be too alkalizing and could exacerbate anxiety and fatigue. The sugar content is high, so it would not be suitable for people with either hypoglycemia or diabetes. It would not be appropriate for adolescents either. Undertaking this fast for 1–2 days would be the limit for safety as there are many other fasts that can achieve better results.

Urine fasting is the practice of drinking one's own urine and water for cleansing. The Jain people practice urine drinking each morning, and this practice has spread worldwide among non-Jain people. The benefit of this fast is in the nutri-ents and NT metabolites available in urine that include a mixture of minerals, salts, enzymes, and hormones, which cleanse the blood. Urea is also put back into the body and acts to cleanse the body of excess mucus.

Benefits

Fasting for a day or two can have positive effects, such as increasing immune health, disease prevention, mental clarity, and improving digestive health. Fasting gives the digestive system a break and allows toxins to be eliminated. The energy that is nor-mally used for digestion can be used for healing and repairing damaged tissues.

Cautions/Deficiencies

Side effects of fasting include headaches, nausea, foul body odor and bad breath, and intense hunger. Nutrient deficiencies can be a problem if fasts are done for long periods of time. Other possible side effects are constipation, dizziness, fatigue, dehydration, and gallstones. Fasting is contraindicated during pregnancy and nurs-ing, and for those on medications or with diabetes, heart disease, cancer, and fevers. Starvation may be induced by strict fasting and could lead to electrolyte imbalances, renal failure, cardiac arrhythmias, and death. People with anorexia nervosa should not fast.

Recommendations/Supplementation

It is important to transition slowly into the fast and out of the fast. Limit fasts to 3 days. Do not use water-only fasts.

Essential Next Steps

Recall that food is to our bodies like fuel is to a car. Some cars can run on any fuel, but others won't unless the mixture is exactly right, and still others do best on one octane while they might limp along on others. Once the basic requirements mentioned earlier are met, diets will differ by their ratios of foods.

- Identify the role of allergies and sensitivities in client mental health.
- Prepare fresh food and avoid packaged foods with preservatives and additives.
- Conduct elimination diets and other tests to assess for sensitivities.
- Work with the client to identify diet types that are optimal.
- Identify the ratio of proteins, carbohydrates, and fats that suits a specific bio-chemically individual metabolism: fast (carnivore), moderate (mixed foods), or slow (vegetarian-based).
- Minimize exposure to toxic heavy metals.
- Undertake periodic cleanses to detoxify.
- Explore the intersection of belief systems and dietary choices, differentiating between close adherence to a specific dietary system for health and orthorexia.

CHAPTER 6

The Kitchen Is Your Pharmacy

Diet Essential: *There is no one right diet for everyone.*

Food as medicine is the foundation for both the prevention and treatment of mental health issues. Foods and their preparation represent an essential part of a complete program for prevention and recovery. Mental health depends on beneficial foods and healthy preparation methods.

In Chapter 3, I explored five essential factors that contribute to mental illness. These are as follows:

1. Chrononutrition imbalance
2. Blood sugar handling and functional hypoglycemia
3. Food allergies and sensitivities
4. Inflammation, oxidative stress, and mitochondrial function
5. Methylation: conversion of folates/folic acid (B9) to l-methylfolate

Next I explore the principles of applying food to prevent and treat these five underlying factors common to all mental illness along with specific categories.

FIVE ESSENTIAL DIETARY PRINCIPLES FOR MENTAL HEALTH

1. *Support chrononutrition.* Chrononutrition refers to the use of certain foods and supplements to regulate circadian rhythm and the specific timing of food intake to effect changes in circadian rhythm. For example, eating protein-rich meals early in the day supports energy and alertness and carbohydrates later in the day enhance relaxation and sleep. Maintaining regular meal times entrains metabolic rhythm, whereas variations of regular meal

times adversely affect fat metabolism and digestion. In Chapter 7, I define four nutritional supplements that are known to help reset the circadian rhythm imbalances, which underlie depression, PTSD, bipolar disorder, and insomnia.

2. *Blood sugar handling and functional hypoglycemia.* Diets that supply moderate to high protein and fat, plant proteins, and low grains will help manage hypoglycemia and sugar handling. Animal proteins combine well with soothing foods like yams and baked potatoes with butter, carrots, corn tamales made with lard, gluten-free pastas with sauces, salads with homemade dressings rich in hemp oil and olive oil—all topped with sea salt, which supports adrenal function and stabilizes blood glucose. Nuts, seeds, and vegetables with some fruit are also beneficial. The timing of food is important; people with unstable blood glucose must eat every 2–3 hours. Glucose tolerance factor and adrenal glandular support recovery.

3. *Decrease food allergies and sensitivities.* The previous chapter explored the methods used to reduce toxins and sensitivities by eliminating "fake" synthetic-rich foods and focusing on the "original," authentic source of food.

4. *Decrease inflammation and oxidative stress and enhance mitochondrial function.* Antioxidants, fruits, vegetables, chocolate, tea, and saturated fats all decrease inflammation and oxidative stress. Eggs, coconut oil, and the anthocyanin-rich blue and purple fruits like blueberries all quench the inflammatory fires that contribute to mental illness.

Fresh whole foods, vegetables and fruits and animal proteins, fuel the little mitochondrial engines. There are a variety of nutrients that act as antioxidants to reduce inflammation and oxidative stress in the brain. Carotenoids found in fruits and vegetables, especially the dark leafy greens and the red orange spectrum, are anti-inflammatory and antioxidant and they improve cognitive health (Johnson, 2012). A number of high-fat foods like avocado or avocado oil significantly increase absorption of the carotenoids, suggesting the benefits of guacamole and tomato salsa to support cognition (Unlu, Bohn, Clinton, & Schwartz, 2005).

5. *Enhance methylation and folates.* Methylation is supported by high-quality foods that emphasize folate, which is found in leafy greens, lentils, sunflower seeds, broccoli, spinach, and almonds. Liver, garlic, onions, beets, and red wine also support the methylation process, as do choline-rich foods like eggs. At least one meal a day, preferably at midday, should include protein and a big bowl of leafy greens to fuel energy and mood throughout the day. The smell of foods also improves mental health as described in Box 6.1.

Box 6.1

Breathe an Orange

More than just nutrients in foods affect our well-being. In fact, the smell of foods affects our mood. The smell of a fresh orange reduces anxiety. Oranges (and other citrus) provide vitamin C, and the white pulp provides bioflavonoids that are powerful antioxidants.

---

13 Essential Foods for Mental Health

- Bone broths
- Raw almonds
- Wild salmon or fatty fish
- Raw butter
- Coconut (meat and oil)
- Sweet potatoes
- Avocado
- Beets
- Cacao (chocolate)
- Oats and gluten-free grains
- Arugula and other bitter greens
- Fresh sauerkraut and other fermented foods
- Coffee/tea (green and black)

FATS AND THE SUBSTITUTION PRINCIPLE

One of the first changes I ask clients to make is to exchange the types of fats they are using. Substituting poor-quality fats for brain-healing fats is easy and one of the top three most beneficial changes people can do first (the other two are replacing refined sugar with better sweet sources and eliminating refined carbohydrates). I have never met anyone who was unhappy when I suggested that they eat more butter and bacon.

Fats are medicine for the brain, so when eating fats consider a selection of raw oils and saturated fats. Eliminate all the Omega-6 oils like corn oil, cottonseed, soybean, canola, and sunflower oil, as well as margarine and butter substitutes. Replace with olive oil, raw organic butter, and for cooking, sesame oil and coconut oil.

Food Sources of Healthy Fats

Seeds and Nuts

Raw seeds and nuts are excellent sources of fats and protein. Avoid roasted nuts due to rancidity. One can lightly roast raw nuts in the oven at a low temperature to engage children who may not like raw nuts. Raw sunflower seeds, sesame seeds, and chia seeds are a rich source of Omega-3 and Omega-6 essential fatty acids. Chia seeds are especially beneficial for their EFAs and also contain a full complement of amino acids as well as a significant amount of digestible fiber. Nuts are best eaten if they are soaked first. Soaking reduces phytic acid that binds calcium absorption in the body. It makes them more digestible, especially for people with intestinal permeability. Peanut butter should be avoided because it carries a fungus called aflatoxin, which is a carcinogen. Better alternatives include hazelnut butter, almond butter, or cashew butter. Nuts can also be ground and used as a flour substitute and made into milk. Walnuts may have beneficial effect in reducing the risk, delaying the onset, or slowing the progression of, Alzheimer's disease (Chauhan et al., 2010). Nut and seed butters are an excellent snack for children at school and adults at work, especially when combined with apples or bananas. Box 6.2 provides an energizing recipe to support mental function and satiety. Soaking almonds, walnuts, and organic dried fruit and placing them in the refrigerator makes a nutritious sweet syrup to cover pancakes or cereal instead of other sweeteners. Box 6.3 provides a recipe for making Coconut Milk Mocha.

Box 6.2
Chia and Nut Butter Smoothie Recipe

Ingredients

1 large ripe banana, peeled and frozen

1 cup unsweetened almond milk

1–2 tablespoons chia seeds

1 tablespoon raw almond butter (can substitute cashew or hazelnut butter)

1 teaspoon of coconut oil (optional)

¼ teaspoon ground cinnamon (optional)

Directions

Put all of the ingredients in a blender and blend until smooth.

Box 6.3

Coconut Milk Mocha

This is my favorite morning or afternoon guilt-free "pick-me-up." It is anti-inflammatory, rich in antioxidants, and provides brain food in the form of the trinity of cognitive function: coffee, cocoa, and coconut. If you prefer, you can substitute organic decaffeinated coffee or just use cocoa when serving to children, replacing the liquid from the coffee with extra coconut milk. Make sure your ingredients are organic and sugar-free.

Ingredients

12 ounces fresh brewed organic coffee, hot

½ cup full-fat, unsweetened coconut milk

2 tablespoons unsweetened organic cocoa powder
(for drinking)

2–5 drops liquid stevia (or to taste)

Coconut cream, unsweetened (optional)

Organic vanilla bean powder (optional)

Directions

Combine all ingredients in a blender at medium speed for a few minutes until frothy. Pour into a mug and top with coconut cream, if desired.

Sea buckthorn is a rich plant source of Omega-7 fatty acids, as well as Omega-3, -6, and -9. Omega-7 monounsaturated fatty acid (MUFA), also called palmitoleic acid, is a nonessential fatty acid that is produced by the body from glucose, which converts to fatty acids. The berries and seeds can be eaten fresh or made into smoothies, and sea buckthorn oil can be used internally and externally for skin, cardiovascular, and gastrointestinal health. It has benefits for cardiovascular health by smoothing arterial walls and reducing C-reactive protein levels, which indicate the amount of inflammation in artery walls. It has twice as much Omega-7 as macadamia nut oil, the next richest plant source of Omega-7. In Table 6.1, you will see the best sources of Omega-3 fatty acids.

Coconut

The coconut (*Coco nucifera*) is a nearly perfect food, rich in fats, protein, and a full complement of B vitamins. Coconuts provide an edible seed, water, and oil. Coco-

TABLE 6.1

Best Sources of Omega-3 Fatty Acids

Food Types	Omega-3 Food Sources
Meat	Grass-fed beef
Fish	Anchovies, caviar, cod, halibut, herring, mackerel, oysters, rainbow trout, salmon, sardines, scallops, shrimp, snapper, striped bass, tuna
Dairy and eggs	Milk and eggs enriched with Omega-3
Legumes and beans	Edamame, miso, tofu
Nuts and seeds	Alfalfa seeds, chia seeds, flaxseeds, walnuts
Land and sea vegetables	Algae, arugula, brussels sprouts, cauliflower, collard greens, green beans, kale, romaine lettuce, spinach, summer squash, turnip greens, winter squash
Oils	Avocado oil, cod liver oil, flaxseed oil, fish oil, hemp oil, walnut oil

nut oil is one of the healthiest and most medicinal of fats and can be incorporated into daily food preparation. Over 50% of the fat in coconut oil is medium-chain triglycerides (MCTs). MCTs enter the body via the portal system without needing the lymphatic system in the intestines or bile salts for absorption. It is easily absorbed and readily available via ketone bodies as an energy source. Coconut fat is used to produce energy, increase satiety, and may help with weight control and a reduction in body fat. Coconut fat does not slow digestion, as most fats do, nor does it circulate in the bloodstream to the degree that other fats do. As a result, it is much less likely to be incorporated into fat cells and does not collect in artery walls or contribute to hardening of the arteries (Felton, Crook, Davies, & Oliver, 1994).

Coconut oil is heat stable and thus an excellent cooking oil. It is slow to oxidize and thus resistant to rancidity. It increases high-density lipoprotein (HDL) levels and, in so doing, improves the cholesterol ratio (Enig, 2000; Norton et al., 2004). When buying coconut oil, look for organic, cold-pressed, unrefined coconut oil. The lipids scientist Mary Enig (2006) recommends blending equal amounts of coconut oil, cold-pressed sesame oil, and extra-virgin olive oil for daily use in cooking. This mixture should be stored in a glass jar at room temperature. In addition to the fat, coconuts contain iron, selenium, sodium, calcium, magnesium, manganese, phosphorus, and vitamins B1,

B3, B5, B6, C, E, and K. Coconut lowers blood sugar, protects the liver, and improves immune function (DebMandal & Mandal, 2011). Coconut water has a naturally sweet flavor and is a healthy refreshing drink. It is low in calories, sodium, sugar, and fat, while providing a rich source of potassium. It supplies the body with electrolytes, increasing energy and lowering blood pressure, and rebuilding lean muscle as well. When buying coconut water, make sure there are no added sugars. The meat of the coconut is especially high in fiber and helps to improve digestion. Dried coconut, also called desiccated coconut, is the dried and grated meat of the coconut. Use it as a topping for curries, desserts, and yogurt, or add it to granola. Buy unsweetened dried coconut with no added preservatives. Learn more about Oats in x 6.4.

Box 6.4
Oats

Oats may be gluten-free or contaminated with gluten. Nevertheless, they are an important addition to the diet, especially for people who are anxious and have insomnia. Steel-cut oats are rich in silicon, phosphorus, and magnesium and provide a calming, nourishing effect. Try sweetening them with a little blackstrap molasses to add iron, copper, magnesium, potassium, and manganese.

Add some raisins and walnuts, and this makes the perfect late-night snack and helps with relaxation and sleep. For people who are not alcohol-contraindicated, a half a cup (4 oz.) of good-quality dark beer made with oats and hops acts as a mild nervine, is anxiolytic and a muscle relaxant, and is also rich in B vitamins.

Cod Liver Oil
Cod liver oil is rich in vitamins A and D, eicosapentaenoic acid (EPA), and docosahexaenoic acid (DHA), which support healthy brain and nervous system function. The best cod liver oil is fermented and enhanced when combined with butter oil or ghee, which adds vitamin K2 .

Butter
Butter is an ideal source of fat and can be used daily. It is best to use raw, unsalted organic butter if possible. Butter contains vitamins A, D, and E, as well as lecithin, iodine, and selenium. One of the reasons butter is so nutritious when added to

vegetables is that vitamins A, E, and K in the vegetables are fat-soluble and thus not well absorbed without the fat.

Bacon

Bacon fat is mostly monounsaturated fat, specifically oleic acid, the same valuable fat in olive oil. Forty percent of the fat in bacon is saturated, which keeps the fats from becoming rancid. Bacon and pork fat contains phosphatidylcholine, which is valuable for brain and liver function. Bacon fat helps to regulate blood sugar, promotes satiety, and reduces sugar and carbohydrate cravings. It serves as a good transition food from high-carbohydrate diets because it is satisfying and provides good amounts of fat and protein.

Ghee

Ghee is butter that has been clarified; it is the oil of the butter separated from the milk solids. Without the milk solids, ghee is free of the hormones and antibiotics found in regular milk products, and it is lactose-free (Gates, 2011). The milk protein casein is almost entirely removed during the clarification process. Ghee is usually tolerated well by those who have lactose intolerance and are unable to handle other milk products.

Hemp Oil

Hemp oil contains a 3:1 ratio of Omega-6 to Omega-3 essential fatty acids, which is ideal for human nutrition. Purchase raw, unrefined, cold-pressed hemp oil. Hemp is best used on salads (not for cooking). It has a nutty flavor and mixes well with olive oil. Try making an oil blend using 50% olive oil and 50% hemp oil, or 75% olive oil and 25% hemp oil.

Lard

Lard is an excellent fat source despite being much maligned. Lard is derived from the pig and is rich in vitamin D and saturated fat. The best quality is called leaf lard, usually available at the local farmer's market or butcher. Do not use vegetable lard or commercial lard. Lard is the perfect fat to combine with coconut fat when baking or making homemade tamales. Lard has a high smoke point and can be used in gentle frying and cooking.

Preparing foods with healthy fats becomes another source of brain/mood support, as you will find in Table 6.2.

TABLE 6.2

Medicinal Fats and Oils for Cooking

Type	"Good" Healthy Fats	Health Benefits
	Butter	Ideal balance of Omega-3 and Omega-6 fatty acids Provides vitamins A, D, and E; iodine; lecithin; and selenium Provides trace minerals such as chromium, copper, manganese, and zinc Supports immune function Increases metabolism Protects against pathogens in the intestinal tract Supports thyroid health Supports brain function and prostaglandin balance Assists with the absorption of fat-soluble vitamins A, E, and K
	Poultry fat (chicken, duck, and goose)	High in vitamin E High in Omega-3 and Omega-6 Supports brain function Prevents cognitive decline
SATURATED	Coconut oil	Anti-inflammatory Antibacterial Antifungal Antiviral Antioxidant Lowers blood sugar Protects the liver Improves immune function
	Clarified butter (ghee)	Helps to heal gastrointestinal inflammation Contains butyric acid, which has antiviral and anticancer properties Helps prevent Alzheimer's disease Promotes digestion and assimilation Provides benefits of butter without the proteins that cause allergies
	Palm and palm kernel oil	Supports healthy brain function, protecting against neurological disorders
MONO-UNSATURATED	Cold-pressed extra-virgin olive oil	Improves brain and nervous system function
	Avocado oil	Helps regulate blood sugar
	Cold-pressed sesame oil	Antidepressant

(continued on next page)

TABLE 6.2

Medicinal Fats and Oils for Cooking (*continued*)

Type	"Good" Healthy Fats	Health Benefits
MONO-UNSATURATED contined	Eggs	Rich in choline, an anti-inflammatory nutrient for the brain and memory Provide calcium, iron, phosphorus, zinc, thiamine, vitamin B6, folate, pantothenic acid, and vitamin B12 Provide the fat-soluble vitamins A, D, and E Provide Omega-3 fatty acids Provide lutein and zeaxanthin for better eye health Cholesterol in eggs is a precursor for production of hormones in the body, including the sex hormones testosterone and estrogen Dietary cholesterol in eggs does not raise blood cholesterol
	Lard (from pigs)	Excellent source of vitamin D Lowers LDL cholesterol
	Tallow (from beef and lamb)	Good source of antimicrobial palmitoleic acid
POLY-UNSATURATED	Walnut oil	Not to be used as cooking oil, only raw Rich in Omega-3 fatty acids Reduces inflammation Supports healthy hormone levels Provides selenium, phosphorus, iron, magnesium, calcium, and zinc Antioxidant
	Cold-pressed flax oil (only use uncooked)	Good source of Omega-3 fatty acids Supplies nutrient-rich lignans Supports healthy cholesterol levels Supports blood glucose levels Rich in alpha-linolenic acid (ALA)
	Pumpkin seed oil	Anti-inflammatory Provides tryptophan Increases good cholesterol Reduces blood pressure
	Grapeseed oil (high cooking temperature)	Can be heated up to 485 degrees F, making it a good cooking oil Rich in linoleic acid Provides polyphenols (flavonoids) Provides vitamin E Anti-inflammatory Antioxidant Antihistamine Adaptogenic (antistress)

PROTEINS

Animal Proteins

Meat Quality

The eating of meat should be limited to humanely raised and slaughtered, grass and organically fed animals. Confined animal feeding operations (CAFOs) are inhumane and produce a lower quality meat with depleted nutrient levels and high levels of contaminants, like antibiotics, hormones, and pesticides. These animals are also fed genetically engineered (GE) corn and soy. Grass-fed beef is superior to grain-fed beef for human health. It is higher in beta-carotene, vitamin E, thiamin, riboflavin, calcium, magnesium, potassium, and total Omega-3s, and it has a healthier Omega-6 to Omega-3 ratio.

Organ Meats

Organ meats are an important source of nutrients, especially for the natural carnivore and balanced metabolizer. Their source must be from grass-fed stock. Many epicurean foods today are made from the glands and organs of animals. Such dishes as liver pâtés, sweetbreads (thymus or pancreas), and dried salami are highly regarded for their contribution to health. Chicken liver pâté and prepared beef or goat lung are prized for their flavor and capacity to rejuvenate. *Menudo* made from tripe or stomach is a prized dish in Mexico, and haggis (sheep stomach stuffed with cooked oats, blood, and organ meat) is still considered a delicacy in Scotland. Blood pudding, kidneys, goat and pork testicles, tongue, heart, pancreas, bone gels, and head cheese (meat gels) all contribute to mental health and support recovery from the addictions. But these traditional foods are increasingly hard to find and their nutritional and ritual value is often forgotten. Adrenal, liver, brain, pituitary, hypothalamus, and thymus glands play an important role in restoring and rebuilding tissue. Despite their healthful benefits, it is often not possible to obtain enough fresh organic organ meats to consume them in the quantities required for medicinal purposes. Most pork, lamb, beef, and sheep glands are available in high-dose, dehydrated form that I discuss further in Chapter 7.

Bone Broth Recipe

Adapted from Allison Siebecker (2005), *Traditional Bone Broth in Modern Health and Disease*. Townsend Letter, February/March. Retrieved from http://www.townsendletter.com/FebMarch2005/broth0205.htm

Bone broth is a traditional recipe that is both medicinal and nourishing. Its high mineral content makes it easy to digest and it is highly nutritious, especially the gelatin obtained from the bones. The broth also supports detoxification of the liver.

Ingredients

Bones (one or more of the following items):
• Bones from poultry, fish, shellfish, beef, or lamb
• Cooked remnants of a previous meal, with or without skin and meat
• Raw bones, with or without skin and meat
• A whole carcass or just parts (feet, ribs, necks, and knuckles)
• Shellfish shells, whole fish carcasses (with heads), or small dried shrimp
Water
Apple cider vinegar or balsamic vinegar (2 tablespoons per quart of water or 2 lb bones)
Vegetables (Optional):
• Celery, carrots, onions, garlic, and parsley, but any will do
• Peelings and scraps ends, tops, and skins or entire vegetable
• If added toward the end of cooking, mineral content will be higher.

Directions

1. Place bones in a Crock-Pot (or stove pot) over a low heat and cover with water. Add vinegar.
2. Heat the broth slowly and once the boil begins, reduce heat to its lowest point, so the broth just barely simmers. Scum will rise to the surface—skim this off.
3. Two hours of simmering is enough to extract flavors and gelatin from fish broth. Larger animals take longer—all day for broth made from chicken, turkey, or duck and overnight for beef broth.
4. To make soup, add vegetables or meat to broth during the last hour or until vegetables are cooked but not mushy.
5. Broth should then be strained. Stock will keep several days in the refrigerator or may be frozen in plastic containers. Boiled down, it concentrates and becomes a jellylike fumée or demi-glaze that can be reconstituted into a sauce by adding water.

Fish

Fish is an excellent source of protein. Only fish from wild sources should be used. Farmed fish is toxic to humans and the environment. An inexpensive source of fish is canned wild salmon and sardines. Fish heads and fish bones make an excellent bone broth to which vegetables are added.

Dairy Products

Bovine (Cow) Milk

Pasteurized, homogenized, and chemical-laden milk is difficult for the body to digest and contributes to an accumulation of mucus in the body. Commercially raised cows are fed a diet of grains, corn, and soy that has been heavily treated with pesticides and herbicides.

If cow milk is to be consumed, the best option is full-fat milk that has not been processed and is from pasture-raised cows. It is highly nutritious, containing calcium, vitamins B6 and B12, CLA (conjugated linoleic acid that protects against cancer), and the fat-soluble vitamins A and D. Natural milk is a complete protein and is high in enzymes, and raw milk provides beneficial bacteria. Goat's milk products are also preferred.

Goat and Sheep Milk

Goat and sheep milk is not as mucus-forming as cow milk, and usually does not have as many antibiotics and drugs in it because goats are cleaner and healthier animals. It is naturally homogenized, so it does not require additional homogenization with machines, and it is more digestible. It has more nutrients because of the rich and varied diet of the goats, and it is often available raw. Goat and sheep milk and cheese should be emphasized instead of cow milk and cheese.

Substitution Principle: Best Dairy Milk Substitutes

Milk substitutes are made from a number of ingredients, including soy, rice, nuts, grains, oats, and seeds. They vary in thickness and flavor, but most milk substitutes can easily be used to replace milk in recipes and on cereals and wherever milk is called for. Nut milks are made with a variety of different nuts, including hazelnuts, cashews, and almonds. They are free of saturated fat, lactose, and cholesterol, while being high in protein and essential nutrients like magnesium, manganese, phosphorus, copper, calcium, fiber, iron, potassium, vitamin E, and zinc. The nutty flavor of these milks makes them perfect for baking.

Coconut milk is tasty, rich, and creamy, and comes as a rich cream in a can or a thinner milk beverage in a carton. It has a high saturated fat content. Canned coconut may be high in bisphenol A (BPA), a toxic chemical used in food packaging, like metal cans.

Rice milk is thin water and rice in suspension with a sweet, subtle rice flavor. It is low-fat, hypoallergenic, and high in niacin and B vitamins. It is a good source of magnesium and helps to regulate blood pressure, and it is also high in manganese and selenium. However, its high carbohydrate content can raise blood sugar levels and is not recommended for those with hypoglycemia or diabetes.

Hemp milk is rich and creamy with a nutty flavor. It provides the perfect balance between Omega-3 and -6 fatty acids, and it is low in saturated fat. It is a good choice for those with nut or milk allergies.

Oat milk is a good source of fiber and protein and is relaxing. Unless it is guaranteed gluten-free it may be problematic for people with gluten allergies.

Soymilk is the most widespread of the milk substitutes, but it is not recommended. This is due to the antinutrients contained in soy (see the section on Food Allergies and Sensitivities).

Cheese

Cheeses contain varying quantities of protein and fat from milk. Most commonly it is made from the milk of cows, goats, and sheep. It is generally high in protein, fat, calcium, zinc, phosphorus, and vitamins A, B12, D3, and K2. Aged cheeses tend to contain less lactose and are more easily tolerated by those with lactose intolerance. Cheese is high in saturated fat. The most nutritious cheese is derived from grass-fed, pasture-raised animals. Raw, unpasteurized cheese contains enzymes and healthy bacteria that improve digestion and also enhance the flavor of the cheese. Organic raw cheese from grass-fed animals is the best choice because it is free of antibiotics and growth hormones and is also higher in nutrients.

Plant Proteins

Hemp Protein

Hemp protein provides a complete protein, making it ideal for vegetarians and vegans, since most sources of plant proteins are incomplete. It also provides both Omega-3 and Omega-6 essential fatty acids in the optimal ratio.

Micro-Algae

Spirulina and chlorella provide a source of protein, chlorophyll, and vitamin K, and they are easily absorbed. Chlorella is an anti-inflammatory and is also a good source of chlorophyll.

Pea (Legume) Protein

Pea protein powder comes from either green or yellow split peas and is a good choice for vegetarians to increase their protein consumption. Yellow peas are rich in amino acids, especially lysine and arginine. Pea protein is also high in iron in a nonheme form (proteins in plants different from animal proteins), which is more easily absorbed by the body. Pea protein is also used in powdered protein mixes instead of rice due to the arsenic levels found in rice.

Whey Protein

Whey is a milk protein that is a by-product of the cheesemaking process. It is a watery liquid that separates from the curds. It is also sometimes separated from casein, the other protein found in milk. It contains all nine amino acids, and its low lactose content makes it suitable for those who are lactose intolerant. Whey protein is an easy source of high-quality protein that can be mixed into smoothies. It contains all nine essential amino acids and is widely available as a nutritional protein supplement. It is rich in beta-glucans and immunoglobulins. Whey is beneficial for recovery from eating disorders.

Hemp Seeds

Rich in complete protein, hemp seeds are a healthy addition to salads, granola, and other dishes calling for nuts. They are high in essential fatty acids with a balanced ratio of Omega-3 and Omega-6. They provide gamma-linolenic acid (GLA). Hemp seeds provide vitamins A, C, and E and beta-carotene, and they are rich in phosphorus, potassium, magnesium, sulfur, and calcium.

For strong mental health, try the recipe for Healthy Mood Salad in Box 6.5.

Box 6.5

Healthy Mood Salad

Every ingredient in this salad is rich and nourishing for the first and second brain. The kale nourishes the microbiome, celery is a natural sedative, the beets and lemon support the gallbladder and mood, sea salt supports adrenal function, and the fats from the avocado, olive oil, and walnuts nourish the mood and cognition. Eat this salad for lunch or dinner or use it as a raw side dish to a hearty stew.

Ingredients

1 bunch lacinto kale

1 teaspoon sea salt

1 stalk celery, finely chopped

2 teaspoons lemon juice

1 avocado, peeled and pitted

2 tablespoons olive oil

1–2 teaspoons fresh minced garlic

½ cup shredded beets

Raw walnuts

Wedge of goat cheese (optional)

Directions

1. Remove stems and chop the kale leaves. Place them in a bowl and add the salt; gently rub the salt into the kale. Add celery and lemon juice and mix.

2. Mix the avocado and olive oil in a bowl with the minced garlic and pour over the salad, mixing well. Top the salad with beets and walnuts. Serve with goat cheese.

Plants Proteins and Green Foods

Plant foods of all kinds, raw and cooked, should be used in the diet daily. Green plants are rich in chlorophyll, the green color of plants that helps to cleanse and build the blood. Chlorophyll is also called "the blood of plants" because its molecular structure is similar to hemoglobin, which is the molecule in red blood cells that transports oxygen through the blood. Chlorophyll inhibits bacterial growth and anaerobic yeasts and fungi in the digestive tract, purifying the body of toxins. It is anti-inflammatory and helps to renew cells and support healthy gut microbiota. Chlorophyll also helps to regulate calcium absorption.

When it is a challenge to integrate fresh greens into the diet, one can use a good-quality green powder rich in chlorophyll and algae. It can be added to a smoothie or to water as a drink. The importance of chlorophyll cannot be overstated for people with gut permeability and colon problems. Chlorophyll is the "deodorizer" food. It is an energizing food important to people with fatigue-related conditions like chronic fatigue syndrome, adrenal fatigue, depression and fibromyalgia, and inflammatory bowel syndrome. Indeed, everyone needs chlorophyll. Chlorophyll works very well in a chocolate smoothie. Remember, while spinach, chard, and beet greens are high in chlorophyll, they are also high in oxalic acid that inhibits calcium absorption. Varying dietary plant foods will provide a balance.

You may wish to try the delicious, mood-elevating recipes in Boxes 6.6, 6.7, and 6.8, that are also easy to prepare.

Box 6.6
Salad Jar Meditation and Brain Bolt Dressing

People often complain to me about the time it takes to prepare fresh salads every day. I try to help them reframe their thoughts about time-consuming food preparation to salad making as meditation. An easy way to prepare salads to have on hand for the week is to make salad jars. Family members, especially kids, enjoy placing vegetables in the jars. A pint-sized or quart-sized Mason jar can be used, depending on the size of the salad you want to make. Fill the jar with all of the salad ingredients that you like. Layer the ingredients so that the dressing is at the bottom of the jar, set the next level with heartier items that can withstand a little soaking, then vegetables, and finally the greens on top. Having the greens separate from the dressing keeps them from getting soggy. Anything that will be improved by soaking in the dressing like a marinade can go on the bottom—things like chicken, fish, tempeh, beans, quinoa, and mushrooms. Be sure to pack the jar tightly so that the ingredients don't shift around too much.

When you're ready to eat the salad, simply shake the jar a little bit, give it a stir, and enjoy!

1. Shop for vegetables from all the colors of the rainbow you will enjoy eating raw.
2. Put some meditation music on to put you in the moment-to-moment mood.
3. Wash all the vegetables and place them on the counter to dry as you prepare to cut them to bite size. Leave the skins on the vegetables unless they are waxed or bitter. Place each type of vegetable in bowls in a "buffet line" with the heavier rooted vegetables like onions, carrots, and celery to the left and work your way up the line so the tomatoes and then the greens like kale, parsley, and lettuce are at the end when finished.

4.   Make your salad dressing.

5.   Place your jars in a line to the back of the vegetable bowls.

6.   Add a layer of salad dressing to the bottom of each jar. Sprinkle different herbs such as dill, parsley, cayenne, or basil on top of the dressing.

7.   Begin adding the heavier items on the left to the bottom of the jar and follow along, adding as you go, until you reach the end.

Note: Items like nuts and seeds may be placed at the bottom to soak in the dressing or added separately when opening the jar.

Brain Bolt Dressing

One of the essentials of mental health is to make your own salad dressing. It can be simple or elaborate, but homemade can be medicine for the brain and store-bought dressings are not. Nearly any dressing will do, but this is one of my favorites. You can make a jar of it and then add some different herbs each day so it is varied for your week of salads.

This recipe makes about 2 cups of dressing.

Ingredients

¾ cup extra virgin olive oil

¼ cup organic hemp oil

10 tablespoons balsamic vinegar

8 tablespoons raw apple cider vinegar

6 tablespoons of dark agave, pure maple syrup, or raw honey

1 teaspoon sea salt

2–3 minced cloves of garlic

Freshly ground black pepper to taste

Directions

Whisk all the ingredients together; store in glass jar. Will keep for 1 week.

Optional add-ins: 4 teaspoons Dijon mustard, 2 teaspoons curry powder

Box 6.7

Baked Kale Chips

Kale chips are a nutritious and incredibly tasty alternative to potato chips and other snacks. Try this basic recipe and then experiment with different spices.

It makes 4–6 servings.

Ingredients

1 bunch of kale

2 cloves of garlic, minced

2 tablespoons extra-virgin coconut oil, melted

Sea salt to taste

Cayenne pepper (optional)

Directions

1. Preheat oven to 350 degrees F.
2. Wash the kale and pat it dry. Remove the thick stems, coarsely tear the leaves, and put the leaves in a bowl.
3. Add garlic, oil, garlic, and sea salt (and cayenne pepper, if using); toss to coat. Alternatively, you can massage the oil and seasonings into the kale by hand. Spread kale out evenly on a baking sheet.
4. Bake for 10–12 minutes, or until kale is crisp at the edges, being careful not to burn it.

Box 6.8

A Delicious Seaweed Salad

This salad uses hijike or arame sea vegetables, which are among the mildest seaweeds. This salad is a good first step in exploring seaweeds in recipes. It is especially beneficial for fatigue, depression, and hypothyroidism.

Ingredients

1 cup of dry arame or hijiki seaweed

3 scallions

1 cup tofu

1 carrot

½ cup peapods

½ of a red bell pepper

½ of an English cucumber

Handful of broccoli florets

¼ cup walnuts or pine nuts

Sprouts (optional)

Dressing

¼ cup toasted sesame oil

¼ cup rice wine vinegar

1 tablespoon wheat-free tamari

Juice from 2 cloves of garlic and a chunk of fresh ginger

Dash of hot red pepper flakes (optional)

Directions

1. Soak the seaweed in warm water for 15 minutes until soft (save the water for soup or to put in your animal companion's bowl).
2. Dice the scallions, tofu, carrots, peapods, red pepper, cucumber, broccoli, nuts, and sprouts (if using) into small (equal size) pieces.
3. Mix all of the dressing ingredients together in a bowl and whisk until well combined.
4. Combine the vegetable mixture with the softened seaweed and pour the dressing over it. Mix and allow to marinate for a few hours. Eat and enjoy!

Sprouts

Sprouts are nutritious, inexpensive, and easy to incorporate into the diet. They provide enzymes and are high in vitamins, minerals, protein, fiber, and antioxidants. The process of making sprouts is easy and fun and children enjoy it.

Try these seeds, beans, and grains for sprouting:

- **Seeds:** Alfalfa, clover, broccoli, radish, fenugreek, sunflower, pumpkin, mustard, and onion seeds
- **Beans:** Mung beans, lentils, and chickpeas
- **Grains:** Millet, wheat, barley, brown rice, quinoa, buckwheat, rye, corn, oats, and wild rice

Alfalfa is a good source of vitamins K and P, carotene, calcium, magnesium, potassium, sodium, iron, phosphorus, sulfur, silicon, cobalt, chlorine, zinc, and chlorophyll.

Broccoli and Cruciferous Vegetables

Glucoraphanin is a constituent of the Brassica vegetables like brussels sprouts with the highest amounts found in broccoli, especially seeds and sprouts. Well-studied and known for its anticarcinogenic effects, it serves as an antioxidant, anti-inflammatory, and increases Phase 2 detoxification. More recently, concentrated amounts of the supplement, many times higher than found in the vegetable alone, have been explored for inclusion in the treatment of autism spectrum disorders and was found to reverse oxidative stress and improve mitochondrial function leading to improved behaviors (Singh et al., 2014). Several products on the market deliver a dose of about 30 mg a day. Eating too many cruciferous vegetables can depress thyroid function.

Seaweeds

Seaweeds are a rich source of vitamins, minerals, proteins, lipids, and amino acids. Seaweeds also contain high amounts of vitamins. They are one of the best foods by which to obtain minerals, including calcium, phosphorus, magnesium, iron, iodine, and sodium. They are especially rich in iodine, which is essential for healthy thyroid function. The high mineral content of seaweeds supports nervous system function, good mental health, and muscle relaxation and function.

There are many varieties of edible seaweeds that can be eaten fresh or dried. They can be added to salads, as seasoning, to wrap sushi and other foods, and to flavor stocks, soups, grains, and beans.

Seaweeds are classified into three types: brown, green, or red. Brown seaweed and kelp tend to be higher in mineral content than red seaweed (Drum, 2013). Brown seaweeds contain alginates that are proactive against ionizing radiation and aid in heavy metal detoxification.

Legumes

Legumes are the edible dry fruits and seeds contained in shells and pods. They include beans, lentils, peas, and peanuts. Beans are a good source of protein and are rich in potassium, iron, B vitamins, and calcium. However, many people have difficulty digesting beans and develop flatulence or bloating after consuming them. Sprouting increases their digestibility and increases their vitamin C and enzyme levels. The sprouting process breaks proteins down into amino acids and starches into simple sugars. Soaking beans before cooking will reduce the cooking time and it begins the sprouting process, which increases their nutritional benefit and reduces their gas-producing enzymes. Cooking beans with fats and oily foods helps to increase their digestibility. Adding seaweed to beans will increase their nutritional benefit, flavor, and digestibility, as well as reducing cooking times. Seaweed, black pepper, fennel, and cumin also reduce their gas-producing effects. Salt should be added only at the end of cooking. Apple cider vinegar can be added at the end of cooking to soften the beans and increase their digestibility (to learn how to soak legumes and nuts, see Appendix S).

Soybeans

Soy should be avoided except in the form of fermented soy products such as miso, shoyu, and tempeh, and then only in very small quantities.

Soy contains very high levels of phytic acid, which suppresses digestive enzymes; it also depresses thyroid function (Fallon & Enig, 1999) and is high in protease inhibitors, which suppress pancreatic enzymes. Phytic acid in soy also inhibits the assimilation of calcium, magnesium, copper, iron, and zinc. Soy also contains trypsin inhibitors that cause problems with protein digestion and may be responsible for pancreatic disorders. Understanding the negative effects of soy phytoestrogens and modulating intake during pregnancy and infancy could prevent neurological damage during critical periods of sensory development (Westmark, Westmark, & Malter, 2013). Soybeans increase the body's need for vitamin B12 and promote the growth of estrogen-dependent tumors. Fermenting soybeans eliminates this problem, so products like miso, tempeh, tofu, and soy sauce are more easily digested. Soy products, like soymilk, soy protein powders, soy isolates, and soy concentrates should be absolutely avoided.

CARBOHYDRATES

Grains

Grains are indigestible—human beings cannot digest grains. We can predigest them though, and all traditional cultures do this by soaking the grains, fermenting the grains, or using a sourdough culture to prepare the bread. Whole grains can be toxic if not prepared properly as they contain phytic acid. Humans do not produce phytase, the enzyme needed to break down phytic acid. Phytic acid inhibits the absorption of calcium, copper, iron, magnesium, phosphorous, silica, and zinc, as well as some amino acids.

Fermenting grains to make sourdough or to sprout them releases and neutralizes the phytic acid and makes them more digestible while increasing their nutrient content.

Adding generous amounts of fat (like butter) to grains protects the gut from fiber damage and increases the absorption of important fat-soluble nutrients in the grains. (To learn how to soak and prepare grains, and prepare a range of delicious grain recipes, see Appendix K.)

Vegetables and Fruits

When I talk with clients about integrating a range of foods, I rarely discuss vitamins at first, but rather, I suggest that if they choose selections from the various colors, then they will obtain the necessary nutrients from food. I provide them with this chart and we review it together and highlight the foods they like and those they would like to try but have not; we also identify the mental health benefits to prioritize.

Diet Essential: *Eat all the colors of the "brainbow."*

Table 6.3 lists all the vegetables and fruits in the "brainbow." Hand this out to your clients to help them make healthy choices.

SPECIAL MENTAL HEALTH FOODS

Bitter Greens

Eat your dandelions; don't spray them! The liver loves bitter plants and foods as an aid to the digestion of fats. Eat some bitter plants like arugula, dandelion, mustard leaves, or watercress each day, especially with a high-fat meal. This will enhance fat digestion.

Root Vegetables

There are so many different types of root vegetables: carrots, turnips, potatoes, celeriac, parsnips, sweet potatoes, and yucca are among the most popular. They are ideal to use as a staple food instead of grains. In Ayurvedic nutrition they are considered emotionally grounding foods that should be used especially by people with addictions, anxiety, and panic.

The Okinawan (Japanese) purple sweet potato is prized for its nutritional value and is considered one of the essential foods contributing to the long life of many Okinawan people (for some delicious root vegetable recipes, see Appendix T).

TABLE 6.3

Colors of the "Brainbow"

Colors	Foods	Nutrients	Benefits
Red	Cherries Cranberries Red cabbage Beets Radicchio Tomatoes Red onions Red bell peppers Red kidney beans Pink grapefruit Red potatoes Rhubarb Red apples and pears Rainbow chard Red grapes Strawberries Raspberries Radishes Red chilies Watermelon	Lycopene (tomatoes, watermelon, pink grapefruit) Anthocyanins (strawberries, raspberries, red grapes) Antioxidants (cherries, cranberries, proanthocyanidins) Anti-inflammatory Vitamin C (red bell peppers, beets, strawberries, tomatoes) Vitamin A (beets, tomatoes) Betaine (beets) Vitamin K (beets) Folate (beets) Quercetin Hesperidin	Improves memory Improves digestion Improves heart health Lowers blood pressure
Orange	Carrots Sweet potatoes Oranges Peaches Pumpkins Apricots Cantaloupe Mangoes Papaya Tangerines Butternut squash Nectarines	Antioxidants (sweet potatoes) Beta-carotene (sweet potatoes, pumpkins, carrots) Vitamin A (peaches, sweet potatoes) Folate (oranges) Vitamin C (peaches, sweet potatoes, oranges) Iron (sweet potatoes) Carotenoids Bioflavanoids Fiber Magnesium (oranges)	Improves digestion Boosts immunity Prevents cellular damage Promotes healthy mucous membranes
Yellow	Yellow bell peppers Lemons Corn Bananas (also white) Pineapple Yellow squash (butterstick, acorn, delicata) Yellow apples and pears Yellow tomatoes	Alpha-carotene Beta-carotene Anthoxanthins Bromelain (pineapple) Carotenoids (yellow peppers) Vitamin A (yellow peppers) Vitamin C (pineapple, yellow peppers)	Improves brain function Improves digestion Boosts immunity

Colors	Foods	Nutrients	Benefits
Green	Cucumbers Leeks Brussels sprouts Arugula Asparagus Kiwi Lettuce Green bell peppers Kale Pumpkin seeds Lima beans Spinach Chard Broccoli Peas Zucchini Green cabbage	Antioxidants (spinach) Lutein (spinach, dark leafy greens, green peppers, cucumber, peas, celery) Indoles (broccoli, cabbage) Folate (kiwi) Glutathione (kiwi) Vitamin E (kiwi) Vitamin C (kale) Calcium (broccoli) Iron (broccoli, spinach, pumpkin seeds, peas, lima beans, kale) Folate (spinach, broccoli) Vitamin A (kale) Vitamin K (spinach, kale) Chlorophyll Calcium (kale)	Detoxification, Oxidative stress reduction, Improves brain function and liver function
Blue/ Purple	Blueberries Green apples Eggplant Blackberries Plums Currants Elderberries Purple grapes Purple carrots Purple cabbage Purple kale Purple potatoes	Anthocyanin (blueberries) Antioxidants (blackberries, blueberries) Fiber Flavanoids Vitamin B (plums) Vitamin E (blueberries) Vitamin C (blueberries, eggplant) Vitamin K (blackberries, plums) Calcium (eggplant) Phosphorus (eggplant)	Improves memory Improves circulation Boosts brain activity Boosts immunity Improves digestion Blood sugar regulation
White	Garlic Onions Cauliflower Potatoes Turnips Jicama Bananas (also yellow) White corn Parsnips Mushrooms Jerusalem artichokes White peaches White nectarines White radishes White beans	Antimicrobial (garlic, onions) Quercetin (onions) Manganese (cauliflower) Vitamin C (cauliflower) Protein (white beans) Iron (white beans) Potassium (white beans, bananas) Vitamin B6 (garlic)	Reduces blood pressure Boosts immunity Cellular protection and recovery New cell growth, circulation, detoxification Lowers blood sugar
Black	Black wild rice Black beans Black lentils	Protein (black rice) Antioxidants / Anthocyanins (black rice, black lentils, black beans) Copper (black rice)	Detoxification Balances cholesterol levels Prevention of Alzheimer's, diabetes

Cherry Juice

Drinking tart cherry juice concentrate increases levels of melatonin (Howatson et al., 2012) and improves sleep (Pigeon, Carr, Gorman, & Perlis, 2010). Cherries are also a powerful anti-inflammatory rich in anthocyanins, and they increase the availability of tryptophan.

Chocolate/Cocoa

Chocolate (without sugar) is anti-inflammatory and high in polyphenols. Cocoa's beneficial effects on the gut are thought to be due to a flavanol called (-)-epicatechin, which increases circulation and blood vessel growth, improving blood flow to the brain and supporting cognitive function and memory. The polyphenols in cocoa have also been shown to improve mood (Pase et al., 2013). Cocoa also stimulates healthy microbiota production in the gut. These microbiota then help to break down the cocoa's undigested fiber into beneficial intestinal butyric, propionic, and acetic acids.

Berries

Berries (raspberries, blueberries, strawberries, and huckleberries) are among the red-blue-purple spectrum of the "brainbow" and are among the most versatile antioxidants. In the summer they can be picked fresh, and during the winter months they can be stored in the freezer. Make them the fruit of choice in smoothies or as toppings to gluten-free pancakes. For a special treat, dip strawberries into stevia-sweetened melted dark chocolate. Goji berries are often available in dry form; they are rich in antioxidants, amino acids, beta-carotene, and vitamins C, B1, B2, B6, and E. Goji berries protect the liver and strengthen the immune system, and they help the body to burn fat. It is a nightshade and some people may be sensitive.

Medicinal Mushrooms

All mushrooms, especially shiitake, are rich in B vitamins, including B6, niacin, choline, and folate, and minerals like selenium, copper, zinc, and manganese. Mushrooms are also rich in beta-glucans, which stimulate immune function. Lion's Mane (*Hericium erinaceus*), also known as yamabushitake, is well known for its ability to support the brain and nervous system, promoting mental clarity, memory, and focus. It supports the immune system and cognitive function. Yamabushitake is effective in improving mild cognitive impairment (Mori, Inatomi, Ouchi, Azumi, & Tuchida, 2009). Reishi (*Ganoderma lucidum*) is known as the "mushroom of immortality" and has a long history of use in Asia. It helps the body respond to stress, and it supports energy and stamina.

Plantains

Plantains are members of the banana family and often overlooked as a food source in the United States. They offer a natural earthy sweetness that can be seasoned as savory or sweet. They are easily digested, which makes them ideal for the elderly or people who are ill. They are a good potato substitute, and they have lower sugar content. Plantains make an excellent addition to the starchy carbohydrate repertoire, especially when eliminating sugar or wheat from the diet. They can be sliced thinly and fried in coconut oil and served as chips, steamed and added to a vegetable dish, or topped with butter. They can be grilled and also used in a curry. My favorite way to eat them is in this soup, in Box 6.9, which also combines coconut and the tang of cilantro (Chinese parsley).

Box 6.9
Plantain Soup

A plantain looks like a very big banana. They can be found in the specialty section of the produce section of your supermarket and at Mexican and Asian food stores. A plantain peels like a banana and should be ripe or moderately soft. It will satisfy the urge for a sweet root vegetable. This recipe combines coconut and cilantro (coriander greens) that enhance brain function.

Ingredients

3 large plantains, peeled and cut into ½ inch slices
Juice from ½ lemon
3 tablespoons unsalted butter
1 medium onion, chopped
5 cloves garlic, minced
4 cups freshly made chicken broth
Sea salt and black pepper, to taste
1 cup coconut milk

Topping

1/3 cup cilantro
1 clove garlic, chopped
1 teaspoon grated orange peel
3 tablespoons lime juice

Directions

1. Place plantains in a bowl; sprinkle with lemon juice to preserve their color.
2. Heat butter in a saucepan on medium heat. Add the onion and the 5 cloves of garlic and sauté until onion is tender, about 5–10 minutes.
3. Add plantains and chicken broth and bring to a boil. Reduce heat to low, add salt and pepper, and simmer until plantains are tender, about 25–30 minutes.
4. Place mixture in a blender and puree just until smooth. Do not overblend. Return to saucepan and add coconut milk. Cook over low heat for 5 minutes to heat through.
5. In a blender or food processor, blend cilantro, garlic, orange peel, and lime juice. After blending, swirl this mixture into the soup and serve.

Another inexpensive food for mental health is the paddles of the prickly pear cactus, known as the Nopal. Have fun with the recipe in Box 6.10 and you will also impress your friends and family.

Box 6.10

Nopales and Eggs

The Nopal cactus (prickly pear cactus) can be found in good supermarkets or Mexican food stores. It is a healthy and versatile food that may be eaten raw or cooked. Rich in fiber and mucilaginous, it is good for digestive problems. Significant research demonstrates that the Nopal cactus reduces blood sugar. This makes it useful for managing mood. This recipe makes a nourishing dish for any time of day. Set aside a half a cup of raw Nopal and use it in your smoothie the next day.

Ingredients

4 paddles Nopal cactus
3 cloves garlic, minced
1 large onion, chopped
1/3 cup olive oil
¼ teaspoon baking soda
5 large eggs
1 pinch pepper, to taste
1 pinch sea salt, to taste

Directions

1. Carefully remove the spines from each Nopal paddle and then julienne it into 1/16-inch slices.
2. Place garlic, onions, and olive oil in a 10-inch fry pan. Cook over medium-high heat until onions are translucent.
3. Add the Nopal to the onion-garlic mixture, then the baking soda, and stir mixture frequently.
4. Whip eggs in a separate bowl.
5. When the Nopal turns lighter green, stir in the whipped eggs.
6. Add pepper and salt to taste. When eggs are set, serve.

Yucca

Yucca, also known as tapioca or cassava, can be used when eliminating potatoes from the diet. It is similar in texture to the potato and makes a good substitute in recipes. The best way to buy yucca is from an Asian market where they sell cleaned cassava in the frozen food section. Remove it from the package, boil it in water for 10–15 minutes, slice it in half, and pull or cut out the tough and stringy core and it is ready for use. Yucca has anti-inflammatory and antioxidant properties.

Watermelon

Use watermelon generously for depression. It is rich in vitamin B6. Only choose watermelons that have seeds. Watermelon rind contains chlorophyll and can be made into pickles. Watermelon is an excellent base for gazpacho. Sweet fruits are a good alternative to refined sugar as a transitional food. In Box 6.11 discover a delicious antianxiety tonic.

Box 6.11
Anti-Anxiety Tonic

It might sound strange to drink apple cider vinegar, but when combined in this drink it is delicious, refreshing, lifts the spirits, quells anxiety, and increases energy. Even children will enjoy this drink. The watermelon is rich in potassium and B vitamins and contains the highest levels of lycopene of all fruits, a powerful antioxidant. The raw apple cider vinegar is acidifying and helps relieve anxiety, depression, hyperventilation, panic, and fatigue. Make a batch and drink 1–2 cups a day for several days. This recipe is adapted from Louisa Shafia's (2013), The New Persian Kitchen (Berkeley, CA: Ten Speed Press).

Makes 5 cups concentrate

Ingredients

3 cups water, plus more to serve
¼ teaspoon sea salt
¼ cup raw organic honey
10 drops liquid stevia
6 cups watermelon, coarsely chopped
1 cup tightly packed fresh spearmint
1 cup raw apple cider vinegar
Ice cubes
Sliced watermelon, sliced unwaxed organic cucumber, and spearmint, for garnish

Directions

1. Bring the water and the salt to a boil in a medium saucepan. Remove from the heat. Add the honey and stir to dissolve.
2. Combine the watermelon and mint in a large bowl. Stir in the honey-water and let cool to room temperature. Add the vinegar and stevia. Steep the mixture in the refrigerator for several hours or up to overnight.
3. Pour the mixture through a strainer. The watermelon chunks can be eaten, if desired. Pour the juice into a clean glass jar and store in the refrigerator for up to 1 week.
4. The juice is very concentrated, so to serve, pour just ¼ cup of the juice into a glass over ice and dilute with ¾ cup water.
5. Garnish with the watermelon, cucumber, and mint.

WHY NOT SUGAR?

Sugar refined from sugar cane and sugar beets depletes B vitamins and immune support minerals, such as zinc, and also reduces the body's capacity to digest and absorb glucose. Refined sugar is also highly inflammatory; it exacerbates pain and raises triglycerides and cholesterol levels. Its use is a major cause of the worldwide epidemic of type 2 diabetes. It is surprisingly common for vegetarians, whose diets are carbohydrate-heavy and often protein-light, to have reactive hypoglycemia and eat a lot of sugar because of their low protein intake.

Fibers and mucilaginous foods, such as edible cacti and slippery elm bark, slow the absorption of sugars in the intestines. Foods high in water-soluble fiber, like flax seed, pectin (from apples), guar gum, and seaweeds, are also highly beneficial at amounts from 80 to 100 grams per day. Research shows that psyllium husk improves glycemic and fat control and reduces cholesterol.

In Box 6.12 learn how to stop the addiction to sugar in 7–10 days.

Box 6.12
How to Stop the Sugar Addiction

Going on a protein-rich diet for 7–10 days can help clients withdraw from sugar and refined carbohydrates. Eat small amounts (2–4 ounces) of protein six times a day (about every 3–4 hours) and one to two servings of a root vegetable, such as a sweet potato or carrots topped with butter, coconut oil, or olive oil, along with raw salads or cooked green vegetables. There is no need to be hungry, so you may eat as often as you need.

Following this change in diet, most people will lose their craving for refined carbohydrates and sugars. From there, small amounts of additional carbohydrates like fruit and grains can be restored to their diet each day.

One of the best ways to engage children and adults alike in giving up candy is to make candy that is healthy and medicinal for mood. Children love making these treats in Box 6.13. Make a double batch and freeze the extra treats.

Box 6.13
Healthy Chocolate-Almond-Coconut Treats

Recipe by Rudolph Ryser

This recipe is medicine. It is a delicious and healthy alternative to commercial candy bars. Making these treats can be a group activity and is especially fun to do with children and adolescents, who can learn about healthy "treats" and the effects of sugar on focus and well-being. The anti-inflammatory properties of both the coconut and dark chocolate make this treat a healthy and effective mood booster.

Makes about 30 pieces

Equipment

Two sheets parchment paper

Half-sheet pan

Ingredients

½ cup blue agave, raw honey, or maple syrup OR 20–25 drops of liquid stevia

2 tablespoons butter

2 cups unsweetened shredded coconut, lightly packed

17 ounces organic dark chocolate (no sugar added), chopped or broken into small pieces

30–35 lightly roasted and unsalted almonds

Directions

1. In a saucepan, bring the agave to a low boil over medium heat. Add the butter and melt it, stirring occasionally. Once fully integrated, remove from heat and let sit for 2–3 minutes. Add the coconut slowly, stirring until it is fully coated.

2. Put a sheet of the parchment paper on a clean cutting board. Pour the agave-coconut mixture onto the parchment, spreading it with a spatula or the flat side of a knife.

3. Spread the mixture to about ½ inch thickness. Form into a rectangle, roughly 9 by 4 inches, and cover with another piece of parchment. Using a rolling pin or bottle, lightly roll the mixture outward until it is about ¼ inch thick.

4. Allow the mixture to cool slightly, remove the top parchment, then sharp cut it into strips about 1-inch wide. Working crosswise cut the strips again into 2-inch rectangles. Slide the coconut squares, still on their parchment, onto a half-sheet pan, allowing them to set while preparing the chocolate. Put the pan in the refrigerator. (TIP: Coat the knife with butter to keep the mixture from sticking.)

5. Place the chopped chocolate into a heat-proof bowl. Set the bowl over a pan of simmering water. Don't allow the bowl to touch the water. Melt the chocolate, stirring constantly with a rubber spatula, until it is smooth. Remove the melted chocolate from the heat.

6. Place the second piece of parchment paper on the cutting board. Working quickly while the chocolate is still warm, spread a thin layer of the chocolate into a rectangle that is more or less the size of the sheet of coconut squares, using only half of the melted chocolate.

7. Remove coconut squares from refrigerator and immediately turn them out onto the sheet of melted chocolate. Press down firmly using your hands. Remove the parchment from the coconut. Using a knife, separate the coconut squares following the cuts made earlier.

8. Top each coconut square with a roasted almond. Using a spoon, ladle the rest of the melted chocolate across the coconut squares, creating an even layer. Refrigerate the pan for 20–30 minutes to allow the chocolate to harden. Recut the squares and refrigerate until ready to serve.

Sugar Substitutes

Stevia is the ideal sugar substitute. It is a hundred times sweeter than sugar and has been shown to reduce blood sugar (Curi et al., 1986). While the powdered form of stevia can tend to leave a bitter aftertaste, the liquid form does not. Either form can be used in drinks or food preparation. Xylitol is another sweetener without side effects. It was first extracted from birch trees and provides a healthy sweet taste that does not raise blood glucose levels or negatively affect dental health. Table 6.4 describes how to convert the amount of sugar used in a recipe into the amount of stevia required.

TABLE 6.4
Stevia/Sugar Conversion

Sugar Amount	Equivalent Stevia Powdered Extract	Equivalent Stevia Liquid Concentrate
1 cup	1 teaspoon	1 teaspoon (24–36 drops)
1 tablespoon	¼ teaspoon	6–9 drops
1 teaspoon	A pinch to 1/16 teaspoon	2–4 drops

COOKING WITH SPICES AND HERBS

Herbs and spices are sources of nutrients, medicine, and culinary pleasure for the brain and mind. Some, like basil and oregano, are best used when fresh, and others, like cardamom and cinnamon, will only be available in dry form. Freeze fresh herbs by chopping them up, or, if you can get a lot of fresh basil during the summer, make pesto and freeze it for the winter months. Always plan your meals for the week that will use up the herb you want to buy so that it does not go to waste.

Dried herbs should be stored in a cool, dry place in tightly sealed containers. You can get creative, making your own spice mixes and substituting one herb for another in recipes.

The Three Sisters: Ginger, Turmeric, and Saffron

Three cooking herbs and spices merit further discussion because they are powerful antioxidants and antidepressants: ginger, saffron, and turmeric.

Ginger as a rhizome is the best form to use. It is a powerful digestive aid and reduces intestinal gas. Ginger aids with protein digestion and reduces problems associated with uric acid in the body. It soothes the gastrointestinal tract and is beneficial for gastrointestinal disorders. Ginger has anti-inflammatory and antioxidant effects, relieving pain and spasms, as well as nausea and menstrual cramps.

Saffron (crocus) is native to Iran and now grows throughout the Mediterranean. The familiar little bright yellow threads are the stigma of the crocus flower. While not commonly used in American or European cooking, it is worthwhile to have in the kitchen for special dishes. A few threads can be added to rice as it is cooking. Research findings indicate it is an antidepressant (Hausenblas, Saha, Dubyak, & Anton, 2013) at a level of 30 mg a day, which equals about 15 threads.

Turmeric is a rhizome related to ginger sold in powdered form and as a fresh root in Asian food markets and some grocery stores with an extensive selection of roots. Both forms can be used for cooking and for making tea. Combined with ginger root for flavor in a tea, its anti-inflammatory benefits are nearly immediate. It is also available in capsules, as a powder, and as a liquid extract. The active ingredient curcumin is a powerful anti-inflammatory, and this "root" can be added to food or may also be used as a supplement.

Turmeric root is protective for the brain and may serve as a preventative for Alzheimer's and Parkinson's disease. It reduces headache pain and supports liver, gallbladder, and digestive health by stimulating bile flow. Try adding turmeric to curries, stir-fries, and sauces. Turmeric and its anti-inflammatory chemical curcumin require black pepper or piperine, a constituent of black pepper responsible for its pungency, to be absorbed (bioavailable) by the body. Whether cooking with turmeric or taking it as a supplement, black pepper should be one of the ingredients to achieve absorption.

When shopping for turmeric supplements, make sure that the brand you choose contains black pepper extract or piperine. A pinch added to any dish will impart a bright yellow color. Box 6.14 combines turmeric in a healthy anti-inflammatory drink for any time of the day. In Box 6.15, a hot drink with turmeric makes a good morning drink or afternoon pick-me-up.

Box 6.14
Inflammation-Fighting Golden Turmeric Smoothie

Ingredients

3–4 ice cubes
1 cup unsweetened, plain coconut milk (or almond, hemp, or rice milk)
½ teaspoon organic turmeric powder
1 teaspoon organic extra-virgin, cold-pressed coconut oil
Generous dash of vanilla extract
Maple syrup, coconut sugar, raw honey, or stevia to taste
Dash of freshly ground black pepper
Dash of cinnamon, nutmeg, ground cloves, or cardamom (optional)

Directions

1. Put the ice in a blender and add the coconut milk, turmeric, coconut oil, vanilla, sweetener of choice, and black pepper.
2. Blend on high for 10–20 seconds until smooth.
3. Pour into a tall cup, sprinkle with your favorite spices, and enjoy!

Box 6.15
Turmeric-Rooibus Brain Chai (Caffeine-Free) *Recipe by Marlene Bremner*

Makes 4 servings

Ingredients

5 cups water
2-inch piece of fresh ginger, coarsely chopped
2-inch piece of fresh turmeric, coarsely chopped
1 tablespoon cardamom pods
1 teaspoon cloves
½ teaspoon black peppercorns
1 cinnamon stick
1–2 tablespoons Rooibus (red bush) tea, to taste
1 cup milk (coconut, almond, or rice, etc.)
1 teaspoon vanilla extract

| 1 teaspoon extra-virgin coconut oil |
| Sweetener of choice (honey, stevia, or agave) |

Directions

1. Place the water, ginger, and turmeric in a medium size pot and bring to a boil. Reduce heat to medium and simmer for 5 minutes. Add the cardamom pods, cloves, black peppercorns, and cinnamon and simmer for another 15 minutes.

2. Strain the liquid into a large bowl, reserving the spices and roots to use for another batch of chai. Add the Rooibus tea to the bowl and cover, steeping for 5–10 minutes.

3. Strain the tea back into the pot. Add the milk, vanilla, and coconut oil and gently heat over medium-low heat for 5 minutes, stirring to combine. Serve in individual cups and sweeten to taste using honey, stevia, or agave nectar.

Contraindications

People at risk of kidney stones or other oxalate-related conditions should avoid large amounts of turmeric. When taking turmeric, use it with food and with probiotics to reduce oxalate levels and use it for 4 weeks and then alternate with another natural anti-inflammatory. Pregnant women should not use it without a doctor's approval. In rare cases, extended use can cause stomach upset or heartburn. Black pepper must not be consumed in excess of 1 teaspoon a day when certain medications like digoxin or phenytoin are used. Table 6.5 lists the mental health benefits of herbs and spices and their special recipes that are found on the book's website: http://nutritionessentialsformentalhealth.com

Sea Salt

Sea salt is an important culinary medicine for the adrenal glands and thyroid. Replace table salt with unrefined sea salt, which contains 80 minerals that support adrenal function and other needs of the body. These include iron, magnesium, potassium, calcium, manganese, zinc, and iodine. While there is less iodine in sea salt than in iodized table salt, it is preferable to rely on sea salt while ensuring that there are other sources of dietary iodine, such as dried seaweed . Most people will benefit from supplemental kelp tablets, along with a diet rich in scallops, cod, shrimp, prunes, eggs, and turkey. Vegetarians and vegans especially are at significant risk for iodine deficiency and should supplement with iodine, as are people with hypothyroidism. Deficiency in iodine causes thyroid problems and learning disabilities. Iodine levels are also influenced negatively by the intake of bromide found in commercial baked goods and pesticides, and fluoride, found in fluoridated water and toothpastes.

Look for the gray sea salt that comes in a larger crystal form or granules, Celtic sea salt, or Himalayan pink salt. These high-quality salts also provide chloride, which helps the body produce hydrochloric acid and improve digestion. Celtic sea salt helps to mineralize and hydrate the body while restoring the sodium-potassium balance. In addition to salt, many types of seaweed can be used in soups or with beans.

Shichimi Togarashi (Seven-Spice Blend)

This spicy seasoning mix is made with Szechuan pepper, red chilies, black sesame seeds, white sesame seeds, seaweed, ginger, and roasted orange peel. Its seven ingredients have given rise to the name *Shichimi*, which means "seven flavors" in Japanese.

FERMENTED FOODS

Fermented foods are a must for everyone but especially for people with anxiety and psychotic disorders, as the fermented foods enhance GABA and minerals in the gut. Fermented foods, like bone broths, are a very inexpensive form of essential brain nutrition. Fermented foods can be used with or instead of supplemental probiotics and are ideal where one's budget will not allow purchases of probiotic supplements. Fermenting food "predigests" the nutrients so they are more easily digested. They are rich in enzymes, lactobacilli, and vitamins. Every culture ferments some kind of food, so the role of fermentation as medicine is well understood.

Start by eating cultured vegetables. Include *raw, unpasteurized* sauerkraut, kimchi (see below), and other pickles, not to be confused with the pasteurized sauerkrauts and pickles sold on grocery store shelves, which are devoid of live cultures and enzymes. Be sure to avoid pasteurized fermented foods, which may claim to have live cultures. Next, I provide the names of some fermented foods, and the recipes for them may be found in Appendix U.

FERMENTED VEGETABLES

Kimchi

Kimchi is the Korean cousin to sauerkraut. It is a fermented vegetable dish that usually includes Chinese (or Napa) cabbage, chili peppers, garlic, radish, green onions, ginger, and salt. Kimchi recipes are similar to sauerkraut but usually call for soaking the cabbage and vegetables in a salty brine, then rinsing the brine off prior to fermenting it. They also include garlic, ginger, onions, and chili peppers (see Appendix U for a Kimchi recipe). Box 6.16 describes a simple method for making your own sauerkraut at home.

TABLE 6.5

Mental Health Benefits of Herbs and Spices

Name	Form	Use	Benefits
Basil	Fresh, dried, or capsules	Mediterranean and Italian dishes, pasta, sauces, dressings, and pesto Recipe: Pesto Dressing	Antioxidant Protects against free radical damage, reduces inflammation Good source of magnesium, vitamin K, and manganese Holy basil, known as Tulsi, is anti-inflammatory, antioxidant, and adaptogenic
Black pepper	Whole or ground	Slightly spicy seasoning for all kinds of foods Recipe: Magic Mineral Broth	Increases hydrochloric acid production in the stomach and improves digestion Required for absorption of curcumin (turmeric)
Cardamom	Ground, seeds, or pods	Tea and coffee, curry, grain dishes, meat dishes, or with winter squash Recipe: Inflammation Fighting Smoothie	Analgesic Good source of calcium, sulfur, and phosphorus Improves digestion and relieves gastrointestinal problems Tea reduces stress and depression
Cayenne pepper	Fresh, dried, and ground	Many dishes from around the world, hot sauces, marinades, or used topically Recipe: Green Soup	High in vitamin A, B6, C, E, as well as riboflavin, potassium, and manganese Promotes healthy liver function and aids digestion Helpful in migraines, heartburn, and allergies Pain reduction (topical)
Cinnamon	Cinnamon sticks or powder, or as an extract	Breads, meats, soups, hot and cold cereal, drinks, and sweets Recipe: Fruity Turmeric Smoothie	Aids digestion and stimulates appetite Rich in manganese and antioxidants Candida treatment Increases glucose uptake Lowers serum glucose in diabetic patients
Cumin	Seeds and ground	Soups, stews, curries, meat dishes, and pickles Recipe: Khichadi	Aids digestion and stimulates appetite

Name	Form	Use	Benefits
Dill	Fresh and dried	Russian, European, Italian, Greek, and African foods; fish, salad dressings, borscht, soups, potatoes, and pickles Recipe: Cucumber-Dill Dressing	Antioxidant Relieves gas Provides vitamin A Antibacterial
Garlic	Fresh, dried, crushed, and capsules	Stir-fries, pastas, marinades, vegetables, meats, dressings, sauces Recipe: Onion-Garlic Soup	Improves immunity, lowers blood sugar, and reduces cholesterol and triglyceride levels Antidepressant and anti-inflammatory
Ginger	Tea, fresh or dried, powdered, and liquid extracts	Stir-fries, Asian food, marinades, desserts Recipe: Anti-Inflammatory Tea	Anti-inflammatory and pain relief Relieves gastrointestinal disorders Boosts immune system Relieves nausea
Oregano	Dried or fresh	Mediterranean and Italian food; savory and/or spicy dishes; marinades, roasted vegetables, casseroles, pasta sauces, and pizza Recipe: Papaya Barbeque Sauce	Rich in vitamin K Antioxidant Relieves gastrointestinal problems and headaches
Rosemary	Fresh or dried	Mediterranean and Italian cuisine; roasted meats, stuffing, roasted vegetables, soups, stews, marinades, and sauces	Provides vitamin A Anti-inflammatory Aids digestion, relieves gas and headaches, and improves concentration Calming
Tarragon	Fresh and dried	French cuisine; salad dressings, fish, and with eggs Recipe: Honeyed Carrots	Antioxidant Rich in vitamins A and C, and B vitamins Provides calcium, manganese, iron, copper, magnesium, potassium, and zinc Stimulates appetite and aids in anorexia Relieves insomnia
Turmeric	Tea, fresh or powdered form, and liquid extracts	Indian food; curry, stir-fries, sauces Recipe: Turmeric-Rooibus Chai	Antioxidant Anti-inflammatory and adaptogenic Relieves pain and depression Improves liver and gallbladder

Box 6.16
Sauerkraut

One of the ways I interest skeptical people in fermented foods (and healthier eating in general) is by the substitution method. Many people like sauerkraut and pickles, but most use bottled products that have no health value. I ask my clients who like their hot dogs to just find some organic all-beef hotdogs, top them with real sauerkraut and homemade pickles, and voila, they now have a healthy recipe. Slowly people will try this approach with other foods as well. Sauerkraut and other fermented vegetables are an excellent source for vitamin U (S-methylmethionine), which helps heal ulcers. This recipe was adapted from Gabriel Cousens, MD, and the Tree of Life Cafe Chefs (2003), Rainbow Green Live-Food Cuisine (Berkeley, CA: North Atlantic Books).

Ingredients

4 cups green cabbage, shredded (reserve 3–5 whole cabbage leaves)

2 cups Napa cabbage, shredded

2 tablespoons ginger, grated

1 tablespoon white miso

2 teaspoons whole caraway seeds

Directions

1. Mix together all ingredients.
2. Spoon mixture into crockpot or gallon-size glass container. Pound the mixture with a wooden spoon to release juices and remove all air. If necessary, add water to cover cabbage if there isn't enough juice to do so.
3. Roll up the reserved cabbage leaves and lay them down across the top of the vegetables.
4. Set a plate on top of the cabbage leaves and weigh down with suitably sized rocks (or other object).
5. Leave sauerkraut in warm (60–70 degrees F) place for 5 days. Do not uncover during this period.
6. After 5 days, remove the covering and scrape away top layer of vegetables. (Do not be concerned if you see mold; remove top layer and the rest is good to eat.) Sauerkraut will become acidic as it ferments, but it takes on a sweeter smell and flavor when it is ready to eat.

Fermented Dairy

Yogurt and Kefir are cultured dairy products containing beneficial microbiota that help to restore balance to the intestinal microbiota. Probiotics contain both beneficial yeasts and bacteria. Kefir is similar to yogurt, but it is more of a liquid and has a tangy flavor. Kefir is considered to be a natural tranquilizer, with a rich supply of tryptophan, calcium, and magnesium. Kefir is rich in B vitamins, including B6, B12, biotin, and thiamin. Eat only full-fat yogurt without additives and artificial sweeteners. It is easy to make yogurt at home as well. Making yogurt and kefir is a great family event and learning process to do with children (for recipes to make yogurt and kefir see Appendix U).

Kombucha

Kombucha originated in China and later spread to Russian and Europe. It is a fermented tea that is effervescent and sour to the taste. It is made using black or green tea that is sweetened with sugar. Then bacteria and yeast are added to ferment it. The tea is left to ferment for at least a week as the microbes feed on the sugar and multiply into a mushroom-like disk that floats on top of the tea. This disk is called a symbiotic colony of bacteria and yeast (SCOBY). The microorganisms in the SCOBY convert sugar into vinegar. Kombucha is very beneficial for the health of the microbiome.

Fermented Soy: Miso, Natto, and Tamari

Miso is a probiotic food made from fermented soybeans or grains. It is a smooth paste that is made from cooked soybeans, salt, a fermenting agent (*Aspergillus oryzae*) and water. It adds beneficial microbiota to the diet and a high dose of protein and several B-complex vitamins, as well as calcium, zinc, iron, copper, and magnesium. Miso can take some getting used to. I recommend a white miso to start because it is the mildest and you can obtain benefits from it easily when it is added to a salad dressing (see Box 6.17).

Box 6.17
Miso Salad Dressing

Miso can be made from soybeans or other grains like barley and rice. If you are new to miso, start with the mild tasting white miso. When using miso, use just a tablespoon or two to achieve a health effect. If you heat it, make sure that it's gently warmed; otherwise it destroys all the beneficial bacteria. It is an ideal food to use for recovery from illness.

Ingredients

1 tablespoon unseasoned rice vinegar

1 tablespoon white miso

2 teaspoons grated peeled fresh ginger

1 garlic clove, minced

½ teaspoon honey or 10 drops stevia liquid (optional)

Pinch of ground black pepper

3 tablespoons sesame or olive oil

Dried red chili pepper flakes, to taste (optional)

Directions

Combine all ingredients; whisk and pour over greens.

Natto is Japanese food made from fermented soybeans. It has a very strong flavor and smell, and it is definitely an acquired taste. It can be added to miso soup (see recipe in Appendix U) or used in small amounts on toast. Natto has been shown in some trials to degrade amyloid associated with dementia (Hsu, Lee, Wang, Lee, & Chen, 2009).

Tamari is a Japanese form of soy sauce generally made with no wheat and traditionally made from miso paste. It is preferable to soy sauce because most commercial soy sauce has wheat and additives. Due to the negative health effects of soybeans, it is important to use fermented Tamari.

Vinegar

Always use raw, organic, unfiltered, and unpasteurized vinegars that have been naturally brewed. Distilled vinegar no longer has the natural enzymes, minerals, and nutrients. Any vinegar that is clear and has no "mother" (the strand-like substance in the bottom of the bottle) has no nutritional value and demineralizes the body. Natural, raw vinegar should be pungent, with a rich, brownish color and a visible "mother." The best choices are apple cider, white wine, rice wine, and umeboshi vinegars. Mix a teaspoon of apple cider vinegar with water and sip throughout the day to boost energy and balance the pH of the body. Apple cider vinegar is especially good for anxiety and depression. A cup can also be added to the bathtub during a long soak to decrease fatigue. Umeboshi vinegar is made from the brine of umeboshi (pickled ume plums and beef-steak leaf). It has a tangy, salty flavor and can be used for dressings, marinades, soups, greens, pickles, and vegetables. Be sure to adjust the amount of salt in dishes when you add umeboshi vinegar because it is quite salty.

JUICING

Juicing vegetables and fruits is a delicious way to intensify their nutritional benefits. Juicing should be used as culinary medicine, not as a beverage. Fresh juices are potent forms of vitamins that can be used for specific purposes. However, juices are missing fiber and should be balanced with whole fruits and vegetables. Juices are an easy way to incorporate chlorophyll-rich vegetables in the diet and children will benefit as well. As a general rule, fruits should be juiced separately from vegetables. Since many fruits are high in fructose, people with sugar handling problems such as prediabetes or diabetes should be careful about the amount of fruits they juice in one setting.

Juice cleanses incorporate the use of fresh vegetable juice for a short period of time, usually 1–3 days. It is used to improve health and to treat specific conditions, and it should be done under the supervision of your health care provider. Carrot and green juice and other vegetable juices can be used in small quantities daily rather than for strict cleanses, providing much of the same benefit. An ideal juice to begin is described in Box 6.18.

Box 6.18
Carrot Juice Jubilee

Serves 2

Ingredients

1 pound organic carrots
1 organic beet
1 organic apple
Small piece of fresh ginger
Optional: 1 teaspoon coconut oil

Directions

Wash and cut all the vegetables and fruits so they pass through the juicer. Keep the skin intact. Strain the juice lightly, keeping some of the pulp.

Green Juices

Green juice is more nutritious than fruit juice, which is high in calories and sugar. The majority of juice should come from greens such as carrots, celery, cucumbers, parsley, cilantro, and other green vegetables. To adjust to the flavor of green juices, try starting with milder vegetables like cucumbers and celery and slowly work up to cabbage, spinach, and lettuce. Bitter greens, like kale, dandelion, and mustard greens, can be added in small amounts. One half to one whole lime or lemon can be added to cut bitter flavors. Other flavor enhancers include cranberries and fresh ginger.

Tips
- Use organic vegetables.
- Use carrots or lemon to improve the flavor of your green juices.
- Always drink juices right after making them to get the most benefit.

SPECIAL TOPIC: ALCOHOL AND DRUG RECOVERY

Based on the specific properties of foods, the diets discussed in Chapter 5 should be enhanced by adding specific types of foods to address the needs of each condition. I explore an example next about how this approach might be applied to people in alcohol and drug recovery.

People in recovery benefit from simple foods, liquid meals, and small meals, and caregivers who ensure they eat and take their nutrients. The use of small amounts of raw honey added to fruit smoothies, to which vitamins are added, can be effective to satisfy sugar cravings. A diet protocol should include animal protein, fat and carbohydrates like root vegetables, and the use of sea salt with each meal. Bitter greens, such as dandelions and arugula, are especially beneficial. Following is an approach to recovery that can be adapted and used for other illnesses. This approach combined with the protocols in Chapter 7 provides a comprehensive nutritional approach to recovery.

Eat smaller meals more frequently (5–6 times a day). Eating the protein first stimulates gastric acid production. Use lots of broths from animal proteins.

Staying well hydrated between meals is important to support proper digestive secretions. Eliminate lentils, peanuts, soybeans, chocolate, tomatoes, grains, and refined carbohydrates, including flours and sugar.

Include fermented foods that are rich in probiotics and prebiotics such as oats, bananas, rye, garlic, asparagus, and leeks; these will feed the healthy gut microflora and improve digestion.

Stimulate liver digestion by including bitter foods like dandelion greens, radicchio, and lemon juice, or take 2–3 teaspoons of apple cider vinegar with meals. Proteolytic enzymes from pineapple and papaya aid digestion. Sauerkraut or cabbage juice, which will stimulate the body to produce hydrochloric acid and improve digestion, should be included.

Foods high in betaine include beetroot, broccoli, and spinach. Betaine increases the synthesis of S- adenosylmethionine (SAM), which is required for liver detoxification, and has been shown to protect against alcohol-related fatty liver.

Increase foods with choline, such as eggs; increase food sources of zinc, such as cashews, ginger, sunflower, and pumpkin seeds; and increase food sources of folate, such as leafy greens.

Healthy sea salts like Himalayan pink salt will support adrenal function and provide the body with chloride.

Sample Food Schedule
- Early morning: protein/carbohydrate/fat
- Mid-morning: protein
- Before lunch: fresh carrot/apple/beet juice
- Lunch: protein/fat/vegetables
- Mid-afternoon: protein/carbohydrate
- Dinner: protein/carbohydrate
- Before bed: carbohydrate and a little protein

WATER

Water should be filtered if it contains impurities. Chlorine in drinking water causes vitamin E deficiency when consumed over the long term and kills beneficial microbiota in the gut. There are different kinds of water purifiers. Activated charcoal filters remove toxins and wastes that are not water soluble, though they will not remove toxins like nitrates, nitrites, and sodium fluoride. Reverse-osmosis purifiers remove nearly all toxins, minerals, and gases and produce almost completely purified water.

Chemicals in plastic can seep out of plastic water bottles when left sitting out for a long time or if they are exposed to heat or sunlight. Even if they are BPA-free, the other chemicals in the plastic are dangerous and could disrupt endocrine function.

COFFEE

Coffee is a drug, not a beverage. So use it like a drug when you need an effect. Using it as a beverage reduces its efficacy and can lead to side effects. Coffee enhances mood, stimulates alertness, and improves mental and physical performance. However, it can also increase anxiety and insomnia. Coffee exacerbates premenstrual syndrome (PMS); indeed, the more caffeine a woman ingests, the more severe her PMS symptoms (Weinberg & Bealer, 2002). Acids in coffee can destroy the villi in the small intestine, causing malabsorption and nutrient deficiencies of important minerals like calcium. People who have GERD do best without coffee or by making cold-brewed coffee, which reduces the acids significantly (see Appendix V for coffee withdrawal protocol and for directions on how to make cold-brewed coffee).

Coffee Substitutes

There are many coffee substitutes made from various roasted grains and seeds. A coffee substitute called *Capomo*, also known as *Ramon*, is made from the breadnut *Brosmium alicastrum*, indigenous to both coasts of Mexico. *Café de capomo* is rich in B vitamins (particularly B6), calcium, vitamin C, and trace minerals; it is so rich in amino acids and folate that it lifts the mood and stimulates breast milk in nursing mothers. Carob tea can also be used to replace coffee. It has a calming effect. Use carob powder mixed with water (1–2 teaspoons per cup of water).

GREEN TEA

Green tea (*Camellia sinensis*) is a traditional beverage in Asian societies and is known for its calming effects. Green tea contains the anxiolytic amino acid L-theanine that counteracts the effects of the caffeine (Yokogoshi, Kobayashi,

Mochizuki, & Terashima, 1998). Dietary theanine supplementation increases a state of alert relaxation. Theanine stimulates GABA and serotonin production and is a relaxing anti-inflammatory beverage. Green tea has at least two important constituents (Epigallocatechin gallate [EGCG] and theanine) beneficial for cognitive health and prevention of Alzheimer's disease (Hyung et al., 2013). Green tea also improves working memory (Schmidt et al., 2014). L-theanine and caffeine in combination appear to significantly improve aspects of memory and attention much more than caffeine alone (Owen, Parnell, De Bruin, & Rycroft, 2008). Add a teaspoon of green tea powder to a smoothie daily to support cognitive function.

Matcha Green Tea

Matcha is a powdered green tea that can be whisked with hot water to make a thick, foamy drink. It is a traditional drink in Japanese tea ceremonies. Matcha is made with the entire green tea leaf that is ground into a smooth powder. It is the only type of tea that uses the entire leaf and therefore Matcha provides more nutrients than other teas. It is high in vitamin C, iron, potassium, and fiber. This delicious powder can also be mixed with steamed or heated milk to make a matcha green tea latte, an invigorating alternative to coffee.

COOKED FOOD OR RAW?

Some foods are best eaten cooked, while others are richest in nutrients when eaten raw or lightly cooked. Raw foods are an ideal way to increase your nutrient intake. Because heating food can decrease the amounts of nutrients and enzymes present in the food, raw foods will often provide more nutritional value to your diet and aid digestion. As a general rule, about 50% of the diet should be eaten raw or slightly cooked. However, raw food is more difficult to digest, so when people are changing their diets, they can begin by adding in small amounts of lightly steamed or raw vegetables and fruits so they can adjust over time. There are a number of ways to enjoy raw foods that range from a simple salad to an apple to sprouting your own nuts and seeds.

Essential Next Steps
Explore the foods of the "brainbow":
- Limit the amount of grains and legumes and possibly eliminate glutens.
- Eat only high-quality, virgin, cold-pressed oils and fats.
- Eliminate refined carbohydrates like flour and sugars.

- Use proteins and root vegetables to stabilize mood and blood sugar.
- Include fermented foods in daily meals.
- Identify new foods to try for their mental health benefits.
- Emphasize organic, farm-raised, hormone-free, and antibiotic-free animal products.
- Try new recipes and share with family and friends.

CHAPTER 7

Best Vitamins, Minerals, Amino Acids, Glandulars, and Special Nutrients for Mental Health

Diet Essential: *Diet is essential but not sufficient.*

A healthy diet is essential for mental health; however, it is not generally sufficient to treat mental illness. Vitamins, minerals, amino acids, special nutrients, and glandulars are also necessary. Foods and supplements contain vitamins, minerals, amino acids, and glandulars that alter the biochemistry of our brain, mind, and body. The effective use of these resources depends upon an individualized approach. These supplements are essential to restoring mental wellness and reducing or eliminating psychotropic medications. Every initial assessment with the client should include a comprehensive list of what nutrients or supplements she or he is taking.

While there are always individual needs arising from biochemical individuality, each person has basic nutritional needs. Adults have consistently responded positively to combining a variety of supplements for mental health, and the combination of amino acids, minerals, and vitamins has shown positive results in children with a bipolar diagnosis (Frazier, Fristad, & Arnold, 2012).

"Can I get all the vitamins and minerals I need from eating food?" is a question my clients frequently ask. There is no simple answer to that question. To prevent or treat an illness, I am convinced the most beneficial approach is to take vitamins, minerals, and nutrients in addition to a selection of healthy, whole foods. The commercially produced food supply in the United States is deficient in vitamins and minerals.

In the pages that follow you will find nutrient combinations designed to treat specific conditions along with dosing recommendations and protocols.

NUTRITIONAL SUPPLEMENTATION AND THE FIVE ESSENTIAL FACTORS

In the previous chapters I have explored the five essential nutritionally-related factors underlying mental illness and have discussed the role of these factors in assessment, as well as the use of food and special diets in their treatment. In this chapter I continue the review of these five essential factors in the content of nutritional supplementation: chrononutrition; blood sugar handling and hypoglycemia; inflammation, oxidative stress, and mitochondrial function; food allergies and sensitivities to gluten and casein; and methylation pathway/folate conversion to L-methylfolate.

Chrononutrition

The most important supplements used to regulate circadian rhythm are lithium orotate, melatonin, phosphatidylserine, and vitamin B12 (methylcobalamin). Combine with bright light exposure in the morning and the use of blue light–blocking glasses at night.

Signs of Chrononutrition Imbalance
- Insomnia
- Depression, especially early-morning waking depression
- Bipolar disorder or labile mood
- Premenstrual syndrome
- Bulimia
- Dementia
- Fibromyalgia

Blood Sugar Handling and Hypoglycemia

The three most important nutrients to support blood sugar levels in the body are B vitamins, glucose tolerance factor, and adrenal glandular.

Signs of Functional Hypoglycemia
- Mood lability
- Irritability
- Shakiness or feeling "rubbery" or about to faint between meals
- Angry
- Inability to concentrate or focus
- Anxious
- Sleepy after meals

Inflammation, Oxidative Stress, and Mitochondrial Function

I have previously discussed the role of inflammation and its effect on depression, anxiety, and cognitive function. Reducing inflammation and oxidative stress and enhancing energy metabolism in the brain are essential to mental health recovery (Jou, Chiu, & Liu, 2009). I have identified healthy anti-inflammatory foods, and there are also vitamins and minerals and special compounds that are powerful antioxidants. Let's review briefly why these are important to mental and physical well-being. Recall the image of a car that is rusting due to its exposure to the elements. This oxidation process is similar to what occurs in our bodies, and it is caused by free radicals.

Free radicals are naturally occurring products created through the process of oxidation in the body. These atoms, or groups of atoms, have an odd number of electrons that steal electrons from other molecules, thereby stabilizing them, but creating a new free radical in the process. This newly created free radical then must steal from another molecule to become stable, and the process continues in a domino effect, causing damage and destruction to the body's cells.

While the oxidative process is necessary for us to obtain energy from our food, if free radicals are excessively produced they are very destructive. Hence, the body has a system of protection through antioxidants, which neutralize free radicals. When oxidation occurs in excess, free radicals are produced in amounts too large for the antioxidants to neutralize them effectively, this leads to "oxidative stress." This, in turn, increases cell destruction and leaves the body vulnerable to mental illness.

A combination of antioxidant foods, such as berries; antioxidant compounds, such as proteolytic enzymes; antioxidants such as vitamin E, lipoic acid, CoQ10 and PQQ are protective against the oxidative process and thus reduce inflammation as an underlying factor in mental illness.

Signs of Inflammation, Oxidative Stress, and Mitochondrial Function

All mental health imbalances have these biological processes underlying them, especially:

- Depression
- Autism spectrum disorders
- Schizophrenia disorders
- Fibromyalgia
- Chronic fatigue
- Dementia

Food Allergies and Sensitivities

I reviewed in depth in Chapter 5 the three essential principles of food allergies and sensitivities. These include: 1) identifying the culprit through elimination diets or specific salivary or serum antibody testing, 2) eliminatimg the exposure, and 3) enhancing digestive function by reducing gut permeability and using digestive enzymes and probiotics.

People can have allergic reactions to vitamins—for example, skin rash in response to Vitamin D2, though these reactions are rare. Most often reactions are a result of the added ingredients to supplements; people who are sensitive or allergic to foods may also be reactive to certain ingredients in nutritional supplements. For these individuals testing one supplement at a time, for 3-7 days, and noting any reaction is important. Then additional supplements may be added one at a time using the same process.

Supplements also have inactive substances and "fillers," like lactose, cornstarch, and preservatives. The best quality supplements limit or eliminate these substances. The poorest quality supplements also include dyes and coloring agents, all of which can trigger reactions. Read the ingredients labels. Some companies advertise as hypoallergenic, meaning they use no fillers or additives that could cause a reaction, others guarantee that they are gluten-free. The list in the resource section of the appendix provides a few of these highest quality companies.

Methylation Pathway/Folate Conversion to Methylfolate

The goal with nutritional supplements includes enhancing methylation. This occurs by increasing doses of vitamins B6 and B12, L-methylfolate, and CoQ10 to support the methylation pathway. Dietary recommendations are provided in Chapter 6.

The Essentials of Nutritional Supplement Dosing

- Treat the individual (age, size, and particular needs), not the disease or symptom.
- Spread the desired effects of supplements across the four broad areas: vitamins, minerals, amino acids, and glandulars.
- Tailor the protocol to client needs and plan for incremental change.
- Start out at lower doses and increase slowly.
- Children's doses are adjusted according to age and body weight.
- Provide the core foundation first: broad-spectrum vitamins, minerals, and amino acids then add in additional, higher doses of specific nutrients as needed.
- Identify the best delivery system for the client based on assessment.

- Use only high-quality, natural form supplements: look for the food sources of the vitamins on the label or 100% natural.
- All vitamins and minerals have cofactors; make sure you use supplements with these cofactors.
- Read labels: lower quality vitamins have additives and fillers and often food coloring.
- Search for a few supplements that combine a variety of vitamins, minerals, and amino acids that will provide most of what you need.

Method of Supplement Ingestion

Most supplements will be taken orally in the form of capsules, pills, or powders. Powders that contain combinations of nutrients may be ideal for mixing in water or smoothies or food, especially for children, the elderly, or people who prefer not to take pills. Some pills can be ground in a spice or coffee grinder and added to applesauce, or capsules may be opened. For example, the mineral magnesium may be absorbed via a lotion or by soaking in it (see Box 7.1), thus reducing the amount of oral magnesium supplementation required. A number of vitamins and nutrients are also available in liposomal form to enhance absorption and bypass the destructive effects of gastric juices.

Box 7.1
Epsom Salt Bath

Epsom salt (magnesium sulfate) baths are a simple way to absorb magnesium, relax muscles, reduce anxiety, and prepare for sleep. Add 1 cup of Epsom salts (magnesium sulfate) to a warm/hot bath and soak for 20 minutes. This bath can be completed 1 hour before bed or can be taken as a foot soak if there is no bathing facility.

Myer's Cocktail Intravenous Nutrient Support

When people are very fatigued, ill, or unable to mobilize to undertake a nutritional program in the early stages of recovery, it can be helpful to obtain the (modified) "Myer's cocktail" by working with a functional medicine physician or nurse. The cocktail contains magnesium, calcium, vitamins B12, B6, and C; it is administered intravenously. People describe a very pleasant feeling as the magnesium courses though the body, bringing with it waves of warming relaxation. It has been found to be effective against migraines, fatigue (including chronic fatigue syndrome), fibromyalgia, and acute muscle spasm (Gaby, 2002; Massey, 2007). Receiving this mixture intravenously is an effective start to any recovery program to boost immunity, strength, and vitality.

Box 7.2 describes a smoothie that has all the ingredients necessary to lift your mood and help children focus (additional smoothie recipes may be found in Appendix W).

Box 7.2

Mood Smoothie

Smoothies are an easy way to ingest nutrients and oils as an alternative to taking pills and capsules. Capsules can be opened and pills can be ground with a mortar and pestle or in a small electric grinder. Experiment with ratios and quantities as well as fruits and base liquids.

For a simple meal or when digestion is impaired, add whey or rice protein powder as an easily digested source of protein; however, ensure it is made without sugar or additives.

Ingredients

4 ounces plain yogurt (goat) or almond or hemp milk or raw milk (without sugar or fruit additives), water, or unsweetened fruit juice
2 teaspoons (heaping) of liquid fish oil (2,000 mg of Omega-3 fatty acids)
¼ frozen banana (peel bananas and place in freezer ahead of time)
¼ cup frozen raspberries, blueberries, mangos, or fruit of choice
3–10 drops liquid stevia (optional to taste)
Green tea powder (1/2 tsp.)
Powdered nutrients
Powder whey protein (optional)

Put ingredients in a blender. Add enough water and ice cubes so that it's either a thin drink or a thick frozen shake.

Tips for Organizing Nutritional Supplements

1. It is easiest to organize enough pills for 3–4 weeks at a time.
2. Place the nutrient bottles in a row.
3. In front of the bottles, place the same number of paper cupcake cups as bottles in a row.
4. Make as many rows as there are times of day. For example, if you take nutrients three times a day, make three rows of cups. Now you have three rows of

cupcake cups: one row for breakfast, one row for lunch, and one for dinner that are 10 cups long.

5. Open one bottle at a time and put one capsule/pill into each cup until each cup is full for that time of day the capsule is called for.

6. Go through each bottle until you have completed all of them. You now have cups filled for 10 days of nutrients. Now repeat this complete process until you have filled enough cups for 3-4 weeks.

7. Obtain small plastic bags and begin to fill a bag one cup at a time and put elastics around one each of your breakfast, lunch, and dinner bags so you end up with 30 packs of bags that will be ready each day.

8. If you will be at the office or on the road, place an extra bag where you might need it.

9. Keep them cool and dry and out of the sun.

ESSENTIAL VITAMINS FOR MENTAL HEALTH

Vitamins are divided into *water-soluble* and *fat-soluble* vitamins. Water-soluble means that they can be dissolved in water and are not stored in the body. The risk of over-dosing is very low. Fat-soluble means they are absorbed by fat and require sufficient dietary fats to be of use; they are stored in body tissues and thus can be overdosed more easily, though this is rare.

Vitamins work synergistically. In this section I review the water-soluble vitamins essential to mental health. The text will highlight essential information about the vitamin and the table will provide complementary information on food sources, benefits, and doses.

Regarding Contraindications and Side Effects

When developing a nutritional protocol, it is essential to include an assessment of the medications and physical diseases the client may have for which certain vitamins, minerals, amino acids, and glandulars may be contraindicated. In cases where clients are on a lot of medications or have co-occurring medical problems, it is useful to coordinate with another health professional and to run the list of medications through a drug-nutrient-herb interaction database (see Appendix Z: Resources). Generally speaking, all of the nutrients identified next have a good record for both efficacy and safety. However, just as we would evaluate whether a client is a candidate for exposure therapy or EMDR or CBT, so shall we evaluate the particulars of each client's requirements, incorporating safety as a criteria. Next I list some of the major cautions or contraindications to consider; however, it is not an exhaustive list.

Among the things to consider are that some nutrients may do the following:

- Slow or increase the metabolism/excretion of certain medications.
- Potentiate or synergize the action of certain medications.
- Exacerbate existing health conditions or be contraindicated for those conditions.

Finally, some nutrients may be mildly stimulating, and others may be mildly sedating; indeed, these are often effects we hope for with our clients. This knowledge should inform the time of day nutrients are delivered. Most vitamins should be taken with food, preferably when at least half the meal has been eaten. The exceptions are amino acids and proteolytic enzymes when used for inflammation. These should be used on an empty stomach.

Water-Soluble Vitamins

B-Complex Vitamin

A B complex is the place to start with vitamin supplementation. Everyone benefits from a B-complex vitamin with comprehensive minerals that is designed to manage hypoglycemia or hyperglycemia. It is ideal for people of all ages with mood, attention, and focus disorders and for alcohol and drug recovery. Roger Williams, the biochemist who named folic acid, identified pantothenic acid, and was the originator of the concept of biochemical individuality, believed that alcoholism was a disease primarily caused by vitamin B deficiency and could be treated with B-complex vitamins and minerals. B-complex vitamins support relaxation, cognition, and neurological health and are cofactors in neurotransmitters. For example, pharmaceutical companies add folate to SSRIs and SSNIs to improve efficacy. When choosing a B-complex vitamin, opt for L-methylfolate instead of folic acid.

Vitamins listed in the following sections are contained in a B complex and may be supplemented individually at higher levels.

Vitamin B1 (Thiamine)

Thiamine deficiency is common as a result of alcohol abuse and can lead to irreversible brain damage, including Wernicke's disease and Korsakoff's psychosis. Adding thiamine to the diet of those who use too much alcohol or are in recovery is essential. Thiamine will benefit people who have had gastric bypass and who have low blood pressure, which leads to complaints of fatigue and just "not feeling well." Benfotiamine, S-benzoylthiamine-O-monophosphate, is a fat-soluble vitamin-B1 (thiamine) derivative that may be absorbed better than thiamine.

Contraindications

Excess B vitamins are excreted in the urine, making it a bright yellow color. If taking chemotherapy medications, consult with your health professional before using B vitamins.

Vitamin B2 (Riboflavin and Riboflavin 5'-Phosphate)

Vitamin B2 is required for the synthesis of folates and vitamin B6. The elderly, people who are chronically ill or who overuse alcohol, and women who are pregnant or on birth control will benefit from supplementation.

Contraindications

Riboflavin is considered very safe.

Vitamin B3 (Niacin, Niacinamide)

Niacin and niacinamide are used for depression and anxiety, and recovery from alcohol addiction. Most people prefer niacinamide because niacin causes (unpleasant) flushing; however, where increased blood flow is beneficial, for example in vascular conditions, niacin flushing may be of help. Niacinamide stimulates the GABA receptors and can be used for mood stabilization and as a sedative. Niacinamide should be a staple for treatment of anxiety, depression, insomnia, dementia, and alcohol withdrawal (Prousky, 2014). Hoffer (1962) conducted research into orthomolecular medicine (the use of micronutrients to treat mental illness) using large doses of niacin and niacinamide for the treatment of schizophrenia. Hoffer found that at least 4 weeks was required to achieve an effect and that treatment reduced the number of days of hospitalization. Lake (2006) suggests adding 15 grams of L-methylfolate (or 500 mg of thiamine t.i.d.) to 3–8 grams of niacinamide, to improve outcomes alongside the use of conventional antipsychotics.

Picamilon (Nicotinyl-γ-Aminobutyric Acid)

This is a special compound that combines niacin and GABA in order to cross the blood-brain barrier and increase blood flow in the brain. It is used for the treatment of depression, alcoholism, migraines, and traumatic brain injury.

Contraindications
When using niacin at doses above 3,000 mg a day, work with a health professional to monitor the response. Nausea and vomiting at high doses are possible. Time-released niacin should not be used as it may cause liver toxicity (elevated liver enzymes, jaundice) at doses of 3 grams/day.

Vitamin B5 (Pantothenic Acid)
Pantothenic acid is essential in the synthesis of neurotransmitters and essential fatty acids and in support of adrenal and digestive function. It is usually included in a complex multivitamin.

Vitamin B6 (Pyridoxine and Pyridoxal 5'-Phosphate)
Vitamin B6, also known as pyridoxine, is necessary to metabolize proteins and essential fatty acids and for the conversion of amino acids into dopamine and nor-epinephrine. Symptoms of vitamin B6 deficiency include fatigue, light sensitivity, and joint pain.

B6 deficiency contributes to insomnia hypertension, PMS, and irritability. It is commonly used for the treatment of depression and anxiety. SSRI formulations often contain added B6.

Supplementation using pyridoxal 5'-phosphate (P5P) is the preferred form. Pyridoxal 5'-phosphate is the active coenzyme form of vitamin B6. To be used by the body, pyridoxine must be converted to P5P by the liver. P5P is necessary in the conversion of tryptophan into serotonin. Some people do not convert pyridoxine efficiently.

Contraindications
If taking antiseizure medication such as Dilantin, consult a health provider before using.

Vitamin B7 (Biotin)
Biotin is a cofactor in the metabolism of energy and fatty acids, and glucose handling. Biotin deficiency could be caused by extended use of oral antibiotics, which negatively affect intestinal flora as does the use of raw egg whites and antiseizure medications. Pregnant women in the United States and smokers may be deficient.

Contraindications
None. Safe at moderate doses in pregnancy and nursing.

Vitamin B8 (Inositol)

Inositol is an important supplement for treatment of bipolar disorder and OCD. It is usually supplemented in addition to B complex. Inositol supports brain health, improves mood, and overall nervous system function. In clinical trials inositol was effective in the treatment of depression, panic attacks, agoraphobia, OCD, bulimia nervosa, and binge eating (Gelber, Levine, & Belmaker, 2001). Inositol reduces OCD symptoms (Levine, 1997), and in one study, it was more effective than fluvoxamine in the reduction of OCD symptoms (Gelber et al., 2001).

Contraindications

High doses can cause upset stomach or nausea. Effects in pregnancy are unknown.

Vitamin B9 (Folate/Folic Acid)

Folate is a natural form of vitamin B9 found in a variety of plant and animal foods. Folic acid is the synthetic form of the vitamin, used in supplements and fortified foods. There is a strong correlation between a deficiency in folate and depression. People with lower folate levels are more depressed and also tend to be nonresponders to antidepressant therapy. A high percentage of the population is deficient in the enzyme that is required to convert folic acid to its active form, 5-methyltetrahydrofolate (5-MTHF). This deficit manifests in high homocysteine levels. Folates can be obtained through food sources (not enriched foods). Bioactive L-5-MTHF can be taken as a supplement, bypassing the need for conversion. It raises folate levels in the blood to a greater degree than folic acid supplements.

Contraindications

L-methylfolate has few to no side effects. However, if systemic inflammation is high, one can experience irritability and insomnia. Start out at a low dose and always include supplemental methyl B12 and niacin.

Vitamin B12

B12 is an essential vitamin used to treat depression, fatigue, anxiety, and psychosis. B12 is a co-factor in the methylation process leading to SAMe. Vitamin B12 is an anxiolytic (Prousky, 2005). Vitamin B12 is the preferred form of methylcobalamin (methyl B12) (not cyanocobalamin). Methyl-B12 is best taken under the tongue (sublingual) for depression, anxiety, cognitive function, and by people who do not eat (a lot of) meat or are over the age of 65.

Vitamin B12 deficiency is common in vegetarian diets and in the elderly with impaired cognitive function (Leyse-Wallace, 2008). Vitamin B-12 deficiencies are also common in people with Crohn's disease, liver disease, chronic stress, a gluten allergy, or malabsorption disorders, as well as people who have had bariatric surgery or who use acid blockers, alcohol, tobacco, or coffee, The diabetes medication Metformin depletes the body of B12, as do birth control pills, and antibiotics.

Contrary to popular belief, tempeh and nutritional yeast are not sources of vitamin B12. Only animal proteins provide vitamin B12.

Contraindications
None. May cause nausea at high doses.

Choline

Choline is found naturally in cell membrane lipids in the brain and is involved in the synthesis of acetylcholine, the "memory" and "learning" neurotransmitter. The three commonly used forms of choline used for mental health are CDP-choline (cytidine-5'-diphosphate choline), also called citicoline, phosphtyidalcholine, and alpha-GPC. Citicoline is broken down into phosphtyidalcholine, and phosphtyidalcholine breaks down into alpha GPC. Use of these forms of choline is potentiated when taken with coffee or tea.

Alpha-GPC choline (glyceryl phosphorylcholine) is a precursor for acetylcholine and GABA and increases the number of hippocampal neurons (Ricci, Bronzetti, Vega, & Amenta, 1992). Studies demonstrate improvement in mild to moderate Alzheimer's at 1,200 mg a day for 6 months. CDP-choline supports acetylcholine, dopamine, and glutamate neurotransmitters, and phospholipid metabolism enhancing the integrity of neuronal membranes. CDP-choline accelerated the recovery in head trauma patients in addition to improving the cognition and memory (Secades & Frontera, 1995). GPC stimulates nerve growth and increases phospholipid synthesis (Aleppo et al., 1994) and thus may be useful in the treatment of schizophrenia.

All these forms of choline are used to protect the brain; to prevent cognitive decline; and to treat stroke and dementia. Phosphatidylcholine is also used for the treatment of alcohol-related fatty liver disease (Knuchel, 1979) and is anti-inflammatory (Buang, Wang, Cha, Nagao, & Yanagita, 2005). Alpha-GPC crosses the blood-brain barrier and is regulated as a prescription drug in Europe used for Alzheimer's disease treatment. A dose of 500 mg CDP-choline twice daily may help reduce cravings for cocaine (Renshaw, Daniels, Lundahl, Rogers, & Lukas, 1999). Choline has been combined with lithium (carbonate) to reduce manic symptoms in bipolar disorder (Lyoo, Demopulos, Hirashima, Ahn, & Renshaw, 2003).

Contraindications
None observed at moderate doses. May be mentally stimulating, so take early in the day.

Vitamin C (L-Ascorbic Acid/Ascorbate)
Vitamin C is an antioxidant found in citrus fruits. It protects the body from oxidative stress, aids in the absorption of iron, and supports the immune system. Vitamin C requirements increase during times of emotional and physical stress. People who smoke, children fed formula, and people with malabsorption are vulnerable to low vitamin C. Deficiencies lead to fatigue and joint pain. A good-quality vitamin C is a *complex* (not just ascorbic acid) and contains bioflavonoids and rutin. Eating some of the pulp of citrus fruits also provides some of these bioflavonoids.

Contraindications
High doses can contribute to kidney stone formation. High doses can cause gas and nausea and diarrhea. High doses should be used at a dose of 1–2 grams every 2 hours for only a day or so to combat infection.

Vitamin U (Methylmethionine)
Vitamin U is the name given to S-methylmethionine because this substance is found in raw cabbage (juice) and it helps heal peptic ulcers (Cheney, 1952), hence U for ulcer. It is also useful in the treatment of GERD and stomach inflammation. Look for a compound that combines vitamin U and chlorophyll.

Contraindications
Should be used for only 1–2 months and then supplementation with hydrochloric acid HCL can begin.

Essential Fat-Soluble Vitamins for Mental Health

Vitamin A (Beta-Carotene)
Vitamin A is comprised of a group of compounds called retinoids. It is fat soluble and supports immune function through the production of thyroid hormones, which can be depressed as a result of chronic stress. Beta-carotene is a precursor to vita-

min A and is also called provitamin A carotenoid. Vitamin A and beta-carotene are stored in the liver.

Beta-carotene is a powerful antioxidant and has been found to prevent memory decline.

Contraindication
People who smoke should consult with their provider prior to supplementation with beta-carotene.

Vitamin D
Vitamin D may be the most important fat-soluble vitamin for the prevention and treatment of depression and chronic pain. Vitamin D receptors in the brain stimulate serotonin production (Holick, 2003) and vitamin D increases endorphin levels in the brain (Vasquez, Manso, & Cannell, 2004) and supports healthy aging. A very high percentage of people in the United States and especially those in the northern regions are vitamin D deficient. People with celiac disease are often vitamin D deficient.

Vitamin D is made up of D2 and D3. It is not a vitamin but rather a neurohormone that helps the body absorb calcium, magnesium, phosphate, iron, and zinc. Cholesterol is a precursor to vitamin D. Vitamin D is produced when sunlight triggers the conversion of provitamin D into vitamin D3. Vitamin D3 can be obtained in the diet. Exposure to sunlight is important in obtaining sufficient vitamin D, though absorption rates drop off with age. At sea level one should aim for 30 minutes a day of exposure to sunlight and expose at least 20% of the skin. Emulsified vitamin D drops are an ideal form that allows for high-dose vitamin D in just a few drops daily.

Contraindications
There are few contraindications. If blood calcium levels are high as in parathyroid disease, consult a practitioner prior to using high doses.

Vitamin E
Vitamin E is comprised of eight fat-soluble antioxidant compounds called tocopherols and tocotrienols. Vitamin E supplementation should always include all the tocopherols and tocotrienols and should always be natural and not synthetic. Several studies have shown high levels of vitamin E are associated with lower risk of cognitive decline and Alzheimer's disease (Mangialasche et al., 2012, 2013). Vita-

min E should be taken with meals and should always be used (400 IU day) when taking fish oil to enhance absorption and prevent oxidation of the oil.

Contraindications

No known contraindications. It is a fat-soluble vitamin and should be dosed accordingly.

Vitamin K

There are two major forms of vitamin K: K1 (phylloquinone) and K2 (menaquinone). They function in different ways. Vitamin K2 is essential for nerve health in the brain; higher levels of K1 are associated with better cognitive function in the elderly (Presse et al., 2013). Supplementation should include K1 and K2. Vitamin K supports bone density by transporting calcium from the blood to the bones, and it plays an important role in blood clotting. Vitamin K1 is found in green vegetables; however, the body does not absorb it easily.

Meat, eggs, and diary products contain vitamin K2, which is more bioavailable than vitamin K1, and it stays active in the body for a longer amount of time. Vitamin K2 promotes cardiovascular health and helps to prevent calcium deposits in the aorta.

Contraindications

People taking anticoagulants (blood thinners) should consult a health provider prior to use.

Table 7.1 is a useful list of the essential vitamins for mental well-being and their food sources and dose ranges.

ESSENTIAL MINERALS FOR MENTAL HEALTH

Minerals and Trace Elements

Minerals are considered the "sparkplugs" (Watts, 2006) of the body. They support the transformation of food into nutrients that can be assimilated by the body.

There are two categories of minerals. The body needs *macrominerals* in larger amounts. These include calcium, phosphorus, magnesium, sodium, potassium, chloride, and sulfur. *Trace minerals* are required in small amounts. These include iron, manganese, copper, iodine, zinc, lithium, cobalt, fluoride, and selenium.

TABLE 7.1

Vitamins for Mental Well-Being

Vitamin	Richest Dietary Sources	Mental Health Benefits	Deficits	Dose Ranges
A (Beta-carotene)	Sweet potatoes, carrots, (raw) dark leafy greens, apricots, butternut squash, red peppers, eggs, peas, parsley, beef liver	Boosts immunity	Increases oxidative stress	Up to 25,000 mg o.d.
B1 (Thiamine)	Beans, blackstrap molasses, bran, brewer's yeast, enriched cereals, enriched rice, fish, lentils, nuts, organ meats, pork, rice, wheat germ, whole grains	Alzheimer's prevention Regulates the nervous system Assists with energy metabolism Reduces stress Boosts immunity	Increases pro-inflammatory cyto-kines, confusion and disorientation, and blood-brain barrier dysfunction Wernicke's encephalopathy resulting from alcohol overuse	4.5–40 mg o.d.
B2 (Ribo-flavin)	Almonds, asparagus, beet greens, meat, dairy products, eggs, fish, leafy greens, liver, legumes, mushrooms (cremini), nuts, spinach, tempeh, turkey, yogurt, leafy greens, mushrooms, almonds, legumes, cheese, liver, kidneys, yeast	Helps memory loss and Alzheim-er's	Depression	2–6 mg o.d.
B3 (Niacina-mide)	Tuna, chicken, turkey, salmon, beef kidney, beef liver, beets, brewer's yeast, dairy products, eggs, asparagus, tomatoes, avocado, sardines, sunflower seeds	Depression, fatigue, and alco-hol recovery Reduces the risk of Alzheimer's disease		Anxiety and fatigue: 500 mg o.d. Schizophrenia: 1,000–4,500 mg o.d. Depression: 500 mg t.i.d. Alcohol recovery: 500 mg o.d. 1,500 mg t.i.d. to 18,000

Vitamin	Richest Dietary Sources	Mental Health Benefits	Deficits	Dose Ranges
B5 (Pantothenic acid)	Avocado, broccoli, cauliflower, cereal grains, chicken, eggs, legumes, lentils, meat, milk, mushrooms (shiitake and cremini), sweet potato, turkey, vegetables, yogurt	Supports neurotransmitters Protects against mental stress and anxiety Reduces depression Balances blood sugar Aids sleep	Fatigue, insomnia, and low mood	500 mg o.d.[a]
B6 (Pyridoxine / Pyridoxal 5'-Phosphate)	Sunflower seeds, pistachio nuts, tuna, turkey, pork, prunes, bananas, avocadoes spinach, black beans, blackstrap molasses, brown rice, cantaloupe, chicken, cod, collard greens, beef, flax seeds, garlic, red bell peppers, salmon, snapper, spinach, strawberries, turnip greens	Relieves depression Essential for neurotransmitter synthesis		Pyridoxal 5'-phosphate: 50–100 mg o.d.
B7 (Biotin) (also called Vitamin H)	Organ meats, (esp. liver), meat, seafood, eggs, almonds, avocado, bananas, nuts, nut butters, berries, sardines, chard	Supports adrenal function Synthesizes fatty acids and amino acids Supports nerve health		500–2,000 mcg o.d.
B8 (Inositol)	Fresh green beans, artichokes okra, eggplant, cantaloupe, citrus fruits	Supports neurological function Improves and balances mood, especially bipolar disorder and OCD		5–20 g o.d. OCD: 4 g[b]

TABLE 7.1

Vitamins for Mental Well-Being (*continued*)

Vitamin	Richest Dietary Sources	Mental Health Benefits	Deficits	Dose Ranges
B9 (Folic acid)	Asparagus, avocado, beef liver, beets, brewer's yeast, brussels sprouts, bulgur wheat, grains, leafy greens, beans orange juice, root vegetables, salmon, spinach, turnips, whole grains, white beans	Supports proper nervous system functioning Reduces homocysteine levels in the blood Supports normal prenatal neural development	Mood disorders, depression, and bipolar disorder	Major depression: 15 mg L-methyl folate, combined with methyl B-12 and niacin Note: Do not use folic acid supplements. Use L-methyl folate
B12 (Methyl-cobalamin)	Beef liver, shellfish (clams, shrimp, scallops), cod, dairy products (esp. yogurt), eggs, fish, salmon, sardines, tuna, animal protein like red meat	Relieves depression Aids cognitive function	Deficiency leads to cognitive decline, Alzheimer's, and brain atrophy	1,000–2,000 mcg o.d. (oral)
Choline	Eggs (yolk), liver and organ meats, nuts, cream, bananas, barley, butter, brussels sprouts, cauliflower, chicken, cod, collard greens, corn, flax seeds, ginseng root, grass-fed beef, lentils, milk, oats, oranges, peanuts, potatoes, salmon, scallops, sesame seeds, shrimp, tomatoes, tuna, wheat germ, whole-wheat bread	Supports acetylcholine in brain Improves brain metabolism and energy Improves memory and attention span Reduces chronic inflammation		CDP-choline (citicoline): 250–500 mg b.i.d. Alpha GPC Choline: 300–600 mg t.i.d.
C	Bell peppers, broccoli, brussels sprouts, cantaloupe, cauliflower, citrus fruits, kiwi fruit, oranges, papaya, pineapple, potatoes, strawberries, tomatoes	Protects against oxidative stress Boosts immunity Promotes synthesis of serotonin and norepinephrine	Depression and schizophrenia	Acute stress periods: 2,000 mg[c]

Vitamin	Richest Dietary Sources	Mental Health Benefits	Deficits	Dose Ranges
D	Oily fish, eggs, sardines, salmon, tuna	Reduces depression and pain Boosts immune function		Depression: 50,000 IU[d] Chronic pain: 4,000 IU o.d.[e] To prevent deficiency: 1,000–4,000 IU o.d.
E	Almonds, spinach, peanuts, turnip greens, asparagus, beet greens, mustard greens, avocado, Swiss chard, sunflower seeds, wheat germ	Improves vascular flow Anti-inflammatory	Increased brain inflammation, depression, poor circulation	400–800 IU o.d.
K1 and K2	Broccoli, brussels sprouts, cauliflower, dairy, fermented soy, leafy greens, liver, meat, eggs, green tea	Anti-inflammatory Protects against cognitive decline Slows progression of Alzheimer's		2,000 mcg o.d.[f]
"U" (Methylmethionine)	Alfalfa, asparagus, beets, cabbage juice (raw), carrots, celery, green tea, onions, parsley, peppers, potato juice (raw), sauerkraut, spinach, tomatoes, turnips	Prevents and relieves GERD Reduces allergies		10–20 mg t.i.d.-q.i.d.[g]

[a]Usually part of a B-Complex or part of "stamina" compounds.
[b]In three divided doses daily.
[c]Every 2–3 hours up to 20,000 mg a day or until diarrhea occurs.
[d]Oral, 1x/week for 8 weeks.
[e]For 5 to 9 months.
[f]Total: 1,000/K1 and 1,000/K2.
[g]For 4–6 weeks at a time. For ulcers, stomach inflammation, and GERD: combine with vitamin A and chlorophyll.
GERD, gastroesophageal reflux disease; OCD, obsessive-compulsive disorder.

An excess or deficiency of macrominerals or these trace elements can affect mental well-being and cognitive function.

The first step for supplementation is to take a *balanced mineral supplement* that includes easily absorbed minerals. All minerals are important, but some may be added to protocols at greater levels to enhance mental health and cognitive function.

Among the most important minerals to supplement for mental heath are calcium chromium, iodine, iron, lithium, magnesium, potassium, selenium, sodium, and zinc.

Chromium

Chromium is an essential mineral that regulates blood sugar by facilitating the glucose-insulin balance. It is the main ingredient of glucose tolerance factor and is best combined with niacin, vitamin B6, and fiber. Chromium is used for depression and mood regulation associated with hypoglycemia and is effective in decreasing carbohydrate cravings and binge eating (Brownley, Von Holle, Hamer, La Via, & Bulik, 2013). Pregnancy, intense exercise, and traumatic injury increase chromium needs. Use the form of chromium picolinate.

Contraindications

Few if any side effects or contraindications have been observed at regular dose levels.

Lithium

Lithium is one of the most important minerals for mental health and should be among the first supplements chosen for mood disorders (Schrauzer & de Vroey, 1994). The mineral lithium provides a very effective alternative to pharmaceuticals when it is part of a complete supplementation program.

Lithium lengthens the circadian rhythm, accounting in part for its positive effect on mood disorders. Lithium is a natural mineral found in some water supplies, including streams and hot springs throughout the hemisphere. Lithium is neuroprotective and anti-inflammatory, increases hippocampal volume, increases brain-derived neurotrophic factor (BDNF), and reduces the risk of the development of Alzheimer's in bipolar patients who take it regularly (Diniz, Machado-Vieira, & Forlenza, 2013).

People with bipolar disorder, depression, cognitive decline, and memory loss (Forlenza et al., 2011; Nunes, Viel, & Buck, 2013), or who are in alcohol recovery and relapse prevention (Sartori, 1986) can all benefit from lithium orotate combined with L-methylfolate, methylcobalamin (B12), and magnesium.

The mineral lithium (orotate or aspartate) should not be confused with the medication lithium carbonate, which is used for the treatment of bipolar disorder. Lithium carbonate has serious side effects and should be avoided. Lithium orotate crosses the blood-brain barrier, whereas the carbonate form does not; thus, lower doses of the former are effective (Lakhan & Vieira, 2008). Dialysis patients are at risk of lithium deficiency.

Contraindications

Not to be taken by pregnant and lactating women. Not to be taken in conjunction with SSRIs or monoamine oxidase inhibitors (MAOIs) unless advised by a health professional. Individuals with bipolar disorder and depression must be monitored closely by a health professional if taking this supplement. It is recommended that individuals taking this supplement have kidney function monitored regularly. Lithium should not be used by individuals with significant renal or cardiovascular disease, severe debilitation or dehydration, or sodium depletion, and by individuals who are taking diuretics or ACE inhibitors. Consult with a doctor before use if taking an antihypertensive, anti-inflammatories, analgesics, or insulin.

Magnesium

Magnesium is among the first choices of mineral supplementation. It is an anxiolytic, antistress mineral and supports healthy cognitive function and mood. Deficiency is common. People who are chronically stressed or abuse alcohol are subject to deficiencies along with people with kidney disease and celiac disease. Telltale signs of magnesium deficiency are body odor, muscle tension, and poor sleep.

Magnesium is a natural sedative; it helps muscles relax and plays an important role in insulin sensitivity, calcium absorption, cardiovascular health, protein synthesis, bone health, and energy metabolism. Magnesium is a quick and simple approach to reduce anxiety, insomnia, and muscle tension. It is effective in depression and bipolar disorder. Magnesium is a smooth muscle relaxant that produces bronchodilation (Stanley & Tunnicliffe, 2008) and is therefore used for asthma. It regulates blood sugar and blood pressure. Magnesium improves serotonin synthesis and reduces, inflammation, and oxidative stress. Supplementing with magnesium is also beneficial for restless leg, fibromyalgia, depression, irritability, and constipation. Magnesium aspartate was found to be as effective as lithium in 50% of severely ill, rapid-cycling bipolar patients (Chouinard, Beauclair, Geiser, & Etienne, 1990).

Magnesium is essential for cognitive health, yet it is not easily absorbed in high quantities and does not cross the blood-brain barrier. The most absorbable forms of magnesium are glycinate and L-threonate, a new form developed to cross the blood-brain barrier. It improves short-term memory (Abumaria et al., 2011) and increases overall cognitive function (Slutsky et al., 2010). Research on L-threonate suggests that it acts as an antidepressant and can dampen traumatic memories (Abumaria, Yin, Zhang, Zhao, & Liu, 2009).

Short-term (4 weeks) supplementation of extra magnesium without additional calcium is acceptable but not for the long term. Magnesium can be taken at night to sleep and during the daytime for mental and muscle relaxation. Dose to bowel tolerance and then reduce dose. Bowel tolerance is found by taking increasing amounts until stools soften and then reducing the dose. Intravenous doses of magnesium are used to alleviate hyperventilation, panic, and asthma.

Contraindications

Monitor magnesium intake levels with kidney disease. Magnesium should be taken separately from bisphosphonate medications.

Potassium

A balanced potassium–sodium ratio is essential in the regulation of blood pressure, heart function and energy production. Alcoholism and the use of diuretics disrupts potassium in the body. The SAD diet is significantly lower in potassium and higher in sodium than the traditional food diets of our ancestors. Early humans consumed about 800 mg of sodium, and 10,000 mg of potassium each day (Eaton & Konner, 1997). The SAD diet averages 4000 mg of sodium and 2500-3400 mg of potassium each day. This imbalance is believed to underlie hypertension which is not evident among people in traditional societies. While people are often instructed to lower salt (sodium) intake, an even more effective health strategy is to increase potassium rich foods and mineral supplementation. Low sodium high potassium diets have been found to improve mood (Torres, Nowson & Worsley 2009).

Potassium deficiency (hypokalemia) can be caused by alcohol abuse, excessive use of diuretics or laxatives, severe vomiting or diarrhea, magnesium deficiency, bulimia, and anorexia (Higdon, 2004). Deficiency can cause depression, mood lability, fatigue, muscle weakness, dizziness, and abdominal pain. When severe, hypokalemia may be fatal due to muscular paralysis and irregular heart rhythms. Dosing range depends upon the type of supplemental potassium. Potassium orotate is very easily absorbed as is potassium citrate.

Contraindications

Dietary and oral potassium is generally safe. High doses can cause dizziness. People who are taking blood pressure medications should consult with a clinician.

Selenium

Selenium elevates mood, reduces inflammation, and supports the thyroid and immune system. Selenium is a component of most multivitamins, and additional selenium can be added for mood support.

Contraindications

Very high doses of selenium can be toxic.

Zinc

Zinc acts as an antidepressant (Levenson, 2006) and is beneficial for cognitive function in the elderly (Maylor et al., 2006). It should always be supplemented in bulimia and purging disorder.

Contraindications

Very high doses of zinc should be avoided as it can contribute to urinary tract infections.

Zinc-Carnosine

Zinc-carnosine is a combination of zinc and carnosine. It is used for the treatment of stomach ulcers (Wollschlaeger, 2003), GERD, and to relieve GI upset, such as bloating, heartburn, nausea, and stomach pain. It promotes the growth of healthy bacteria and increases healthy mucus secretion.

When supplementing HCL for the treatment of depression and anxiety, first use with Gastrazyme™ (vitamin U and chlorophyll) and zinc carnosine to treat GERD prior to HCL supplementation.

Contraindications

No side effects or contraindications. However, high doses can disrupt copper and iron metabolism.

Sodium

Sodium is essential for nervous system function. It keeps minerals soluble in the blood and stimulates the adrenal glands.

While processed foods have too much sodium and can be detrimental to health, too little sodium is also harmful. Severe reduction of salt can lead to too little sodium in the diet.

Supplementing sodium is best done in the form of mineral-rich sea salt, which is beneficial for adrenal stress and fatigue.

Contraindications

Sodium supplements are unnecessary. Avoid table salt and avoid too much sea salt if you have high blood pressure or are salt sensitive. Salt-sensitive people are often dehydrated and benefit from more water.

Calcium

Calcium is an essential mineral used in the growth and maintenance of healthy bones. It also plays a role in muscle contractions, blood coagulation, hormone and enzyme release, and blood flow. Calcium absorption is supported by vitamin D. Overuse of calcium supplements, for example by postmenopausal women, can lead to fatigue, exhaustion, headaches, depression, anxiety, and insomnia (Watts, 2006). Overconsumption of calcium may inhibit zinc, phosphorous, and copper absorption. SSRIs have been shown to inhibit calcium absorption into bones, thus increasing risk of fracture.

Foods rich in calcium often contain these other nutrients, so eating calcium-rich foods or balanced supplements is generally not a problem. Calcium hydroxyapatite, which is derived from animal bones, is highly absorbable and the preferred form of calcium followed by calcium citrate-malate, which is absorbed with or without food. Avoid calcium carbonate. If taking a calcium supplement, take at least an equal amount of magnesium and supplement with vitamins D and K.

Box 7.3
Recipe for Calcium-Rich Soup

Calcium can be absorbed when obtained from calcium-rich food. Too often we think children (and the elderly) need milk for calcium. Cow milk is best avoided. However, this recipe is an ideal way to obtain calcium and it takes about 10 minutes to prepare for the Crock-Pot. Throw in everything early in the morning and by evening you have a nourishing soup enjoyed by children and adults alike.

Add 8 cups of bone broth (and a marrow bone or two if you have it) to the crock, add 2 cups of dry pinto beans, and then add 3 tablespoons of blackstrap molasses, a head of chopped broccoli including stems, 4 potatoes (cubed), a bunch of chopped kale, and a pinch of your favorite seaweed. Cook on low for 8 hours and add a pinch of sea salt and black pepper before serving. You can top it with walnuts.

Copper

Copper regulates cellular energy production and neurotransmission. A deficiency of copper may be caused by a high dietary or supplemental zinc intake, or a high-sugar diet, and this can cause neurologic disorders. High copper levels are linked to depression and may be a result of drinking well water. Antacids interfere with the absorption of copper.

Copper gluconate is the preferred form for supplementation. Always combine with zinc supplementation.

Contraindications

High levels of copper are associated with depression. As a trace mineral, use it in micro doses.

Boron

Boron is used in very small amounts and appears to enhance brain function and cognitive performance (Penland, 1994).

Contraindications

There are no apparent contraindications or side effects.

Iodine

Iodine deficiency can result in brain damage, hypothyroidism, goiter, and growth and developmental disorders (Higdon, 2003). Goiter (enlargement of the thyroid) is an early sign of iodine deficiency. Vegetarians and athletes are more susceptible to iodine deficiency. Food sources of iodine include seafood, seaweed, and iodized salt. Supplementation can benefit fatigue, ADHD, and ASD.

Contraindications

Supplementation should be done under the guidance of a health practitioner.

Iron

Iron is a main component of hemoglobin and is responsible for transporting oxygen throughout the blood, energy production, brain development, and immune function. Iron deficiency increases the risk of mood disorders, autism spectrum disorder, attention-deficit/hyperactivity disorder (Chen et al., 2013), fatigue, anemia, poor cognitive function, and developmental disorders. Iron deficiency is very common; women who are menstruating or pregnant are more at risk for iron deficiency. Excess iron can be very toxic and even lethal. Iron should be obtained from both animal foods and plant foods. Low HCL in the stomach can prevent the breakdown of iron. Anemia is often due to missing cofactors (vitamin B12, vitamin B6, and folates) and not iron per se. Vitamin C improves iron absorption. Ferric pyrophosphate is a more absorbable form of iron supplement. When supplementing with iron, include iron (gluconate), zinc (gluconate, aspartate), vitamin B12, and copper (gluconate, aspartate).

Dosing
Iron should only be supplemented under the advice of a health professional. Iron is best obtained via the diet.

Manganese
Manganese is important to mental health because excess exposure via environmental or occupational exposure is associated with cognitive decline in working memory and the dysregulation of dopamine. People at high risk for exposure should be evaluated. Higher levels of manganese increase the negative mental effects of alcohol abuse. Table 7.2 lists the essential minerals required for mental well-being and their food sources and dose ranges.

Special Nutrients/Supplements

Apoaequorin
Apoaequorin (āpoe-ēkwôr-ĭn) is a calcium-binding protein derived from jellyfish (*Aequorea victoria*). It has been shown to improve cognitive function by addressing calcium imbalance inside the brain cell by functioning like a "surge protector," regulating the influx of calcium into the cells. Calcium dysregulation in brain cells is posited as a significant cause of cognitive decline. Apoaequorin use demonstrates significant memory improvements in adults who reported mild memory problems (Underwood, Sivesind, & Gabourie, 2011).

Contraindications
It is well tolerated, though headaches may occur at high doses in some people.

Cannabis
Cannabis is widely used to self-medicate by people with chronic pain, neurological diseases, PTSD, and schizophrenia. The two major constituents of cannabis are

TABLE 7.2

Minerals for Mental Well-Being

Mineral	Dietary Sources	Mental Health Benefits	Deficits	Dose Ranges
Calcium	Dairy products, spinach, fortified breakfast cereals and nondairy milks, greens	Nervous system communication Depression with excessive intake	Irritability, anxiety, and depression	Younger adults: 500–1,000 mg o.d.[a]Ages 50+: 1,200 mg o.d.[a]
Chromium	Brewer's yeast, liver, mushrooms, whole grains	Helps regulate blood sugar levels Regulates and improves mood Reduces carbohydrate cravings		Binge eating disorder and depression: 600–1,000 mcg o.d.[b]Hypoglycemia and mood regulation: 200 mcg b.i.d.-t.i.d.[b]
Copper	Seafood (esp. oysters and lobster), kale, avocado, asparagus, chocolate, grains, molasses, mushrooms nuts, sesame seeds/tahini, nuts	Causes weakness, fatigue, reduced immunity, and thyroid problems Toxicity may cause fatigue, premenstrual syndrome, anorexia, depression, anxiety, allergies, autism, schizophrenia, and postpartum depression		For those taking 50 mg or more of zinc daily, and/or consuming high amounts of sugar: 1–2 mg/week
Iodine	Eggs, iodized salt, fish, milk, mozzarella cheese, sea vegetables, shellfish, strawberries, yogurt	Promotes production of thyroid hormones	Developmental delays Depression Brain damage and cognitive decline	12-25 mg./day. Short term use. Consult with clinician if using for hypothyroidism.
Iron	Beef and beef liver, chicken and chicken liver, clams, halibut, mollusks, mussels, oysters, sardines, turkey, ham, veal, lentils, spinach, beans, fortified breakfast cereals, tofu, pumpkin seeds, sesame seeds	Boosts immunity	Fatigue Reduced work performance	Best obtained from diet

(continued on next page)

TABLE 7.2

Minerals for Mental Well-Being *(continued)*

Mineral	Dietary Sources	Mental Health Benefits	Deficits	Dose Ranges
Lithium	Mineral water, sugarcane, seaweed, lemons, eggs			Brain antiaging: 10–20 mg o.d. (lithium orotate or aspartate) PTSD and TBI: 50 to 150 mg o.d. (lithium orotate) 45 mg/day[c]
Magnesium	Almonds, avocado, black beans, cashews, fortified foods, legumes, oatmeal, nuts, peanuts, seeds, spinach, whole grains, yogurt	Promotes healthy blood sugar and blood pressure levels Reduces oxidative stress Reduces inflammation		400–1,200 mg o.d.[d]
Manganese	Almonds, brown rice, cloves, garbanzo beans, oats, peanuts, pecans, pineapple, pinto beans, pumpkin seeds, rye, tempeh, spinach, sweet potato	Antioxidant Helps to metabolize carbohydrates, amino acids, and cholesterol. Important for fat metabolism	Low manganese is associated with, but does not cause, poor glucose tolerance, skin rashes	Normally 1-2 mg. as part of a multivitamin. Rare to supplement additionally
Potassium	Bananas, beets and beet greens, blackstrap molasses, carrots, clams, cod, halibut, prunes, turkey, salmon, spinach, sweet potatoes, tomatoes, tuna, winter squash, yogurt	Electrical conductivity of the brain and nerves Transports serotonin in the brain Delivers oxygen to the brain, improving cognitive function	Depression, anorexia, insomnia, mental fatigue, anxiety, mood swings, psychosis, nervous system disorders, and confusion	99 mg Potassium Orotate

Mineral	Dietary Sources	Mental Health Benefits	Deficits	Dose Ranges
Selenium	Sardines (and fish skins), garlic, onions, bananas, prunes, turkey, beets, spinach, salmon, organ meats, grains, brazil nuts, raw dairy products, eggs, and meat	Elevates mood Supports normal thyroid function	Cognitive decline and Alzheimer's	10–50 mg o.d.
Silicon	Almonds, apples, artichokes, asparagus, beans, beets, celery, cherries, cucumbers, grapes, greens, lettuces, onions, oranges, peanuts, peas, plums, pumpkin seeds, radishes, raisins, sunflower seeds, whole grains		Cognitive decline and Alzheimer's	Obtain by drinking mineral water rich in silicon.
Sodium	Table salt, baking soda, baking powder, soy sauce, bananas, cheese, seafood	Sea salt supports adrenal function especially under stress and fatigue May increase high blood pressure	Lethargy, fatigue, confusion, irritability, and hallucinations	Add mineral-rich sea salt to the diet Ensure adequate potassium intake
Zinc	Beef, cashews, garbanzo beans, grains, lamb, lentils, nuts, oysters, poultry, pumpkin seeds, quinoa, sesame seeds, shrimp, turkey	Promotes immune function and insulin production Anti-inflammatory Antidepressant Antioxidant Digestive aid	Depression, autism, schizophrenia, aggression, ADHD, learning difficulties, impaired memory, and seizures	Binge eating disorder and bulimia/purging: 25 mg b.i.d.

[a]Avoid calcium carbonate.
[b]Obtaining chromium as part of a glucose tolerance factor formula of chromium/fiber/B6 is optimal.
[c]From Shealy (2006).
[d]Dose to bowel tolerance.
ADHD, attention-deficit/hyperactivity disorder; PTSD, posttraumatic stress disorder; TBI, traumatic brain injury.

THC, the psychoactive component, and cannabidiol (CBD). Cannabidiol (CBD) is a major phytocannabinoid present in the Cannabis sativa plant. It lacks the psychotropic effects of the main plant compound (THC) and has antipsychotic-like properties (Zuardi, Crippa, Hallak, Moreira, & Guimarães, 2006), targeting the metabolic, inflammatory, and stress-related components of schizophrenia (Robson et al., 2014). It is unresolved whether cannabis contributes to the progression of psychosis in young people; however, it is likely that it is the THC that contributes to side effects. Smoking strains of cannabis containing CBD in addition to D9-THC may be protective against the psychotic-like symptoms induced by D9-THC alone (Morgan & Curran, 2008), and high-CBD-content medical cannabis may provide an alternative for the one-third of people who do not respond to conventional antipsychotic medication (Robson, Guy, & Di Marzo, 2014) and the many others who experience intolerable side effects. Cannabis use is associated with a lower rate of type 2 diabetes and lower insulin levels. There is evidence that essential fatty acids positively affect the endo-cannabinoid system in the brain, reinforcing the idea of supplementation for people who wish to decrease or eliminate recreational cannabis use. Hemp oil is a good fat of choice, along with fish oil, borage oil, and butter.

The psychoactive component of cannabis THC may be beneficial in Alzheimer's disease because it inhibits the enzyme acetylcholinesterase (AChE) as well as prevents AChE-induced amyloid ß-peptide buildup (Eubanks et al., 2006). Significant evidence supports its use as an antidepressant and anxiolytic.

Cannabis increases serotonin and dopamine levels; some research suggests that at low doses cannabis decreases depression but at high doses increases it (Bambico, Katz, Debonnel, & Gobbi, 2007). Many people with inflammatory bowel disease use cannabis, and research demonstrates that the phytocannabinoids decrease and reverse intestinal permeability associated with inflammation (Alhamoruni, Wright, Larvin, & O'Sullivan, 2012).

Contraindications

People under the age of 18 should use cannabis with caution. Where medical cannabis is available, specific strains should be identified with a specialist for the correct CBD/THC content.

Coenzyme Q10

Coenzyme Q10 (CoQ10) is a vitamin-like, fat-soluble substance that is found in the mitochondria. It is available in two forms, ubiquinol and ubiquinone, and both are equally effective. CoQ10 is an important nutrient beneficial for the treatment of bipolar disorder, depression, fatigue, fibromyalgia, and schizophrenia.

Contraindications
CoQ10 can reduce the body's response to blood thinning (anticoagulant) medicine, and CoQ10 can decrease insulin requirements in people with diabetes.

Garum Armoricum (Stabilium®)
Garum Armoricum is derived from an extract of Blue Ling (*Molva dypterygia*). It is found off the coast of the Armorican Peninsula of France and is rich in amino acids and neurotransmitter peptides, fatty acids, and vitamin E. It reduces stress and anxiety (Dorman et al., 1995) and improves mood and sleep. Stabilium is an alternative to lactium if there is casein sensitivity.

Theanine
Theanine is an amino acid found in both green and black teas. It crosses the blood-brain barrier, where it acts as an anxiolytic. It increases relaxation via increasing alpha wave activity and enhances levels of brain-derived neurotrophic factor (BDNF), improving learning and memory (Lardner, 2014).

Lactium (Milk-Derived Biopeptides)
Developed in France, lactium is the generic name of bioactive milk-derived peptides. They are amino acid chains concentrated from casein, derived from cow milk, that act on GABA receptors. Lactium reduces stress and cortisol levels while inducing relaxation and improving mental function, digestion, cardiovascular health, and social interactions (Kim et al., 2007; Messaoudi, Lefranc-Millot, Desor, Demagny, & Bourdon, 2005). It also improves sleep (Clare & Swaisgood, 2000; Delini-Stula & Holsboer-Trachsler, 2009; de Saint-Hilaire, Messaoudi, Desor, & Kobayashi, 2009). It is an effective alternative to medication for anxiety and insomnia.

Contraindications
Casein sensitivity may preclude usage.

Lipoic Acid
Lipoic acid serves several functions as an antioxidant and has been shown to slow the progression of mild Alzheimer's disease (Maczurek et al., 2008). There are two

forms of lipoic acid; one is the "R" form, which is the biologically active component, and the S form. The R form is the preferred supplement.

Contraindications

It may lower blood sugar and thyroid hormones, so consult with a health provider if taking medication for diabetes or thyroid hormone replacement.

Melatonin

Melatonin is a hormone synthesized as the final metabolite by the tryptophan-serotonin pathway. The use of tryptophan or 5-HTP may eliminate the need for melatonin supplementation directly. It should always be used with caution, starting with a dose of .05 mg.

Contraindications

Some people do not respond to melatonin and others may experience side effects, such as feeling tired in the morning. The alpha- and beta-blocking drugs used for hypertension can disrupt sleep by decreasing melatonin release (Stoschitzky et al., 1999). For this reason, it is preferable to manage high blood pressure without medication, when possible, by using potassium, magnesium, taurine, CoQ10, garlic, hawthorn extract, and fish oil, along with CBT and neurofeedback.

Nattokinase

Nattokinase (nat-oh-KY-nase) is a product derived from the Japanese fermented food from soybeans called Natto. Natto has been shown in some trials to degrade amyloid associated in dementia (Hsu, Lee, Wang, Lee, & Chen, 2009). Natto is also high in PQQ and reduces fibrin in the blood and has beneficial effects on circulation and cardiovascular health.

Contraindications

People who take anticoagulant medications should consult with their health provider prior to using.

Phosphatidylserine

Phosphatidylserine (PS) is a phospholipid, a key component of the cell membrane, and is essential for the transfer of biochemical messages into the cells within the brain and central nervous system. PS regulates cortisol levels via the HPA axis and increases acetylcholine in the brain; it supports memory in chronic stress, depression, ADHD, PTSD, and traumatic brain injury (TBI). Egg yolks and liver are rich PS sources.

Phenibut

Phenibut (beta-phenylgamma-aminobutyric acid hydrochloride) is a derivative of GABA that acts on both GABA and dopamine receptors. Developed in Russia, it is a powerful anxiolytic and mild sedative. It is a good alternative to benzodiazepines and is useful for the short-term treatment of anxiety and drug and alcohol withdrawal. While GABA is sometimes used as an anxiolytic, it is not as efficient at crossing the blood-brain barrier as phenibut (Lapin, 2001).

Contraindications

Phenibut should be used with caution as dependence can develop. People using MAO inhibitors or epilepsy medications like carbamazepine or oxcarbazepine should consult with their prescriber before using phenibut. To avoid a habit-forming effect, use three times a week only and alternate with lactium.

Pregnenolone

Pregnenolone improves cognition and long-term memory, and it may also prevent stroke and improve memory formation. Pregnenolone has been suggested for the treatment of schizophrenia (Marx et al., 2011), based on its ability to decrease inflammation. It is also used to treat opioid addiction (Concas et al., 2006.) and cannabis withdrawal.

Contraindication

Pregnenolone may affect levels of other hormones, such as progesterone, estrogen, testosterone, and/or DHEA. Do not take this product if you have a history of seizures. Do not take this product if you have breast cancer, prostate cancer, or other hormone-sensitive diseases.

Probiotics

Everyone needs a healthy microbiome, and this can be achieved with a combination of a diet rich in fermented foods and probiotic supplementation. Supplementation is essential for people with a history of digestive problems, intestinal permeability, inflammation, alcohol and drug overuse, and people who have used antibiotics. Probiotics decrease anxiety (Rao et al., 2009), increasing levels of brain-derived neurotrophic factor (BDNF). Eating kimchi is associated with decreased depression and anxiety (Bested, Logan, & Selhub, 2013).

Choose supplements that contain Lactobacillii and Bifidobacteria. *S. boulardii* is also used as a yeast probiotic.

Supplemental probiotics can be expensive and many require refrigeration. Probiotic quality is measured by colony forming units (CFUs), which is an estimate of the number of viable bacteria in the sample. Fresh, good-quality fermented foods are an alternative.

Proteolytic Plant Enzymes

Proteolytic enzymes include papain (from the papaya) and bromelain (from the pineapple). Bromelain inhibits the cyclooxygenase enzyme and inhibits the synthesis of prostaglandin 2. It also breaks down fibrin and reduces swelling. They should form the foundation of anti-inflammatory treatment and be used for pain and fibromyalgia (with CoQ10) in particular. When used with food, they are digestive aids. When absorbed from the gastrointestinal tract, they reduce inflammation and stimulate immune function.

Contraindications

Proteolytic enzymes and EFAs can act as blood thinners; hence, people on blood thinners may need to adjust their doses downward under the guidance of their health provider.

Pyrroloquinoline Quinone

Pyrroloquinoline quinone (PQQ) is a micronutrient that improves mitochondrial function. It reduces inflammation based on C-reactive protein levels (Harris et al., 2013), acting as an antioxidant and anti-inflammatory, especially targeting energy production within the mitochondria. It improves fatigue, anxiety, and sleep (Nakano, Ubukata, Yamamoto, & Yamaguchi, 2009). Combine with CoQ10 for optimal benefit. PQQ is especially high in parsley, green peppers, kiwi fruit, papaya, and tofu.

Contraindications

People with kidney or liver disease should consult with their health provider before use.

S-adenosyl-L-methionine

S-adenosyl- L-methionine (SAMe) is synthesized in the body from the amino acid methionine. It plays an important role in methylation and the synthesis of serotonin and dopamine, acting as an antidepressant. It has been well studied in clinical research and has excellent efficacy for depression. It has also been used to improve survival or delay liver transplantation in patients with alcoholic liver cirrhosis (Mato et al., 1999).

Use with co-factors: L-methylfolate, betaine, vitamin B6, and vitamin B12.

Contraindications

People with bipolar disorder should use SAMe at much lower doses and with caution under supervision of a health professional, as it could trigger mania. High doses can lead to some digestive distress. Some people do not react well to SAMe and often know this soon after taking it. SAMe use is contraindicated with antidepressant medication, dextromethorphan, meperidine (Demerol), and Levodopa due to added serotonergic effects. However, if used with professional guidance, it may be used as part of the strategy outlined in Chapter 8 to reduce or eliminate SSRIs and other psychotropics.

Uridine-5' monophosphate

Uridine-5' monophosphate (UMP) is the basic building block of RNA, DNA, and brain fats necessary for healthy neuronal membrane function. It supports CDP choline and acetylcholine levels required for memory. It is found in beer. When combined with DHA, it has a synergistic benefical effect on memory (Sakamoto, Cansev, & Wurtman, 2007). It is usually part of cognitive support formulae containing several nutrients for brain function and memory.

Contraindications

Uridine may lower levels of vitamin B12, suggesting extra supplementation is beneficial.

Table 7.3 describes special nutrients that are essential for mental well-being along with their sources and dose ranges.

ESSENTIAL FATTY ACIDS

Generous use of essential fatty acids supports brain structure and synaptic communication. DHA, a constituent of fish oil, improves communication between synapses and increases dendritic spines on postsynaptic neurons; higher blood levels of fish oil are associated with increased brain volume (Pottala et al., 2014). Lewis, Ghassemi, and Hibbeln (2013) have used 20 grams daily of fish oil for the treatment of traumatic brain injury.

TABLE 7.3

Special Nutrients and Their Mental Health Benefits

Nutrient	Benefits	Dose
Apoaequorin	Improves cognitive function and memory	10-40 mg./day
Cannabis	Reduces pain Lowers rate of type 2 diabetes Lowers insulin levels May be beneficial in Alzheimer's disease Antidepressant Anxiolytic Decreases and reverses intestinal permeability associated with inflammation	Obtain cannabidiol (CBD)-rich strains versus strains high in tetrahydrocannabinol (THC). THC is the psychoactive substance. CBD targets symptoms of psychosis, anxiety and depression. Work with an informed prescriber.
CoQ10	Cellular health Cardiovascular support	300–1,200 mg o.d.
De-Stress (Lactium: milk biopeptides)	Reduces stress Reduces cortisol levels Induces relaxation Improves mental function, digestion, cardiovascular health, and social interactions	Anxiety: 150–300 mg o.d. Sleep problems: 450–600 mg o.d.
Galantamine	Improves cognitive function in Alzheimer's disease	Alzheimer's patients: 24 grams o.d. For enhancing memory, TBI, or dreams: 4 mg o.d.
Glucose tolerance factor		
Green tea/ EGCG/theanine	Improves cognitive health Prevents Alzheimer's Reduces anxiety Improves learning and memory	
Lipoic acid	Antioxidant Slows the progression of mild Alzheimer's	
Melatonin	Regulates circadian rhythm Antioxidant Induces sleep Improves sleep quality	0.05 mg to 2 mg o.d. For OCD: 0.3–5 mg (sometimes up to 10 mg)
Phenibut	Anxiolytic Mild sedative Short-term treatment of anxiety and drug and alcohol withdrawal	

Nutrient	Benefits	Dose
Phosphatidyl-serine (PS)	Improves memory and cognitive function Regulates cortisol levels Supports memory in chronic stress, depression, PTSD, and TBI	100 mg t.i.d.
Pregnenolone	Anxiolytic Improves cognition and long-term memory	50 mg o.d.
Probiotics	Improves digestive problems Reduces intestinal permeability Reduces gut inflammation Increases healthy gut microbiota Reduces anxiety	
Proteolytic enzymes	Relieves depression, pain, schizophrenia, and fibromyalgia	500-1,000 mg every 4–6 hr[b] Proteolytic enzymes containing Nattokinase and Serrapeptase and/or Bromelain/Papain: 500–1,500 mg o.d.
Pyrroloquino-line quinone (PQQ)	Improves mitochondrial function Antioxidant and anti-inflammatory Improves fatigue, anxiety, and sleep	20 mg o.d. For cognitive function: Combine with CoQ10
SAMe	Relieves depression Improves survival or delays liver transplantation in patients with alcoholic liver cirrhosis	400–600 mg o.d.c
Stabilium (Garum armoricum)	Reduces stress and anxiety Improves mood and sleep	200–400 mg o.d.d
UMP (uridine-5' mono-phosphate)	Increases CDP choline in the brain; improves memory	50–100 grams o.d.

[a]Take before bed.
[b]Take away from food.
[c]Brown, Gerbarg, and Bottiglieri (2000).
[d]Daily and then reduce to every other day.
OCD, obsessive-compulsive disorder; PTSD, posttraumatic stress disorder; TBI, traumatic brain injury.

Table 7.4 describes medicinal fats and oils used in supplementation and their purpose and dose range.

AMINO ACIDS

Amino acids are the building blocks of proteins and precursors to neurotransmitters provided in good-quality proteins and supplements. The use of amino acid therapies serves as an alternative to psychotropic pharmaceutical medications. Pharmaceutical-grade amino acids may be compounded according to the specific biochemical needs of the individual to provide the building blocks that support specific NT production and neuronal communication.

Modes of Administration

When using amino acid supplements, follow the principle I discussed earlier. Use smaller doses of many nutritional supplements rather than high doses of only a few. Amino acids are delivered via the proteins in food and via capsules, powders, and intravenous therapy. Take amino acids away from the meal by 30 minutes so it does not compete with the amino acids in food. Dosing should be done in conjunction with a health professional to avoid overdosing. In Chapter 8, I provide a table of amino acid alternatives to medication.

Amino acids are available in powder or liquid form and can be added to water or a smoothie for ease. There are special amino acid combinations available in liquid drops that are designed for maintaining blood sugar and mood during the day. I suggest children and adults with ADHD, hypoglycemia, and adrenal stress carry a little dropper bottle and take 10–30 drops under the tongue during the day if they feel their energy, mood, or focus drop, until they can eat some food.

Intravenous Amino Acid Therapy

A health professional (most often a naturopath or integrative medicine physician or nurse) can deliver IV amino acids intravenously. It is designed to supply high-dose amino acids, combined with vitamins and minerals therapy, for fatigue and chronic mental illness. This approach can be implemented during initial stages of recovery from drug and alcohol abuse, during transition off medications, during acute stress, or during obstacles to self-care that prevent oral administration of amino acid nutrients.

TABLE 7.4

Medicinal Fats and Oils Used in Supplementation

Type	Fat/Oil	Benefits	Dose Range
EPA & DHA	Fish oils	Lowers blood pressure DHA (docosohexaenoic acid) supports learning ability with its role in brain development and growth Anti-inflammatory Cognitive performance, memory, depression, PTSD, bipolar disorder, and ADHD Can reduce psychotic symptoms For acute and chronic TBI	1 gram b.i.d. 2–3 grams t.i.d. 3 grams b.i.d. TBI: Up to 20 grams o.d.
	Cod liver oil (must be fermented)	High in Omega-3 fatty acids Supplies DHA, supporting brain and nervous system health Anti-inflammatory Supports the immune system Rich in vitamins A, D	Children: 1 teaspoon o.d. (4,000 IU of vitamin A) Adults: 2 teaspoons o.d. Pregnant women: 3 teaspoons o.d.
ALA	Cold-pressed flax oil	Good source of Omega-3 fatty acids Supplies nutrient-rich lignans Supports healthy cholesterol levels Supports blood glucose levels Rich in alpha-linolenic acid (ALA)	Organic Flax may be used in salad dressings or ground and added to smoothies
GLA	Black-currant seed oil	Relieves uterine cramping (PMS) Alzheimer's disease	
	Borage oil	Reduces inflammation and pain Improves nerve transmission Reduces depression	
	Evening primrose oil	Anti-inflammatory Relieves headaches Regulates hormones Boosts nerve transmission and may benefit Alzheimer's disease Relieves withdrawal symptoms from alcohol	

ADHD, attention-deficit/hyperactivity disorder; PMS, premenstrual syndrome; PTSD, posttraumatic stress disorder; TBI, traumatic brain injury.

Free Amino Acid Therapy

The use of amino acid therapy is an essential component for mood regulation. People with mood lability, anxiety-focusing ADHD, and memory and cognitive concerns will all benefit from a free amino acid blend. Nearly everyone will benefit from a supplement with free amino acids as the foundation for neurotransmitter function. Amino acids should be delivered by increasing all the amino acids in the form of free amino acids. This prevents increasing one at the expense of another. Too often people take 5-HTP alone or a GABA precursor, but most people require support for all amino acids. Once all the amino acids are provided, additional amounts of single amino acids may be delivered as necessary.

Contraindications

People with tardive dyskinesia should not take phenylalanine supplements. Kidney or liver disease patients should consult their primary care practitioner before taking high amounts of amino acids.

Individual Amino Acids

See Table 7.5 to review the major amino acids used for additional supplementation.

N-Acetyl Cysteine

N-acetyl-cysteine (NAC) is derived from the amino acid cysteine. NAC is a precursor to the antioxidant glutathione and taurine. It may reduce oxidative stress in schizophrenia. NAC shows promise in the treatment of the addictions, compulsive and grooming disorders, schizophrenia, and bipolar disorder (Dean, Giorlando, & Berk, 2011).

L-Glutamine

L-Glutamine is not an essential amino acid since the body makes it; however, under stress the body may require additional glutamine. Glutamine supports immune, brain, and digestive function and is often included in compounds of vitamins and amino acids to restore gut function. Glutamine improves energy and is frequently combined with curcumin and phosphatidylcholine to enhance digestive function and heal gut permeability. Matthews and colleagues (2012) suggest adding high-dose glutamine to a TBI protocol.

Glycine

Glycine is an inhibitory amino acid that antagonizes norepinephrine. It is the amino acid of choice for use during acute panic. Glycine added to antipsychotic medication improved the negative symptoms of schizophrenia (Heresco-Levy et al., 1999; 1994).

Dose

Take sublingually in doses of 2–10 grams. Place 2 grams under the tongue every few minutes in cases of acute panic (Prousky, 2005).

Contraindications

If using clozapine, do not take glycine except on the advice of a prescribing clinician.

DL-phenylalanine

DL-phenylalanine and tyrosine support dopamine and are used to increase energy and reduce fatigue and depression. DL-phenylalanine converts to tyrosine and may be better absorbed. Use DL phenylalanine when pain co-occurs with depression.

Taurine

Taurine is an antioxidant that supports glucose management and reduces blood pressure. A dose of 500 mg two times a day reduces blood pressure associated with stress; it is also beneficial for alcohol-related liver disease and should be used during recovery.

L-Theanine

Theanine is often paired with 5-HTP for treatment of depression and anxiety. It is an analog of glutamine. It is a natural anxiolytic, and it is found in large quantities in green tea. This is why it moderates the energizing effects of caffeine in green tea, making it a "relaxing stimulant." L-Theanine is found in green tea and promotes relaxation by crossing the blood-brain barrier and stimulating the production of the inhibitory neurotransmitter, GABA. GABA helps shift brain waves from the stressed beta waves to the relaxed alpha waves. It also increases concentration, learning ability, and memory. It also reduces the negative effects of stress, anxiety, caffeine, and other things that raise norepinephrine (adrenaline). L-theanine is good for the immune system and may reduce the side effects of chemotherapy.

TABLE 7.5

Essential, Nonessential, and Conditional Amino Acids

Amino Acids		Richest Food Sources	Benefits	Dose Range
Essential amino acids	Histidine cofactors	Bananas, buckwheat, cauliflower, cheese, corn, dairy, eggs, fish, kidney beans, meat, mushroom, potatoes, rice, rye, soybeans, spirulina, tofu, wheat	Supports transmission of nerve messages from brain to organs Prevents nerve damage May prevent Alzheimer's and Parkinson's Strengthens the immune system Anti-inflammatory Reduces allergy symptoms Psychological disorders may result from excess histidine	0.5 and 20 grams o.d.
	Isoleu-cine	Almonds, black beans, cashews, cheese, chicken, dairy, eggs, fish, lentils, liver, meat, pinto beans, soy protein isolate	Assists in muscle recovery Regulates blood sugar Regulates energy levels Depression, irritability, hypoglycemia, and confusion may result from deficiency	
	Leucine	Almonds, beans, beef, brown rice, chicken, chickpeas, corn, fish, lentils, milk, whey	Supports healthy muscle mass Improves cholesterol levels	
	Lysine	Beans, brewer's yeast, cheese, dairy products, eggs, meat, nuts, spirulina	Supports immune system Increases calcium retention and absorption Maintains lean body mass Relaxation Balances hormonal stress response Deficiency may cause nausea, fatigue, dizziness, agitation, and slow growth	800 mg o.d.
	Methio-nine	Almonds, beans, brazil nuts, broccoli, chickpeas, eggs, fish, garlic, lentils, meat, oats, onions, pumpkin seeds, sesame seed, yogurt	Supports detoxification Supports joint health Helps liver to process fats Lowers cholesterol levels Reduces histamine levels; may help with schizophrenia Deficiency may cause dementia	

Amino Acids		Richest Food Sources	Benefits	Dose Range
Essential amino acids continued	DL-Pheny-lalanine	Anchovies, beef, bison, catfish, chard, cheese, chicken, chocolate, cod, cured ham, eggs (whites), fish, lamb, mackerel, milk, pork, poultry, rainbow trout, salmon, sesame seeds, spinach, sunflower seeds, trout, turkey, watermelon, yogurt	Improves mental energy levels Increases production of neurotransmitters, including epinephrine, norepinephrine, and dopamine Increases production of thyroid hormones May reduce depression Deficiency causes depression, impaired memory, reduced alertness, confusion, low energy, and reduced appetite	
	Threonine	Beans, cottage cheese, eggs, dairy, fish, grains, leafy greens, lentils, meat, mushrooms, nuts, sesame seeds, wheat	Fat metabolism Improves intestinal disorders Improves indigestion Boosts immune system Improves depression Supports central nervous system function	
	Tryptophan	Avocado, beef, black walnuts, cheese, chicken, chocolate, cod, cottage cheese, duck, eggs, granola, fish, lamb, nuts, oat bran, pork, pumpkin seeds, ricotta, sesame seeds, soy, tahini, tofu, turkey, wild game, yogurt	Required to produce serotonin and niacin Improves sleep by regulating the sleep-wake cycle Reduces stress Improves mood	500–1,500 mg[a,b]OCD Insomnia, binge eating, and bulimia
	Valine	Bananas, beans, beef, broccoli, brown rice, cheese (cottage cheese in particular), eggs, fish, milk, oranges, potatoes, poultry, seaweed, sesame seeds	Supports liver and gallbladder health Improves sleep May benefit brain trauma Supports cognitive function Supports immune and nervous system health Stimulating Regulates blood sugar Supports muscle repair and growth Deficiency may cause reduced cognitive functioning, insomnia, and myelin sheath damage	

(continued on next page)

TABLE 7.5

Essential, Nonessential, and Conditional Amino Acids *(continued)*

Amino Acids		Richest Food Sources	Benefits	Dose Range
Nonessential Amino Acids:	Alanine	Avocado, beans, brewer's yeast, brown rice, corn, dairy, eggs, fish, legumes, meat, mushroom, nuts, poultry, seeds, spirulina, watercress, whole grains	Supports central nervous system function Aids in the formation of neurotransmitters Provides energy for brain and central nervous system Supports the immune system Regulates blood sugar	
	Aspara-gine	Asparagus, beef, chicken, dairy, eggs, fish, soy, whole grains	Supports healthy immune system function Reduces fatigue Protects the liver Supports neuronal health and transmission of nerve signals Deficiency may cause depression and confusion	
	Aspartic acid	Almonds, beef, eggs, flaxseeds, garbanzo beans, lentils, molasses, ricotta cheese, salmon, shrimp, walnuts	Supports hormone production Supports healthy nervous system function Promotes healthy metabolism Plays an important role in the production of ATP Increases cellular energy May reduce fatigue Detoxifying	
	Glutamic acid	Beans, dairy, eggs, fish, leafy greens, kombu, lentils, meat, poultry	Metabolizing sugars and fats Utilized in the production of GABA Detoxifies ammonia from the brain Improves behavioral disorders Improves epilepsy	
	Taurine	Meat, seafood	Reduces blood pressure Seizure prevention Supports glucose management Helps prevent and treat alcohol-related liver disease	500–1,000 t.i.d.

Amino Acids		Richest Food Sources	Benefits	Dose Range
Nonessential Amino Acids:	L-Theanine	Green tea	Improves sleep quality, mood Can reverse liver damage caused by alcohol	
Conditional Amino Acids:	Arginine	Almonds, brazil nuts, cashews, crab meat, eggs (yolks), hazelnuts, lentils, lobster, meat, pecans, pistachios, red meat, salmon, shrimp, spinach, tuna, walnuts	Aids with hormone secretion Supports the immune system Stimulates the release of insulin Relaxes blood vessels by stimulating the release of nitric oxide Ammonia detoxification	
	Cysteine	Broccoli, chicken, cottage cheese, eggs, garlic, leafy greens, lentils, oats, onion, pork, red pepper, turkey, wheat, whey, yogurt	Detoxifying Supports gastrointestinal health Protects cells from radiation Assists with weight loss Protects brain and liver from damage	OCD and cocaine craving: N-Acetyl-Cysteine 1,200–1,800–3,600/mg o.d.[c]
	Gluta-mine	Beans, beef, cabbage, cottage cheese, milk, parsley, pork, poultry, ricotta cheese, seafood, spinach, yogurt, whey	Precursor for the brain neurotransmitter glutamate Improves inflammatory bowel disease Use for intestinal permeability	500–5,000 mg o.d.[d]
	Glycine	Bone broth, bananas, beans, burdock root, cabbage, cauliflower, cheese, cucumber, dairy, fish, kale, kiwi, legumes, meat, pumpkin, spinach	Detoxification Calms the brain Promotes growth Supports deeper sleep Improves attention and memory Immune booster Used to treat schizophrenia	2–10 grams o.d.[e] Acute panic: 2 grams[f]
	Ornithine	Dairy, eggs, fish, meat	Reduces physical fatigue Detoxifying Speeds physical recovery from injuries	
	Proline	Asparagus, avocados, bamboo shoots, broccoli rabe, brown rice bran, cabbage, chives, dairy, eggs, fish, legumes, meat, nuts, seafood, seaweed, seeds, spinach, watercress, whey	Supports collagen production Supports tissue repair Regulates blood pressure Supports collagen production Prevents arteriosclerosis	

TABLE 7.5

Essential, Nonessential, and Conditional Amino Acids *(continued)*

Amino Acids		Richest Food Sources	Benefits	Dose Range
Conditional Amino Acids continued:	Serine	Almonds, asparagus, beef, cheese, chickpeas, dairy, flaxseeds, lentils, meat, sesame seeds, soybeans, walnuts	Fat metabolism Tissue growth Supports immune system function Aids in the synthesis of tryptophan Regulates blood sugar	
	Tyrosine	Almonds, avocados, bananas, bison, cheese, chicken, dairy products, eggs, fish, mustard greens, pork, pumpkin seeds, salmon, sesame seeds, shrimp, spirulina, steel-cut oats, tuna, turkey, watercress, yogurt	Metabolism Precursor to the mood regulating neurotransmitters norepinephrine and dopamine Precursor to thyroid hormone, thyroxin Improves mood Deficiency causes norepinephrine deficiency and depression Supports adrenal, thyroid, and pituitary gland health Reduces stress and fatigue May improve depression and anxiety	Tobacco withdrawal: 500 mg b.i.d.[g]

[a] Take away from food.
[b] Take before bed.
[c] Dean, Giorlando, & Berk (2011).
[d] Combine with curcumin for gut function.
[e] Sublingually.
[f] Sublingually every few minutes (Prousky, 2005).
[g] Two weeks before the quit date and for at least 2 months following: 500 mg b.i.d. building up to 2,000 mg o.d.
OCD, obsessive-compulsive disorder.

L-Tryptophan and L-5-Hydroxytryptophan

Tryptophan is an essential amino acid that converts to L-5-hydroxytryptophan (5-HTP), serotonin, and melatonin. Tryptophan improves mood and sleep and helps to regulate stress. It may be used at night to aid sleep. 5-HTP is derived from the amino acid L-tryptophan. It is able to cross the blood-brain barrier and is then converted to serotonin. 5-Hydroxytryptophan (50 mg) is a good choice for additional amino acid supplement for depression, insomnia, anxiety, and intestinal problems.

Use with synergistic cofactors including vitamin B6 (10 mg), niacinamide (50 mg), and L-theanine (50 mg).

Contraindications

Tryptophan can aggravate asthma and should be avoided in pregnancy and in individuals with lupus (Prousky, 2007). Taking excessive doses of 5-HTP may lead to excess serotonin levels, a condition known as serotonin syndrome. This can also result from the combination of 5-HTP with serotonergic drugs like Prozac, Zoloft, MAOIs, SSRIs, weight-loss medications, and St. John's wort. However, as discussed in Chapter 8, 5-HTP is a viable alternative to use when reducing SSRI dose under the guidance of a health professional. Pregnant or lactating women, and those with cardiovascular disease, should avoid taking 5-HTP. Those taking serotonin 5-HT or receptor agonists (naratriptan, sumatriptan, zolmitriptan) should not take 5-HTP.

Tyrosine

Tyrosine is an energizing and mood-elevating amino acid that increases dopamine levels. It is used for low mood, pain, and for people withdrawing from dietary stimulants like coffee. Do not take after 3 p.m., as it can be stimulating. If one becomes jittery, lower the dose.

Contraindications

Do not take L-tyrosine or DL-phenylalanine with Grave's disease, phenylketonuria, or melanoma.

Supplemental amino acids and their application and doses are described in Table 7.5.

GLANDULARS

Glandulars provide some of the most potent nutritional therapies available and should be part of every mental health nutritional protocol. Using glandulars is like refurbishing parts on your car because they have worn down or no longer function efficiently. Glands are the "replacement parts" coming to aid our organs and glands.

The use of fresh and dried animal glands as nutritional therapy has a long history. Our ancestors and indigenous peoples who hunt for food today consider the glands among the most prized and medicinal part of the animal. Organ meats and glands are more nutritious than muscle meats and until modern practices started to eliminate access to these glands and organs, they were considered most nutritious. Glands were part of the medical repertoire until synthetic hormones were developed, and we see vestiges of the use of glandulars today in medicine, such as porcine thyroid hormone or pancreas. Gourmands, "foodies," and peoples who continue to follow authentic diet traditions relish these rare sources of nutrition. While glands and organs in the form of whole food are healthy, one cannot always obtain them, nor eat a sufficient amount to provide medicinal benefit when ill; this is when the use of dehydrated (lyophilized) glandulars and organs is required.

Glandular supplements are purified extracts derived from mammal organs, endocrine glands, and tissues. They are usually harvested from cattle, pigs, or lamb and freeze dried. They contain large amounts of DNA and RNA from the cell's nucleus. They help to regenerate organs, glands, and tissues by targeting the same gland in the human through the action of peptides, minerals, lipids, and nutrients that are present in the glands themselves (Bland, 1980).

Glandulars are harvested from neonatal animals and are hormone-free as required by law, so adrenal glandular contains no cortisone and thyroid glandular contains no thyroid hormone. Glandular supplements are affordable and nontoxic (if taken from animals not treated with antibiotics and hormones). Glandulars can neutralize antigen-antibody reactions that occur in gut permeability and in celiac disease. Specific glandulars target the organ at risk. Hence, the use of dehydrated liver glandular for the person recovering from alcohol abuse; brain glandular for the shrinking of tissue in TBI, PTSD, and dementia and depression; hypothalamus and pituitary for chronic stress disorders; and thymus to support depressed immune function.

Brain

This is useful for all mental health conditions, especially depression, cognitive decline, dementia, PTSD, and TBI. Brain glandular combines well with hypothalamus and adrenal glandular. Thus, it is advisable to combine adrenal glandular with hypothalamus glandular for the treatment of stress-related illnesses. Since the hypothalamus is involved in regulating dreams and sleep, using hypothalamus glandular can increase vivid dreams, which can restimulate traumatic nightmares in sensitive individuals. In these cases, reduce the dosage if the dreams are intolerable.

Liver

As the major detoxifying organ of the body, almost everyone can benefit from liver glandular, but especially individuals with a history of pharmaceutical or substance use, people in alcohol recovery, or those with chemical sensitivities.

Pancreas

The pancreas glandular is very useful for inflammation, detoxification, and digestion. Note, when taken with food, pancreas glandular assists the digestive process; when taken away from food, it scavenges inflammatory cells and toxins in the body.

Pituitary

This specialized gland is essential to the endocrine system, which releases a variety of hormones under the influence of the hypothalamus for cognitive function and in chronic stress.

Table 7.6 describes how to use glandulars for mental well-being.

TABLE 7.6
Glandular Supplementation

Glandular	Benefits	Dose Range
Adrenal	Helps the body respond to stress Supports immune function Supports metabolism and physiological function of adrenal glands Addresses fatigue, sugar metabolism, and weight loss	100 mg b.i.d.a or 200 mg t.i.d.[a]
Adrenal cortex	Helps to support a healthy stress response.	250 mg (1, t.i.d.)
Brain	Supports HPA axis depression	250 mg (1–2, t.i.d.)
Hypothalamus	Supports HPA axis depression Very useful for the treatment of TBI	500 mg (1–3, t.i.d.)
Liver	Alcohol recovery	400 mg (1–2, t.i.d.)
Lung		400 mg (1–2, t.i.d.)
Pancreas	Support digestion May support and modulate the immune function May support blood glucose within normal limits Supports pancreatic function and fat digestion	425 mg (1–3, t.i.d.)
Pituitary	Supports HPA axis depression	250 mg. (1, b.i.d.)
Thymus	Immune function	1,000 mg (1–2, t.i.d.)
Thyroid	Low thyroid function	40 mg (1–2, 3x/day)

[a]Take before 4 p.m.
TBI, traumatic brain injury.

Thymus

This powerful gland is located in front of the heart behind the sternum and supports immune response. There is a tradition in many traditional nutrition cultures of eating the thymus, often called sweet breads.

HORMONES

Bioidentical hormones can be beneficial for maintaining cognitive function in men and women. Estrogen deficiency in postmenopausal women reduces semantic memory. Adequate testosterone levels improve cognitive ability in both men and women.

Low levels of dehydroepiandrosterone (DHEA) in response to stress lead to cognitive decline in both men and women. Many studies demonstrate that progesterone is neuroprotective in TBI and brain injury (Wei & Xiao, 2103). It is also a sedative (Arafat et al., 1988; Söderpalm, Lindsey, Purdy, Hauger, & de Wit, 2004). Oral micronized progesterone in pre- and perimenopausal women may be useful at night to aid relaxation and sleep onset.

MENTAL HEALTH DISORDERS

In Tables 7.7–7.25, I offer detailed sample protocols that may be adjusted according to the needs of the client. Each contains core essential nutrients and additional nutrients that target specific symptoms or deficits.

These protocols include vitamins, minerals, amino acids, glandulars, and special nutrients that comprise the core nutrients along with the requisite co-factors that synergize their action. Adjunctive options are also provided to address the special variations in each condition. Because each person is an individual, a range of doses has been provided based on the scientific literature.

Essential Next Steps
- Educate your client about the role of nutritional supplementation in their well-being.
- Prioritize core nutrients for the client; identify what will come from supplements or foods (e.g., probiotics supplements or fresh fermented foods or both).
- Review the assessment findings and match specific modes of ingestion: for example, smoothies, capsules, liquids, IV, and so on.

- Refer to Appendix Z: Resources to apply the drug/nutrient interactions database as you consider protocol design.
- Consider if a consultation with a prescribing clinician is necessary.
- Develop the Core and adjunct nutrient protocol.
- Identify obstacles or challenges to adherence that will be addressed using methods outlined in Chapter 9.

TABLE 7.7

Protocol for Depression

Nutrients	Dose
Complex vitamin and minerals with L-Methylfolate	Dose varies t.i.d.
Omega-3 fish oil	1–3 grams o.d.
Gamma linoleic acid (GLA)/borage or evening primrose oil	1,000 mg o.d.
Free amino acids	Dose varies b.i.d.[f]
Probiotics	100+ billion CFUs o.d.
Vitamin D	50,000 IU[a] 2,000–4,000 IU o.d.[b]
Glucose tolerance factor	1–2 capsules t.i.d.
Vitamin B6	10 mg q.i.d.
Niacinamide	50 mg b.i.d.
Methylcobalamin	1–2 mcg o.d.
Lithium orotate	50–150 mg o.d.[c]
Magnesium	400 mg[d,e]
5-HTP	50–100 mg o.d.
5-HTP or tryptophan	50–100 mg[d]
L-Tyrosine	250–500 mg b.i.d.[f]
Adrenal glandular	100–200 mg t.i.d.
Hypothalamus glandular	500–1,500 mg b.i.d.
Melatonin	0.5–1 mg o.d.[d]
Lactium	300–450 mg[d]
Orthophosphoric acid	30 drops o.d.[e]

[a]Oral, 1x/week for 8 weeks (for deficiency).
[b]For maintenance.
[c]Combined with folate.
[d]Take before bed.
[e]Take in the morning in water.
[f]Take away from food.
[g]Take magnesium to bowel tolerance. More magnesium at bedtime aids sleep.

TABLE 7.8

Protocol for Bipolar Disorder

Nutrients	Dose
Complex vitamin and minerals with L-methylfolate	Dose varies t.i.d.
Omega-3 fish oil	1–3 grams o.d.
Gamma linoleic acid (GLA)/borage or evening primrose oil	1,000 mg o.d.
Free amino acids	Dose varies b.i.d.
Probiotics	100+ billion CFUs o.d.
Vitamin D	50,000 IU (oral, 1x/week for 8 weeks) for deficiency 2,000–4,000 IU o.d. for maintenance
Glucose tolerance factor	1–2 capsules t.i.d.
Magnesium	200 mg t.i.d.
Lithium orotate	100 mg b.i.d.
CDP-choline	500 mg b.i.d.
CoQ10	200 mg t.i.d.
Inositol	1,000–2,000 mg b.i.d.

TABLE 7.9

Protocol for Seasonal Affective Disorder

Nutrients	Dose
Complex vitamins and minerals with L-methylfolate	Dose varies t.i.d.
Omega-3 fish oil	1–3 grams o.d.
Gamma linoleic acid (GLA)/borage or evening primrose oil	1,000 mg o.d.
Free amino acids	Dose varies b.i.d.
Probiotics	100+ billion CFUs o.d.
Vitamin D	50,000 IU (oral, 1x/week for 8 weeks) for deficiency 2,000–4,000 IU o.d. for maintenance
Glucose tolerance factor	1–2 capsules t.i.d.
Vitamin B6	50–100 mg o.d.
Tryptophan	500 mg o.d. at night
Melatonin	0.5–1 mg o.d. at night
SAMe	400–600 mg o.d.
Whey protein	2 heaping tablespoons o.d.

TABLE 7.10

Protocol for Anxiety

Nutrients	Dose
Complex vitamins and minerals with L-methylfolate	Dose varies t.i.d.
Omega-3 fish oil	1–3 grams o.d.
Gamma linoleic acid (GLA)/borage or evening primrose oil	1,000 mg o.d.
Free amino acids	Dose varies b.i.d.[a]
Probiotics	100+ billion CFUs o.d.
Vitamin D	50,000 IU (oral, 1x/week for 8 weeks) for deficiency 2,000–4,000 IU o.d. (maintenance)
B6 pyridoxal phosphate	50 mg b.i.d.
B-12 methylcobalamin	1,000 mcg o.d.
Niacinamide	500 mg b.i.d.
Magnesium L-threonate or glycinate	100–400 mg[b]
Alpha GP-choline	600–1,000 grams o.d.
Tryptophan	500 mg[c]
Lactium	150–450 mg as needed 450–600 mg for sleep
Orthophosphoric acid	30 drops o.d.[d]

Adjunct Protocol for Anxiety

Nutrients	Dose
Lithium orotate (Depression and mood lability)	45 mg o.d. (Shealy, 2006)
Taurine (High blood pressure or gallbladder issues)	500–1,000 mg t.i.d.
Glycine strips(Acute panic)	2 g (sublingually) every few minutes (Prousky, 2005)
Phenibut	250–500 mg o.d.[e]
Adrenal glandular stress	100 mg b.i.d. or 200 mg t.i.d.
Stabilium (Garum armoricum) (Use if casein allergy)	200–400 mg o.d.[f]
Oral micronized progesterone (Prescription only for menopausal women)	50–100 mg o.d.
Phosphatidyl serine (Posttraumatic stress disorder)	100 mg t.i.d.

[a]Take magnesium to bowel tolerance. More magnesium at bedtime aids sleep.
[b]Take before bed.
[c]Take in the morning combined with water.
[d]Take away from food.
[e]1 day on 1 day off for 1 month only as needed for acute anxiety.
[f]After 1 month, reduce to every other day.

TABLE 7.11

Protocol for Obsessive-Compulsive Disorder

Nutrients	Dose
Complex vitamins and minerals with L-methylfolate	Dose varies t.i.d.
Omega-3 fish oil	1–3 grams o.d.
Gamma linoleic acid (GLA)/borage or evening primrose oil	1,000 mg o.d.
Free amino acids	Dose varies b.i.d.
Probiotics	100+ billion CFUs o.d.
Vitamin D	50,000 IU (oral, 1x/week for 8 weeks) for deficiency 2,000–4,000 IU. o.d. for maintenance
Glucose tolerance factor	1–2 capsules t.i.d.
Vitamin B-12	Injections until blood level reaches 900 g/mL; thereafter sublingual levels of B-12: 1 mg
L-theanine/lactium	100–400 mg o.d.
Melatonin	0.5 mg at night
N-acetylcysteine (NAC)	1,200–2,400 mg o.d.
Glycine	1–3 grams t.i.d.
5-HTP	25–100 mg b.i.d.
L-tryptophan	500 mg at night
Inositol	1,000–3,000 mg t.i.d.

For trichotillomania, add the following: tyrosine 500 mg b.i.d.

TABLE 7.12

Protocol for Alcohol Addiction

Nutrients	Dose
Complex vitamins and minerals with L-methylfolate High-dose phosphorylated thiamine B-vitamin-mineral complex	Dose varies t.i.d. 1–2 mcg o.d.
Omega-3 fish oil (DHA/EPA)	1–2 grams t.i.d
Gamma linoleic acid (GLA)/borage or evening primrose oil	1,000 mg o.d.
Free amino acids	Dose varies b.i.d.[a]
Probiotics	100+ billion CFUs o.d.
Vitamin D	50,000 IU[b] 2,000–4,000 IU o.d.[c]
Glucose tolerance factor	1–2 capsules t.i.d.
CDP-choline	500 mg b.i.d.
Liver glandular	400 mg t.i.d.
Adrenal glandular	200 mg, t.i.d.
Hypothalamus glandular	500 mg t.i.d.
Niacinamide	500 mg
Magnesium	400–1,200 mg o.d.[d]
Potassium	99 mg o.d.
Lithium orotate	45 mg o.d.
5-HTP	25–100 mg o.d.
Tryptophan	500 mg[e]
Melatonin	0.5–1 mg[e]

Adjunct Protocol for Alcohol Addiction

Nutrients	Dose
Phenibut (Anxiety)	250–500 mg o.d.[f]
Phosphatidylcholine	800–1,200 mg b.i.d
SAMe	400 mg b.i.d.
Lactium (Anxiety)	150–300 mg o.d.

[a]Take away from food.
[b]Oral, 1x/week for 8 weeks, for deficiency.
[c]For maintenance.
[d]Take magnesium to bowel tolerance. More magnesium at bedtime aids sleep.
[e]Take before bed.
[f]1 day on 1 day off for 1 month only as needed.

TABLE 7.13

Protocol for Cannabis Withdrawl

Nutrients	Dose
Complex vitamins and minerals with L-methylfolate	Dose varies t.i.d.
Omega-3 fish oil (DHA/EPA)	1–2 grams t.i.d
Gamma linoleic acid (GLA)/borage or evening primrose oil	1,000 mg o.d.
Free amino acids	Dose varies b.i.d.[a]
Probiotics	100+ billion CFUs o.d.
Vitamin D	50,000 IU[b] 2,000–4,000 IU o.d.[c]
Glucose tolerance factor	1–2 t.i.d.
CDP-choline	500–1,000 mg b.i.d.
Liver glandular	400 mg (1–2, t.i.d.)
Adrenal glandular	100 mg b.i.d or 200 mg t.i.d.
Hypothalamus glandular	500 mg (1–3, t.i.d.)

Adjunct Protocol for Alcohol Addiction

Nutrients	Dose
Phenibut (Anxiety)	250–500 o.d.[d]

[a]Take away from food.
[b]Oral, 1x/week for 8 weeks, for deficiency.
[c]For maintenance.
[d]1 day on 1 day off for 1 month only as needed.

TABLE 7.14

Protocol for Cocaine Addiction

Nutrients	Dose
Complex vitamins and minerals with L-methylfolate	Dose varies t.i.d.
Omega-3 fish oil (DHA/EPA)	1–2 grams t.i.d
Gamma linoleic acid (GLA)/borage or evening primrose oil	1,000 mg o.d.
Free amino acids	Dose varies b.i.d.[a]
Probiotics	100+ billion CFUs o.d.
Vitamin D	50,000 IU[b] 2,000–4,000 IU o.d.[c]
Glucose tolerance factor	1–2 t.i.d.
CDP-choline	500–1,000 mg b.i.d.
Liver glandular	400 mg (1–2, t.i.d.)
Adrenal glandular	100 mg b.i.d or 200 mg t.i.d.
Hypothalamus glandular	500 mg (1–3, t.i.d.)

Adjunct Protocol for Cocaine Addiction

Nutrients	Dose
Phenibut (Anxiety)	250–500 o.d.[d]

[a]Take away from food.
[b]Oral, 1x/week for 8 weeks, for deficiency.
[c]For maintenance.
[d]1 day on 1 day off for 1 month only as needed.

TABLE 7.15

Protocol for MDMA/Ecstasy Recovery

Nutrients	Dose
Complex vitamins and minerals with L-methylfolate High-dose phosphorylated thiamine B-vitamin-mineral complex	Dose varies t.i.d. 1–2 mcg o.d.
Omega-3 fish oil (DHA/EPA)	1–2 grams t.i.d
Gamma linoleic acid (GLA)/borage or evening primrose oil	1,000 mg o.d.
Free amino acids	Dose varies b.i.d.[a]
Probiotics	100+ billion CFUs o.d.
Vitamin D	50,000 IU[b] 2,000–4,000 IU o.d.[c]
Glucose tolerance factor	1–2 t.i.d.
CDP-choline	500 mg b.i.d.
Liver glandular	400 mg (1–2, t.i.d.)
Adrenal glandular	100 mg b.i.d or 200 mg t.i.d.
Hypothalamus glandular	500 mg (1–3, t.i.d.)
Beta-carotene	25,000 IU
Bioflavonoids	500 mg t.i.d.
Vitamin E	400 IU b.i.d.
Selenium	500 mcg
CoQ10	300 mg b.i.d.
L-ascorbic acid	2–3 grams t.i.d.
L-carnitine	1–2 grams b.i.d.
N-acetylcysteine (NAC)	3 grams b.i.d.
L-tyrosine	500 mg b.i.d.

Adjunct Protocol for MDMA/Ecstasy Recovery

Nutrients	Dose
Phenibut (Anxiety)	250–500 mg o.d.[d]

[a]Take away from food.
[b]Oral, 1x/week for 8 weeks, for deficiency.
[c]For maintenance.
[d]1 day on 1 day off for 1 month only as needed.

TABLE 7.16

Protocol for Methamphetamine Addiction

Nutrients	Dose
Complex vitamins and minerals with L-methylfolate	Dose varies t.i.d.
Omega-3 fish oil (DHA/EPA)	1–2 grams t.i.d
Gamma linoleic acid (GLA)/borage or evening primrose oil	1,000 mg o.d.
Free amino acids	Dose varies b.i.d.[a]
Probiotics	100+ billion CFUs o.d.
Vitamin D	50,000 IU[b] 2,000–4,000 IU o.d.[c]
Glucose tolerance factor	1–2 t.i.d.
CDP-choline	500 mg b.i.d.
Liver glandular	400 mg (1–2, t.i.d.)
Adrenal glandular	100 mg b.i.d. or 200 mg t.i.d
Hypothalamus glandular	500 mg (1–3, t.i.d.)
Brain glandular	250 mg (1–2, t.i.d.)
Phosphatidylserine	100 mg t.i.d.
DL-phenylalanine	500–1,000 mg t.i.d.

[a]Take away from food.
[b]Oral, 1x/week for 8 weeks, for deficiency.
[c]For maintenance.
[d]1 day on 1 day off for 1 month only as needed.

TABLE 7.17

Protocol for Opiate Addiction

Nutrients	Dose
Complex vitamins and minerals with L-methylfolate	Dose varies t.i.d.
Omega-3 fish oil (DHA/EPA)	1–2 grams t.i.d
Gamma linoleic acid (GLA)/borage or evening primrose oil	1,000 mg o.d.
Free amino acids	Dose varies b.i.d.[a]
Probiotics	100+ billion CFUs o.d.
Vitamin D	50,000 IU[b] 2,000–4,000 IU o.d.[c]
Glucose tolerance factor	1–2 t.i.d.
CDP-choline	500 mg b.i.d.
Liver glandular	400 mg (1–2, t.i.d.)
Adrenal glandular	100 mg b.i.d. or 200 mg t.i.d.
Hypothalamus glandular	500 mg (1–3, t.i.d.)
Selenium	10–50 mg o.d.
N-acetylcysteine (NAC)	3 grams b.i.d.
DL-phenylalanine	500–1,000 mg t.i.d.

Adjunct Protocol for Opiate Addiction

Nutrients	Dose
Phenibut (Anxiety)	250–500 o.d.[d]

[a]Take away from food.
[b]Oral, 1x/week for 8 weeks, for deficiency.
[c]For maintenance.
[d]1 day on 1 day off for 1 month only as needed.

TABLE 7.18

Protocol for Tobacco Addiction

Nutrients	Dose
Complex vitamins and minerals with L-methylfolate	Dose varies t.i.d.
Omega-3 fish oil (DHA/EPA)	1–2 grams t.i.d
Gamma linoleic acid (GLA)/borage or evening primrose oil	1,000 mg o.d.
Free amino acids	Dose varies b.i.d.[a]
Probiotics	100+ billion CFUs o.d.
Vitamin D	50,000 IU[b] 2,000–4,000 IU o.d.[c]
Glucose tolerance factor	1–2 t.i.d.
CDP-choline	500 mg b.i.d.
Liver glandular	400 mg (1–2, t.i.d.)
Adrenal glandular	100 mg b.i.d or 200 mg t.i.d.
Hypothalamus glandular	500 mg (1–3, t.i.d.)
Lung	400 mg (1–2, t.i.d.)
Vitamin B complex	
Vitamin C	1,000 mg t.i.d.
Vitamin E	400 mg b.i.d.
Beta-carotene	25 IU
Niacinamide	1,000–3,000 mg o.d.
Thiamine	4.5–40 mg o.d.
5-HTP	50–100 mg b.i.d.
Tyrosine	500 mg t.i.d.
Pregnenolone	50 mg b.i.d.

Adjunct Protocol for Tobacco Addiction

Nutrients	Dose
Phenibut (Anxiety)	250–500 o.d.[d]
Taurine (Optional)	500 b.i.d.
Tincture of CBD medical cannabis (Optional)	p.r.n.

[a]Take away from food.
[b]Oral, 1x/week for 8 weeks, for deficiency.
[c]For maintenance.
[d]1 day on 1 day off for 1 month only as needed.

TABLE 7.19

Protocol for Autism and Neurodevelopmental Disorders

Nutrients	Dose
Complex vitamins and minerals with L-methylfolate	Dose varies t.i.d.
Omega-3 fish oil (EPA-rich)	1–2 grams b.i.d.
Gamma linoleic acid (GLA)/borage or evening primrose oil	500–1,000 mg o.d.
Free amino acids	Dose varies b.i.d.[a]
Probiotics	100+ billion CFUs o.d.
Vitamin D	50,000 IU (oral, 1x/week for 8 weeks) for deficiency 2,000–4,000 IU o.d. for maintenance
Glucose tolerance factor (GTF)	1–2 capsules t.i.d.
NAC	900 mg o.d.–t.i.d.
Glucoraphanin/sulforaphane	p.r.n.
Cholesterol supplementation	p.r.n.
Phosphatidylcholine	30–60 mg o.d.

Adjunct Protocol for Autism and Neurodevelopmental Disorders

Nutrients	Dose
Pregnenolone (Adults, irritability)	50 mg o.d.
Tryptophan (Adults)	500 mg[b]

[a]Take away from food.
[b]Take before bed.

TABLE 7.20

Protocol for Cognitive Decline, Dementia, and Traumatic Brain Injury

Nutrients	Dose
Complex vitamins and minerals with L-methylfolate	Dose varies t.i.d.
Omega-3 fish oil (DHA-rich)	2-3 grams b.i.d.–t.i.d.
Gamma linoleic acid (GLA)/borage or evening primrose oil	1,000 mg o.d.
Free amino acids	Dose varies b.i.d.[a]
Probiotics	100+ billion CFUs o.d.
Vitamin D	50,000 IU (oral, 1x/week for 8 weeks) for deficiency 2,000–4,000 IU o.d. for maintenance
Glucose tolerance factor	1–2 capsules t.i.d.
Methylcobalamin	2,000 mcg o.d.
Vitamin E	400–600 IU b.i.d.
Lithium orotate	45 mg o.d. (Shealy, 2006)
Magnesium L-threonate	
CoQ10	300–600 b.i.d.
PQQ	20 mg o.d.
Acetyl L-carnitine	850 mg b.i.d.
CDP-choline	300–1,000 mg b.i.d.
Phosphatidyl serine (PS)	100 mg t.i.d.
RNA/DNA	200–400 mg o.d.
Huperzine	50–200 mcg o.d.
Vinpocetine	10–20 mg t.i.d.
Pregenolone	50 t.i.d.
Curcumin	80 mg o.d.
R-lipoic acid	0.5–2 mg o.d.
Brain glandular	250 mg (1–2, t.i.d.)
Hypothalamus glandular	500 mg (1–3, 3x/day)
Pituitary glandular	250 mg o.d.
Adrenal glandular	100 mg b.i.d. or 200 mg t.i.d.
Apoaequorin/prevagen	20–40 mg o.d.

TABLE 7.20 (continued)

Protocol for Cognitive Decline, Dementia, and Traumatic Brain Injury

Adjunct Protocol for Cognitive Decline, Dementia, and Traumatic Brain Injury

Nutrients	Dose
Melatonin	0.05–5 mg p.r.n.
Bioidentical progesterone, estrogen, and testosterone (for women)	
Testosterone (for men)	
Fish oil may be dosed as high as 20 grams during acute phase under the direction of a prescriber	
Progesterone may be used for men and women with TBI under direction of prescriber	

[a]Take away from food.

TABLE 7.21

Protocol for Attention-Deficit/Hyperactivity Disorder

Nutrients	Dose
Complex vitamins and minerals with L-methylfolate	Dose varies t.i.d.
Omega-3 fish oil	Adult: 1–3 grams o.d. 4–6 years: 500 mg t.i.d. 7–14 years: 1–2 grams b.i.d.
Gamma linoleic acid (GLA)/borage or evening primrose oil	1,000 mg o.d.
Free amino acids .	Dose varies b.i.d.
Probiotics	100+ billion CFUs o.d.
Vitamin D	2,000–4,000 IU o.d.
Glucose tolerance factor	1–2 capsules t.i.d.
Vitamin B6	50–100 mg o.d.
Magnesium threonate	100–400 mg o.d.
Zinc	25 mg b.i.d.
L-tyrosine	500 mg b.i.d.

TABLE 7.22

Protocol for Sleep/Wake Disorders

Nutrients	Dose
Complex vitamins and minerals with L-methylfolate	Dose varies t.i.d.
Omega-3 fish oil	1–3 grams o.d.
Gamma linoleic acid (GLA)/borage or evening primrose oil	1,000 mg o.d.
Free amino acids	Dose varies b.i.d.
Probiotics	100+ billion CFUs o.d.
Vitamin D	50,000 IU (oral, 1x/week for 8 weeks) for deficiency 2,000–4,000 IU o.d. for maintenance
Glucose tolerance factor	1–2 capsules t.i.d.
B-12 methylcobalamin	1 mg o.d.
Magnesium threonate	100–400 mg o.d.
Lithium orotate	1.5 mg o.d.
Alpha-lipoic acid	200 mg o.d.
Melatonin	0.5–1 mg night
Lactium	450–600 mg o.d.
5-HTP (optional)	25–100 mg o.d.
Phenibut (optional)	250–500 mg o.d. (reduce after 1 month to every other day)

TABLE 7.23

Protocol for Psychosis/Schizophrenia

Nutrients	Dose
Complex vitamins and minerals with L-methylfolate	Dose varies t.i.d.
Omega-3 fish oil	1–3 grams o.d.
Gamma linoleic acid (GLA)/borage or evening primrose oil	1,000 mg o.d.
Free amino acids	Dose varies b.i.d.
Probiotics	100+ billion CFUs o.d.
Vitamin D	50,000 IU (oral, 1x/week for 8 weeks) for deficiency 2,000–4,000 IU o.d. for maintenance
Glucose tolerance factor	1–2 capsules t.i.d.
Glycine	4–8 grams b.i.d.
Glutamine	5 grams o.d.
N-acetylcysteine (NAC)	300–600 mg b.i.d.
Pregnenolone	50 mg b.i.d.
Glutamine (optional)	500–5,000 mg o.d.
CBD-rich cannabis (optional)	p.r.n.
Proteolytic enzymes (optional)	500–1,000 mg every 4–6 hr (away from food)

TABLE 7.24

Protocol for Anorexia

Nutrients	Dose
Complex vitamins and minerals with L-methylfolate	Dose varied t.i.d.
Omega-3 fish oil	1–3 grams o.d.
Gamma linoleic acid (GLA)/borage or evening primrose oil	1,000 mg o.d.
Free amino acids	Dose varies b.i.d.
Probiotics	100+ billion CFUs o.d.
Vitamin D	50,000 IU (oral, 1x/week for 8 weeks) for deficiency 2,000–4,000 IU o.d. for maintenance
Glucose tolerance factor	1–2 capsules t.i.d.
Vitamin E	400 IU o.d.
Vitamin K	1,000 mcg o.d.
Beta-carotene	25,000 mg o.d.
Potassium	99 mg o.d.
Zinc	25 mg b.i.d.
Tyrosine	500 mg o.d.
Inositol	1,000–3,000 mg b.i.d.
SAMe	400 mg t.i.d.

TABLE 7.25

Protocol for Bulimia and Binge Eating Protocol

Nutrients	Dose
Complex vitamin and minerals with L-methylfolate	Dose varies t.i.d.
Omega-3 fish oil	1–3 grams o.d.
Gamma linoleic acid (GLA)/borage or evening primrose oil	1,000 mg o.d.
Free amino acids	Dose varies b.i.d.
Probiotics	100+ billion CFUs o.d.
Vitamin D	50,000 IU (oral, 1x/week for 8 weeks) for deficiency 2,000–4,000 IU. o.d. for maintenance
Glucose tolerance factor	1–2 capsules t.i.d.
Vitamin B6	50–100 mg. o.d.
Magnesium threonate	100–400 mg. o.d.
Zinc	25 mg. b.i.d.
5-HTP	50 mg t.i.d.
Lactium	150–300 mg. o.d.
Inositol	2,000 mg. t.i.d.
Whey protein	2 heaping tablespoons o.d.

CHAPTER 8

Medications: Side Effects and Withdrawal

Diet Essential: *Choose healthy foods and nutrients over alcohol and drugs to alter consciousness.*

Pharmaceutical medications alter consciousness and brain chemistry along with nutritional well-being. The theme of this chapter is summarized in the words of the pioneering orthomolecular physician and scientist Carl Pfeiffer: "For every drug that benefits a patient, there is a natural substance that can achieve the same effect." In this chapter I describe the effects of medications on nutritional status within the framework of mental health and some of the side effects and dangers of psychotropic medications. I also provide strategies to reduce and ultimately withdraw from powerful pharmaceutical medications.

My clinical practice is devoted to helping people reduce and eliminate psychotropic and other medications. I have successfully guided thousands of individuals in the withdrawal from pharmaceuticals, and there are many clinical practitioners doing the same. I am against the use of psychotropic medications as a rule because I believe that they are more dangerous than helpful, leading to debilitating side effects that are often worse than the original symptom, and because there are better and safer alternatives. Among other critics of psychotropic medications are Breggin (2013), Whitaker (2010), and Kirsch (2010). Even the director of the National Institute of Mental Health, Insel (2013), has questioned the efficacy of long-term use of antipsychotics. While mental health practitioners frequently prescribe psychotropic medications, clients routinely use other prescription medications for digestion, pain, and other illnesses. Some of these medications are necessary, but most are not. All of these medications have significant interactive side effects. Pharmaceutical medication side effects are directly responsible for more than 100,000 deaths each year in the United States (Vukadin, 2014).

Why psychotropics are used so widely is less a result of need and efficacy and more a response to pharmaceutical marketing and the "quick fix" mentality that is often instilled in the minds of patients who cannot afford therapy and the considerable care that is regularly required for mental health. The problem is multilevel: (1) pharmaceutical companies do not always reveal the results of negative studies, (2) marketing strategies downplay the side effects (Vukadin, 2014), and (3) marketing methods include incentives for prescribers and materials that obscure the side effects and dangers. Added to these issues is the decreased time allowed for the clinician to treat complex problems, and advertising targeting consumers actively encouraging them to request certain medications from their providers. Finally, many instructors, clinicians, and their agency administrators have been conditioned into thinking medications are the answer and the go-to response for every symptom.

Attitudes and institutional impediments underlie in part the "whys" of psychotropic use more than treatment efficacy. Many people cannot afford psychotherapy and other forms of therapies, or good nutrition. Insurance company policies are an added complication since most do not pay for the nonpharmaceutical therapies. Medications should not be the default response because social supports, food security, and health care are generally inadequate.

People can successfully withdraw from all kinds of medications and drugs but not everyone will choose to do so, and it is important to understand this when working with clients. The approaches outlined in this chapter will not be suitable for everyone. Not everyone is willing to use or can afford practical alternatives. Severely ill individuals require care and help from others to apply these methods. Applying the information in this chapter (and the previous ones) will make sure they receive the proper nutrition and nutritional protocols as well as care during the stage of acute withdrawal. People are often fearful of eliminating medications. Withdrawal and personal maintenance is feasible notwithstanding these obstacles.

To withdraw and eliminate psychotropics, one benefits from using nutrient-dense foods and nutritional supplements to ease the withdrawal and address the underlying needs of the brain and body. This chapter advances the discussion of protocols defined in Chapter 7 by identifying effective approaches for achieving balance and nourishing the brain, mind, and body while liberating oneself from the use of toxic drugs.

Finally, clients need to believe that they can withdraw and stay off psychotropic medications, and to do so they require the support of a clinician who also believes this is not only possible but also preferable. Clinicians and clients alike need to decondition from the consensus trance, and clinicians will benefit from releasing their own fears about psychotropic withdrawal and drug-free maintenance.

ESSENTIAL STRATEGIES FOR WITHDRAWAL

Philosophical Preparation

An important part of the withdrawal process is recognizing that many people have been conditioned to believe that taking medication is necessary and usually the only option. People adhere to what Tart calls the "consensus trance" or social dissociation, when it comes to pharmaceutical use. While we often treat clinical dissociation associated with traumatic events and substance use, people often experience a social dissociation when it comes to medication use; they often do not question it when recommended, and they often actively seek it in response to social media and advertising or peer pressure. This same type of disconnection occurs in regard to diet and the dissociation from how and what one eats affects one's mental and physical well-being and consciousness. While not easily changed, like any conditioned response, understanding these forces provides the basis for engaging the client in the questioning process. Another level of brainwashing occurs, according to Breggin (2013), who suggests that once people have been on psychotropics for some time, they experience medication spellbinding as a result of chronic brain impairment that results from chronic use of psychiatric medications. Breggin (2013) suggests that people on psychotropics lose the ability to recognize symptoms of their own impairment or drug intoxication. Hoffer (2008) also referred to "tranquilizer psychosis" among people prescribed antipsychotics.

Elements Essential to Psychotropic and Medication Withdrawal

- Psychoeducation
- Self-care plan
- Prescribing clinician
- Withdrawal schedule
- Clinician availability contract
- Nutritional supplementation protocol
- Social support team
- Therapeutic supports
- Sleep regulation
- At-home detoxification methods

Psychoeducation

I spend time during each session reviewing with the client her or his decision to withdraw, providing support and hope, and exploring fears, concerns, and potential obstacles, including the opinions of family members, friends, or others. I review the variety of side effects she may be experiencing or that are known to occur with the medication and also review the process of withdrawal and what to expect over what period of time. Breggin (2013) does not use the term "dependence" for addiction or "discontinuation" to mean withdrawal, suggesting that these terms are euphemistic expressions implying that the difficulties people experience during withdrawal are not the return of symptoms but the toxic effects of the medication.

Self-Care Plan

I work with the client for 4–12 weeks or more to prepare for withdrawal and elimination. In my experience, unless the client has a consistent plan of self-care in place, withdrawal and maintenance are unlikely to be successful. The self-care plan consists of good-quality food, a tailored nutritional protocol as outlined in the previous chapter, and daily exercise and other therapeutic supports like acupuncture and massage. Soon after the initial assessment, I begin a client on Omega-3 fatty acids (minimum of 2,000 mg/day) and full-spectrum vitamin E (400–800 IU/day) and B Complex including vitamins B12 and B6 to militate against the damaging effects of the current medication regimen. Following the development of a withdrawal plan, a core nutrient program is established that will include vitamins, minerals, amino acids, and glandulars that support brain function, support sleep and relaxation, and reduce inflammation and oxidative stress. Skill building to tolerate discomfort should be included.

Prescribing Clinician

I ask the client to communicate this plan to the prescriber and engage support and recommendations. I may also call or write them. If they will not cooperate, it is important to understand why they are against the proposed process, and it may be beneficial to conduct a team conference call or meeting. If following a discussion of the approach, the clinician still does not wish to join the support team, then a new provider should be identified prior to the withdrawal process. This is assessed case by case. I work with a team of prescribing professionals (MD, ARNP, ND) and a compounding pharmacist (RPh). Once a schedule is delineated, one can also work directly with the compounding pharmacist if necessary to create a liquid formula.

Developing a Withdrawal Schedule

The client and I (and other team members) develop a calendar that includes the timeline for tapering off the medication. We fill it in together, define the therapeutic supports and what they provide and at what specific intervals. This can be integrated into a notebook or digital or web-based shared calendar.

The withdrawal schedule will be designed based on the following:

- The "half-life" of the specific medication or drug
- How many different drugs people are taking and which order is prioritized
- How many months/years the client has been using the medication(s)
- What the client and clinician identify as optimal and achievable
- Stress levels in the client's life, including acute perturbations
- Social supports that are in place to carry out the plan

The 2:1 Rule

As a general rule, the longer one has been on a drug, the longer she or he will take to withdraw. I use a 2:1 rule, although this has to be adjusted to individual needs. If someone has been taking Prozac for 6 months, then we use about 3 months to slowly taper the dosage. Someone on medication for 2 years would take 1 year to withdraw. Rarely does the pace of withdrawal go evenly, however. I suggest that clients reduce dosage slowly by milligram or microgram per milliliter depending on the medication, and then stabilize at that level for at least 1–2 weeks. I have worked with many individuals who reduce their medication by half and then stay there for a month or more. Some people reduce Prozac by 35 mg and remain on 5 mg for a year. The complexity of withdrawal includes the mindset of the individual, her or his fears (and the client's family's fear), and concerns about the return of symptoms. People who have been labeled and medicated for years need time to change their identity and beliefs along with their biochemistry during this process.

First Steps

Month 1

Prior to withdrawal of medications and drugs:

- Eliminate gluten and casein, food additives.
- Initiate Omega-3 and Omega-6 fatty acids, free amino acids, vitamin E, vitamin B complex, minerals, and probiotics.
- Initiate daily skin brushing and twice weekly sauna baths.

Month 2

- Begin the withdrawal process with a titration schedule appropriate for the specific drug/medication.
- Additional nutrients include amino acids targeting the appropriate receptors that the medication targets.
- Continue psychotherapeutic support for the emotional ups and downs of the withdrawal process.
- Provide nutritional support to ease withdrawal.
- Provide nutritional support to treat the original nutrient deficits or causes such as inflammation and oxidative stress.
- Stabilize at each new dosage level before reducing further.
- Educate about detoxification strategies for use at home.

I review via phone or e-mail how the client is coping and adjust her or his program as often as required. This might be daily at first and then taper off after the first month. I engage family and friends in the treatment meetings, and I work with the prescribing clinician to adjust dosages. I will also adjust supplements up or down and support adherence to carrying out the necessary work to eat fresh food, get daily exercise, and take nutrients. Wilma's story in Box 8.1 helps us understand the process of withdrawing from medication.

Box 8.1
Wilma's Story

Wilma was a 36 year old single professional who had been on 40 mg daily of Prozac for depression and 75 mg of trazadone to help with sleep for 7 years. She wanted to withdraw from these medications. She felt the side effects of weight gain and diminished libido, and she was unsure of the current benefit. She also wanted to try to become pregnant. We had worked together in counseling for depression and bulimia for 12 months, and she said that she felt ready to withdraw and use some alternatives. In our work together we reviewed Wilma's current self-care program of exercise, healthy mineral-rich proteins, fats, and non-grain carbohydrate food and a supplementary protocol of Omega 3 EFAs, B-complex with L-methylfolate, magnesium, and lactium. I suggested that she add 50 mg lithium orotate to support her mood and free amino acids, which would provide 100 mg a day of 5-HTP. As she began to decrease the Prozac, she could increase the amino acids and lactium as needed. Because she took 75 mg of trazadone to help her sleep, we agreed that she would reduce the trazadone first and support her improved sleep and then begin to reduce the

Prozac by 3–4 mg a month or 1 mg a week. We developed the schedule together by which she would reduce the trazadone first by 5 mg a night and we would supplement her at night with 450 mg of milk biopeptides and 400 mg of magnesium. At 3 months she felt stable and wanted to reduce the medications more quickly and increased the reduction to 5 mg a month. After 9 months she had withdrawn from all her medications, and we turned our attention to supporting her mental health and well-being as she prepared for pregnancy.

Social Support Team

Identifying the client's social supports is essential. Hold a meeting in person or via conference call to educate everyone about the process and to engage their support for participating in specific tasks. Withdrawing from psychotropics should be undertaken much like any drug addiction. There may be intensive stages requiring full-time care and then supports for relapse prevention and care. I make myself available by phone or e-mail as needed, even if it is daily, to receive communications from the client or family members. During the planning stages I create an "availability contract" so the client knows that she or he can reach me between our sessions, if necessary. They may require education, emotional support or "cheerleading," and words of hope and confidence in the process. If the individual lives alone, it is important that someone is with her or him at all times. Or, if the individual can move in with a friend or family member during the first intensive weeks, this may be ideal. While we focus on nutritional support, the support of friends, family, and health providers is essential; mental illness involves disrupted attachment either as a primary or secondary outcome. Providing support for attachment behaviors during this time is essential for success.

Therapeutic Supports

Therapeutic supports that aid the withdrawal process can be instituted during the preparation stage and intensified as needed. This can take the form of a spa-like atmosphere of self-care both in the home and outside, including reflexology and acupuncture. If the client works and can take time off, or at least reduce the workload during the initial withdrawal phase, this is advisable.

Regulate Sleep

Most people on psychotropics have disrupted circadian rhythm and disrupted glucose handling (hypoglycemia or hyperglycemia). Nut butters, cheese, or an egg and crackers will often help one to get through the night. Cranial electrical stimulation can also support withdrawal as does acupuncture. Upon awakening in the middle of the night, another dose of lactium can be administered. Light therapy and vigorous exercise during the day and blue light–blocking glasses before bed can help reset circadian rhythm along with nutrients defined in the previous chapter. Box 8.2 describes strategies for insomnia that synergize the nutrient protocol.

Box 8.2

Strategies for Insomnia and Sleep Disorders
When Coming Off Medications and Drugs

- Cognitive-behavioral therapy
- Electroencephalography biofeedback, neurofeedback
- Bright light therapy in the a.m.
- Exercise before 4 p.m.
- Magnesium sulfate bath 30 minutes before bed
- Room should be totally dark with no light source
- Blue light-blocking glasses at night
- Regulate ambient bedroom temperature to between 60 and 67 degrees F adjusted to personal need/preference

---

At-Home Detoxification Methods

There are two interrelated processes in detoxification. The first is to eliminate and reduce exposure to harmful or toxic substances in food or the environment. The second is to engage actively in specific detoxification activities that support excretion of waste though the many organs of the body.

Methods that support the elimination of toxins from the body will ease the physical and emotional burden of withdrawal. While these methods will help with all medications, as well as drugs and alcohol, they may not be powerful enough to support, for example, opiate withdrawal alone and should be considered adjunctive. These methods should be started prior to the withdrawal start date and continued as part of daily or weekly routines to restore health.

Detoxification Strategies

There are many natural approaches to enhancing the elimination of toxins from the body and enhancing the function of the major organs of elimination: the skin, liver, kidney, and colon. Integrating these methods will ease discomfort due to circulating waste and aid in relaxation and sleep. These methods also have the added benefit of contributing to self-care rituals and decreasing dissociation. Among the detoxification methods I recommend for use at home and that I have written about extensively elsewhere (Korn, 2013) are as follows:

- Coffee enemas
- Skin brushing
- Liver flush
- Fiber flush
- Magnesium sulfate (Epsom salt) baths
- Vinegar baths
- Sauna and sweatbaths
- Acupuncture/acupressure
- Castor oil packs

HOW PHARMACEUTICAL USE AFFECTS NUTRITIONAL STATUS AND MENTAL HEALTH

Whether or not one uses or withdraws from psychotropics, they, along with most all pharmaceuticals, affect nutrition status by creating nutrient deficits. People who take medications are more likely to have nutritional deficits and side effects. This, in turn, worsens physical and mental health problems.

These effects suggest the following prevention and treatment strategy:

- Identify the effects of the pharmaceutical on nutrient status.
- Supplement with the identified vitamins, minerals, or other nutrients to counteract the effects of the pharmaceutical.
- Work with an integrative medicine clinician to find an alternative to the pharmaceutical or to reduce dosage and eliminate over time.

In addition to the nutritional effects of pharmaceuticals used for psychotropics, drugs used for medical conditions also produce side effects. Likewise, some pharmaceuticals can affect the sense of smell, which in turn can affect food intake, leading to nutritional deficits.

PSYCHOTROPIC MEDICATIONS, NUTRITIONAL STATUS, AND STRATEGIES FOR WITHDRAWAL

Medications and drugs affect nutrition in two ways: The primary result occurs when the medication or drug interacts with nutritional behaviors of the client, leading to poor dietary habits, such as failure to eat, eating too much, or eating too much of the wrong food. Medications that cause nausea or are stimulants are among these, and opiate use frequently leads to excessive sugar consumption. The second type of effect is the metabolic response of a drug or medication on the body, leading to secondary effects such as nutrient deficits. For example, statins deplete CoQ10, which is essential for mitochondrial function. This occurs because the same enzyme that statins inhibit in order to reduce cholesterol is the same enzyme responsible for the production of CoQ10. Both primary and secondary malnutrition should be considered when evaluating nutritional and mental health status. I discuss some major categories of psychotropics and their effects on nutrient status next.

During the assessment process, the clinician has reviewed all substances the client is using and, before designing a supplement program, a drug–nutrient interaction analysis should be conducted.

THE USE OF NUTRITION AND DIET DURING WITHDRAWAL

The application of diet and supplementation begins prior to withdrawal and intensifies at each stage, according to the ability of the client and the support team. Because psychotropic medications target the NT system, Table 8.1 may be used to identify the most beneficial foods and nutrients to use to support that system as psychotropic medications are withdrawn. Keep in mind that amino acid supplements are best absorbed away from food.

Antipsychotics

Antipsychotics for Bipolar Disorder

These include Aripiprazole (Abilify, Aripiprex), Asenapine (Saphris, Sycrest), Chlorpromazine (Thorazine), Olanzapine (Zyprexa, Zypadhera and Lanzek), Quetiapine (Seroquel), Risperidone (Risperdal), and Ziprasidone (Geodon, Zeldox, and Zipwell).

Effects on Nutritional Status

Bipolar disorder and schizophrenia are metabolic disorders. Antipsychotics appear

TABLE 8.1

Food and Nutrient Sources of Neurotransmitters to Support Mood

Neurotransmitters	Amino Acids/Nutrients	Foods
GABA	Glutamine, taurine, milk-derived neuropeptides, lithium orotate, phenibut	Walnuts, oats, spinach, beans, liver, mackerel
Serotonin	Tryptophan, 5-HTP, B vitamins, especially B12, B6, niacinamide, folic acid	Salmon, beef, lamb, figs, bananas, root vegetables, brown rice
Dopamine	Tyrosine, DL-phenylalanine, B12, B6	Coffee, tea, eggs, pork, dark chocolate, ricotta cheese
Norepinephrine	Tyrosine	Meats, fishes, cheese
Epinephrine	Tyrosine (increases)	Caffeine increases/Camomile tea decreases
Acetylcholine	GPC choline, phosphatidylserine, acetyl-L-carnitine, huperzine-A	Eggs, liver, salmon, shrimp, nut butters, coffee
Glutamate	Glutamic acid	Caffeine, fermented foods, chicken, eggs, dairy
Endogenous opioids	Milk biopeptides	Casein (milk), gluten (grains), spinach, fat, fasting
Cannabinoids	Fish oil, lactobacilli	Hemp seeds/hemp oil

to exacerbate the glucose management, which is already a challenge in these disorders. People taking resperidone and other atypical antipsychotics are at a greater risk for developing hyperglycemia and diabetes (Leyse-Wallace, 2008). They also reduce the B vitamins, in particular B2.

Antidepressants

Monoamime Oxidase Inhibitors
These include tranylcypromine sulfate (Parnate), phenelzine sulfate (Nardil), and isocarboxazid (Marplan).

Tricyclic Antidepressants
These include clomipramine hydrochloride (Anafranil), amitriptyline hydrochloride (Elavil), desipramine hydrochloride (Norpramin, Pertofrane, and others), nortriptyline hydrochloride (Pamelor), doxepin hydrochloride (Sinequan), trimipramine maleate (Surmontil), and imipramine (Tofranil).

Selective Serotonin Reuptake Inhibitors

Citalopram hydrobromide (Celexa), escitalopram oxalate (Lexapro), fluvoxamine maleate (Luvox), paroxetine hydrochloride (Paxil), fluoxetine hydrochloride (Prozac), sertraline hydrochloride (Zoloft), venlafaxine (Effexor), venlafaxine XR (Effexor XR), and duloxetine (Cymbalta).

PTSD With Depression Medications

These include nortriptyline (Aventyl or Pamelor), amitriptyline (Elavil), doxepin (Sinequan or Adapin), and clomipramine (Anafranil).

Other Antidepressant Medications

These include duloxetine hydrochloride (Cymbalta), venlafaxine hydrochloride (Effexor), mirtazapine (Remeron), and trazodone (Desyrel).

Weight gain and depression of sexual function are common side effects with most psychotropic medications, including antidepressants, mood stabilizers, and antipsychotic drugs (Ruetsch, Viala, Bardou, Martin, & Vacheron, 2005). Long-term use of antidepressants can permanently desensitize postsynaptic neurons (Kharrazian, 2013). These medications reduce metabolic rate and alter both appetite and cravings (for sweet foods). They also increase blood alkalinity, which ironically can exacerbate depression and anxiety. This may account for why some people do worse than others on these medications. Suicidality and aggression are also associated with SSRIs; children and teens are more susceptible to suicidality (Breggin, 2013). Antidepressant medications may increase the risk of developing *Clostridium difficile* infection (CDI) (Rogers et al., 2013).

Use of antidepressant medications is widespread and also used for many other symptoms, including pain, premenstrual syndrome disorder, and eating disorders. The benefits and risk of side effects remain controversial, with a number of researchers concluding that the effects of SSRIs that are observed for the treatment of depression are based on placebo response (Kirsch, 2010) and that long-term efficacy in particular has not been established. Breggin (2013) suggests that long-term studies of every class of psychiatric drugs show no proof of efficacy. Kirsch et al. (2008) found that both patients receiving placebo and an antidepressant improved, and the difference among those using the antidepressant was below the level of significance.

A meta-analysis of the benefits of antidepressant medications compared with placebo shows the beneficial effects are minimal to nonexistent for patients with mild or moderate symptoms, and have substantial benefits for patients with very severe depression (Fournier et al., 2010). The largest study conducted on antidepressants, the Sequenced Treatment Alternatives to Relieve Depression, showed only 2.7% of patients had a remission lasting more than 12 months (Breggin, 2013). Another study showed that the risk of relapse is greater for those taking medication once they stop than for those who take no medication. The return of the depression leaves patients in a cycle in which they need to continue taking antidepressants (Breggin, 2013). Use of antidepressants in the elderly also carries an increased vulnerability and risk of suicide (Crumpacker, 2008), which contrasts with literature suggesting that antidepressants reduce the risk of suicide in elders.

Effects on Nutritional Status

People who take SSRIs for long periods may have deficiencies in betaine, folate/folic acid, and vitamin B12 (Kharrazian, 2013). Amitriptyline reduces riboflavin, sodium, and CoQ10; and Trazadone can also deplete vitamin B2 and selenium.

Barbituates, Benzodiazepines, and Opiates

Barbiturates

These include amobarbital sodium (Amytal Sodium), phenobarbital (Nembutal), secobarbital sodium (Seconal Sodium Pulvules), butabarbital sodium (Butisol), and mephobarbital (Mebaral).

Effects on Nutritional Status

Barbiturates deplete biotin, folic acid, and vitamins D and K.

Barbiturates have been largely replaced by benzodiazepines but are still used for some treatment of migraines.

Benzodiazepines

These include clonazepam (Klonopin, Rivotril), diazepam (Valium), estazolam (Prosom), flunitrazepam (Rohypnol), lorazepam (Ativan), midazolam (Versed), nitrazepam (Mogadon), oxazepam (Serax), triazolam (Halcion), temazepam (Restoril, Normison, Planum, Tenox, and Temaze), chlordiazepoxide (Librium), and alprazolam (Xanax).

Effects on Nutritional Status

Benzodiazepines deplete melatonin levels, calcium, biotin, folic acid, and vitamins D and K.

Benzodiazepines target the GABA receptors and are used for anxiety. Benzodiazepines increase the risk of falling and fracture in elderly women, while withdrawal from them decreases the risk of falling (Salonoja, Salminen, Vahlberg, Aarnio, & Kivelä, 2012). They exacerbate nightmares and deep sleep. They should only be used for very short-term acute treatment, if at all. Withdrawal must be very slow (with the exception of triazolam [Halcion]) and is aided by switching from short-acting to long-acting benzodiazepines.

GABA-acting nutrients for anxiety provide effective alternatives to benzodiazepines and other sedatives and hypnotics for sleep—in particular, 5-HTP or tryptophan, phenibut, and milk biopeptides. Nutrients that target the GABA receptors are most useful along with substitution of Kava, an effective botanical anxiolytic (Korn, 2013). Ashton (2002) is a leading expert on benzodiazepine withdrawal and provides comprehensive withdrawal schedules for each specific drug type. For people who are also taking antidepressants, withdraw from the benzodiazepine first. Prousky (2005) suggests the use of melatonin (1 mg) to promote sleep and niacinamide (400 mg 4–6 times a day) up to a total 1,500–2,500 mg/day divided throughout the day.

Opioids

These include codeine (codeine sulfate); oxycodone hydrochloride and ibuprofen (Combunox); oxycodone and acetaminophen (Endocet); oxycodone and acetaminophen (Percocet); aspirin, oxycodone hydrochloride, and oxycodone terephthalate (Percodan); oxycodone hydrochloride (Roxicodone); methadone (Dolophine, Methadose); and propoxyphene (Darvon, Darvocet-N).

The term "opioid" refers to all opioids and opiates including natural opioids called endorphins; opium-derived alkaloids like morphine and codeine; semisynthetic opioids such as heroin, oxycodone, hydrocodone, and buprenorphine; and synthetic opioids like methadone. Heroin is also an opioid. Opiates impair digestive function, and prolonged use impairs the body's capacity to reduce pain. People addicted to opiates (or on methadone treatment) are at risk for increased sugar intake (Mysels & Sullivan, 2010), leading to obesity, hypoglycemia, and diabetes.

Effects on Nutritional Status

Opiate use is associated with increased sugar intake and B-vitamin deficits.

Strategies for Withdrawal

It takes 7–10 days for many opiates to leave the system, though some longer acting drugs require 30–40 days. Substitute less dangerous alternatives for opiates. Deaths due to opiate use were reduced by 25% in states that provide medical cannabis for the treatment of pain (Bachhuber, Saloner, Cunningham, & Barry, 2014). Some current approaches include hybrid inpatient/outpatient programs using naltrexone detoxification over 3–5 days. Naltrexone can cause liver damage and digestive problems. Research demonstrates that cannabis users adhere to their naltrexone treatment better than nonusers, and there are a variety of studies demonstrating cannabis may serve as an "exit drug" out of opiate addiction.

Stimulants for the Treatment of ADHD

Short-Acting (Immediate-Release) Forms
These include extroamphetamine sulfate (Dextrostat, ProCentra, Dexedrine) and methylphenidate (Ritalin, Methylin, Equasym XL).

Intermediate-Acting Forms
These include mphetamine and dextroamphetamine (Adderall), dextroamphetamine sulfate (Dexedrine Spansule), methylphenidate hydrochloride (Metadate ER), and methylphenidate (Methylin ER, Ritalin SR).

Long-Acting Forms
These include amphetamine and dextroamphetamine (Adderall XR), methylphenidate (Concerta), methylphenidate (Daytrana), methylphenidate hydrochloride (Metadate CD, Ritalin LA, Quillivant XR), and lisdexamfetamine dimesylate (Vyvanse).

Effects on Nutritional Status
Children with attention and focus challenges are already starting out with nutritional deficits such as Omega-3 fatty acids and often B vitamins. Stimulants can contribute to poor appetite.

Mood Stabilizers

Anticonvulsants That Act as Mood Stabilizers
These include carbamazepine (Tegretol), divalproex (Epival), lamotrigine (Lamictal), gabapentin (Neurontin), and topiramate (Topamax). Carbamazepine (Tegretol) is an anticonvulsant used for irritability, aggressiveness, and for mania and mixed states instead of lithium.

Mood Stabilizers for Bipolar Disorder
These include lithium (Eskalith, Lithobid).

Valproic Acid/Valproate

These include Depakene, Depacon, Stavzor, Depakote, and Valproic.

Effects on Nutritional Status

Tegretol depletes vitamin D, biotin, calcium, and folic acid. The combination of mood stabilizers and antipsychotics causes more weight gain. Lithium inhibits the production of inositol, and valproic acid causes deficits of the amino acid carnitine, which can lead to liver problems. It also leads to folate/folic acid, vitamins D and E, and selenium deficits. Long-term usage of Depakote can result in vitamin D deficiency.

COMMONLY USED MEDICATIONS AND THEIR EFFECTS ON NUTRITIONAL STATUS AND MENTAL HEALTH

Antibiotics/Antifungals

Examples

These include gentamycine (Garamycin, Gentak), neomycine (Neo-Fradin), penicilin (Permapen), tetracycline (Diabecline, Acnecycline, Dyabetex, Tetra-abc), and cephalosporins.

Effects on Nutritional Status

The major effects of antibiotics are on the healthy gut flora because they kill all bacteria in the gut. This leads to digestive problems, poor absorption of nutrients, and the potential for antibiotic resistance. Antibiotics in general can deplete the B vitamins and vitamin K, particularly the tetracyclines, affecting the absorption of minerals such as calcium and magnesium. Even when one does not use antibiotics orally in the form of pharmaceuticals, there are antibiotics in commercial animal feed production (80% of all antibiotics used in the United States). Antibiotic-resistant bacteria are the result. This suggests that one should avoid mass-produced animal products inoculated with antibiotics unless absolutely necessary or if there is no alternative. When antibiotics have been consumed, reinoculate the gut with probiotic-rich foods and supplemental bacteria.

Floroquinolones are among the most dangerous antibiotics. These medications should be used only as a last resort and never in children under the age of 18. These medications include ciprofloxacin (Cipro), levofloxacin (Levaquin), gemifloxacin (Factive), moxifloxacin (Avelox), norfloxacin (Noroxin), and ofloxacin (Floxin). These antibiotics are associated with side effects that include psychosis, suicidality, anxiety, and physical illnesses, including permanent peripheral neuropathy (Cohen, 2001). Antibiotic use leads to deficiencies in folate; vitamins B1, B2, B6, and B12; calcium; magnesium; potassium; and vitamin K.

Alternatives

There are certainly medical necessities for the use of antibiotics. However, they are often prescribed when other alternatives might also be effective and would also avoid the side effects. Among these are chronic childhood ear infections, colds or flu, and urinary tract infections, especially in the elderly. Barring emergency situations, consider the use of garlic and onions, which are rich in sulfur (see Appendix X for Garlic and Onion Soup recipe), and oil of oregano; all have mild antibiotic properties.

Anticonvulsants.

Examples

These include pregabalin (Lyrica), gabapentin (Neurotin), phenytoin (Dilatin), carbamazepine (Carbatrol, Epitol, Equetro, Tegretol, Tegretol XR), valproate (Depacon, Depakene, Depakote, and Eliaxim), lamotrigine (Lamictal), oxcarbazepine (Trileptal), and topiramate (Topamax).

Effects on Nutritional Status

Anticonvulsants are used for seizure control and are also used as psychiatric medications. Over time, these medications can deplete vitamin D, calcium, vitamin B12, vitamin K, copper, selenium, and zinc. Chronic use can lower immunity, exacerbate depression, and cause muscle weakness.

Alternatives

Fish oil and B vitamins are widely used, along with ketogenic and grain-free diets. Consultation with an integrative neurologist is essential prior to medication change for seizure control. There is some (controversial) use of medical cannabis for children with severe seizure disorder.

Anti-Inflammatories

Examples

These include aspirin, ibuprofen (Advil, Genpril, IBU, Midol, Motrin, Nuprin), diclofenac, and naproxen (Aleve, Midol Extended Relief, Naprelan 375, Naprosyn).

Effects on Nutritional Status

Nonsteroidal anti-inflammatory drugs (NSAIDs) include aspirin, ibuprofen, and naproxen; they can be very dangerous, especially when used over the long term. NSAIDs contribute to depression and interfere with antidepressant efficacy. NSAIDs are also associated with damaging joint cartilage and gut and kidney damage.

NSAIDS deplete folic acid, B6 and B12, vitamin C, calcium, and magnesium. The use of an NSAID should be employed only after reading contraindications and as an emergency response to acute pain that cannot be managed otherwise. NSAIDs are often used to manage chronic pain, and an alternative, integrative approach to pain management can be very successful (Korn, 2013).

For localized pain compounding, pharmacists can formulate topical creams or gels that contain compounds that are very effective. These might include a cream containing ketaprofen (NSAID), ketamine, and capsaicin for neurological pain. Because it is applied topically, the NSAID does not become systemic and thus does not cause the types of side effects that oral use causes. Nevertheless, it is designed as a powerful intervention for short-term use. Fibromyalgia creams containing capsaicin at a higher dose are also available.

Alternatives

Integrated nutrition for pain management includes proteolytic enzymes, amino acids (DLPhenyalanine), to support analgesia, vitamin D, natural herbal cyclooxygenase-II enzyme inhibitors (COX-2 inhibitors) and lipoxygenase (LOX-inhibitors), Omega-3, and GLA oil.

Blood Pressure Medications/Antihypertensives

Examples

These include methyldopa (Aldomet), ramipril (Altace), verapamil (Calan), doxazosin (Cardura), losartan (Cozaar), benazepril (Lotensin), and enalapril (Vasotec).

Calcium Channel Blockers

Examples
These include amlodipine (Norvasc), nifedipine (Procardia), verapamil (Calan, Verelan, Covera-HS), and diltiazem (Cardizem, Dilt-cd).

Effects on Nutritional Status
Among these medications, ACE inhibitors deplete zinc, calcium channel blockers deplete potassium, and the beta-blockers deplete CoQ10. Propranolol (Inderal) and atenolol (Tenormin) are also used for social anxiety and can lead to CoQ10 and choline deficits.

Alternatives
Fish oil has been shown to reduce blood pressure. Use together with garlic, taurine magnesium, CoQ10 at 100 mg b.i.d.

Corticosteroid Medications

Examples
These include hydrocortisone (Solu-cortef, Locoid, Cortef, Anucort-hc, Cortifoam, Pandel, Proctocort, Westcort, Colocort, Hytone, Alacort, Caldecort, Texacort, Procto-Kit, Theracort, MiCort-HC, CortAlo, A-hydrocort, U-cort, Poli-A, Maximum-H), cortisone, and prednisone (Deltasone, Rayos, Sterapred).

Effects on Nutritional Status
Cortisone, hydrocortisone, and prednisone are used commonly for the treatment of inflammatory conditions and autoimmune diseases in inhalers. Commonly used in inhalers for the treatment of asthma or as anti-inflammatories. Short-term use can reduce symptoms of inflammation and pain but also carry significant mood-altering side effects such as euphoria and hypomania (Warrington & Bostwick, 2006). Corticosteroids can induce anxiety and insomnia associated with use of inhalers for the treatment of allergies and asthma. Clients should be monitored for mood changes or elevated anxiety soon after beginning steroidal treatment. Corticosteroids can decrease potassium and calcium, zinc, selenium, vitamins D and K, and folic acid, and can cause sodium retention and increase blood pressure.

Alternatives

Corticosteroids are available in both natural and synthetic forms. Because the adrenals are a major organ involved in managing inflammatory processes, chronic inflammation and pain are often signs of adrenal insufficiency due to chronic stress. Supporting adrenal function through food and nutrients is central to prevention and recovery. Animal proteins, sea salt, adrenal glandulars, phosphatidylserine, and licorice root are a few of the first options. Naturopathic physicians also work with compounding pharmacists to provide low-dose physiologic cortisol (5–25 mg/day) for short-term use. A compounding pharmacist can be helpful for formulating an alternative to synthetic steroids. The alternatives to steroid use follow.

Pain and Inflammation

These include adrenal glandular, curcumin, proteolytic enzymes, and medical cannabis.

Joint Pain

In addition to the above nutrients and herbal medicines for acute and chronic pain, treatment with prolotherapy, stem cell, platelet-rich plasma (PRP), and hyaluronic acid injections should be investigated.

Dermatological Treatment

A variety of options are available for topical treatment depending on the skin problem. Corticosteroids are often prescribed for rashes. For shingles (Herpes zoster) a licorice root gel is available.

Allergies/Asthma

Identify food allergies/sensitivities, especially gluten, diary, and mucus-forming foods.

Increase Omega-3 fatty acids and gamma linoleic acid; acidify diet; use hydrotherapy: ice packs between the shoulder blades.

Autoimmune Disorders

Identify food allergies/sensitivities, especially gluten and diary.

Increase Omega-3 fatty acids, GLA, and nattokinase.

Antiviral Medications

Examples

These include azidothymidine (AZT), zidovudine (Retrovir), acyclovir (Zovirax, Sitavig, Cyclovir, Herpex, Zoral, Xovir, Imavir), amantadine (and interferons (Roferon A, Multiferon, Avonex, Cinnovex, Pegasys).

Effects on Nutritional Status

There is a broad range of antiviral drugs most often used for serious diseases. If these medications are required, then an active program of supplementation can often improve efficacy as well as counteract nutrient loss. Among these medications are AZT (azidothymidine) and Retrovir for HIV/AIDS, and Acyclovir (herpex), which is used for treatment of herpes infections. Amantadine and interferon are used for treatment of Hepatitis B and C.

Tamiflu is commonly used for the treatment of flu (influenza) in spite of data demonstrating virtually no effect on prevention or treatment; it carries a risk of side effects in 1 out of 94 people (Vasquez, 2004), including psychiatric and kidney problems in adults, nausea, and vomiting in adults and children (Jefferson et al., 2014).

Most of these medications reduce carnitine, copper, zinc, vitamin B12, calcium, magnesium, and potassium.

Alternatives

These include thymus glandular, selenium, vitamins D and E, lysine, probiotics, and CoQ10.

Diabetes

Examples

These include metformin (Glumetza, Fortamet, Riomet, Glucophage), sulfonylurea (Glibenclamide, Glimepiride, Glipizide, Tolbutamide, Chlorpropamide, Tolazamide, Glyburide/Metformin, Glipizide/Metformin, Pioglitazone/Glimepiride, Rosiglitazone/Glimepiride), and insulin (Humalog, NovoLog, Humulin R, Levemir, Apidra, Exubra, Lantus).

Effects on Nutritional Status

Metformin can cause low vitamin B12 levels leading to a type of anemia that results in nerve damage. Take a B-complex vitamin and B12 lozenge, consume red meat, or obtain vitamin B12 shots to prevent anemia if taking metformin long term.

Alternatives

Glucose tolerance factor increases chromium, vitamin B6, and fiber; aloe, CoQ10, and vanadium all improve blood sugar control.

Diuretics

Examples

These include furosemide (Lasix), caffeine (Vivarin, Cafcit, Alert), indapamide (Lozol), pamabrom (Aqua-Ban, Diurex Aquagels, Diurex Water Capsules, Aqua-Ban with Pamabrom), and loop diuretics (Furosemide, Bumetanide, Torsemide, Etacrynic acid, Co-amilofruse).

Effects on Nutritional Status

Diuretics can lead to reduction in calcium, magnesium, the B vitamins, and especially potassium and sodium.

Alternatives

Diuretic alternatives include celery, dandelion greens, and parsley (salad of these three things). Supplement with potassium-rich minerala and a B vitamin–rich multivitamin.

Female Hormones

Examples

These include estrogen (Cenestin, Divigel, Femtrace, Ogen, Menest, Vagifrm, Elestrin), progestin (Makena, Plan B, My Way, Megace, Prometrium, Mirena, Skyla), and contraceptives (Nordette, Zeosa, Triphasil, Loestrin, Falmina, Rivora).

Effects on Nutritional Status

Hormone replacement and oral contraceptives can lead to reduced B vitamins, folate, and magnesium.

Alternatives

These include bio-identical hormones and nonpharmaceutical contraceptives.

Laxatives

Laxatives reduce vitamin and nutrient absorption.

Alternatives
Adding fiber to the diet, eating 3-4 organic dried prunes, and the judicious use of herbal laxatives like senna and casacada sagrada can eliminate the use of OTC laxatives.

Lipid Lowering/Statins

Examples
These include atorvastatin (Lipitor), simvastatin (Zocor), rosuvastatin (Crestor), pravastatin (Pravachol), lovastatin (Altoprev, Mevacor), ezetimibe/simvastatin (Vytorin), and fluvastatin (Lescol).

Effects on Nutritional Status
Statins lead to lower cholesterol, and they can increase anxiety and rarely suicidality.

One side effect of the statin group is muscle tenderness, pain, or weakness. Very rarely, this can progress to severe muscle breakdown, or rhabdomyolysis, which causes severe kidney damage. Other side effects are headache, nausea, flatulence, and constipation. Statins reduce CoQ10 levels.

Alternatives
One alternative is red rice yeast.

Nasal Decongestant

Examples
These include pseudoephedrine (Sudafed, Suphedrine, Wal-Phed, SudoGest), phenylephrine (Dimetapp Cold Drops, Nasop, Nasop12, Sudafed PE, Sudafed PE Children's Nasal Decongestant, Sudogest PE), and ephedrine (Bronkaid Dual Action Formula).

Effects on Nutritional Status
Decongestants should not be combined with MAO inhibitors as they can raise blood pressure.

Proton-Pump Inhibitors and Antacids

Examples
These include meprazole (Prilosec, Omesec), pantoprazole (Protonix), and esomeprazole (Nexium).

Effects on Nutritional Status
Chronic use of proton-pimp inhibitors (PPIs) interferes with the absorption of

nutrients; long-term use of PPIs may reduce the efficacy of nonsteroidal anti-inflammatory drugs, antithrombotic, and bisphosphonates. PPIs are particularly dangerous for the elderly, and they increase the risk of pneumonia, malnutrition, infections, and fractures (Maggio et al., 2013).

Antacids inhibit the absorption of vitamin B12 and can lead to a vitamin B12 deficiency, causing anemia, psychiatric problems, dementia, and nerve damage (Lam, Schneider, Zhao, & Corley, 2013). Antacids deplete vitamin B12, vitamin D, folic acid, calcium, iron, and zinc.

Nutritional Alternatives

These include vitamin U, chlorophyll (Gastrazyme), zinc carnosine, hydrochloride, and betaine supplements.

Essential Next Steps

- Identify current medications and their side effects.
- Identify medications' effect on nutritional status.
- Develop an enhanced self-care plan with the client.
- Plan a schedule for withdrawal in cooperation with the prescribing clinician.
- Conduct a family/social support session to identify specific areas of support or obstacles.
- Identify inpatient or at-home withdrawal processes.
- Discuss the timeline of your availability to the client during withdrawal and create an "availability contract" with the client so the client can reach the clinician.
- Engage (para) professional supports for food and nutrient administration where necessary.
- Begin nutritional protocols at least 2–4 weeks prior to initiating withdrawal.

CHAPTER 9

Putting It All Together: Making Recommendations for Success

Diet Essential: Integrate behavioral change strategies with the principle of substitutions.

The concept of biochemical individuality describes how each individual has unique nutritional requirements specific to her or his genetic makeup based in biological, cultural, environmental, and familial heritage. The essential concepts and methods I presented throughout the preceding chapters describe and explain the ways our clients can improve their well-being and reduce medication use.

Identifying the best nutritional approach for our clients, combined with determining how to best support behavioral changes while we engage their strengths to overcome obstacles, is the essence of mental health nutrition.

One of the first goals of a program for your clients is to help them to make the connection between what they eat and how they feel in order to overcome the nutritional dissociation they experience. What clients choose to eat frequently reflects a complex interplay between personality, emotions, family history, culture, and beliefs; all of this is bidirectionally influenced by biochemistry—their first and second brains. NT levels affect food choices and behaviors; some people use tryptophan-rich foods, fats, or sugar to self-medicate. The microbiome also influences food choices, as bacteria demand their nourishment. The brain depends on fats to communicate and the carotenoids (from carrots) affect how fast the brain processes information. The capacity to even adhere to a nutritional plan depends in part on NT levels; low dopamine may make it more difficult for a client to adhere to a nutrient program (Kharrazian, 2013), suggesting that we start with these clients by enhancing dopamine, the "pleasure" NT.

There will also be special issues that arise based on the mental health challenges facing each individual. Restoration of high-quality foods and delivery of nutrients is central to recovery from the psychotic disorders, though often fraught with challenges because self-care and adherence to a therapeutic program is very challenging with this population. For example, there are several avenues of nutritional intervention which have been demonstrated to improve and treat the schizophrenias and psychotic disorders. Factors affecting medication adherence depend heavily on patient support and therapeutic alliance along with client insight and the attitudes about and side effects toward medication (Kikkert et al., 2006). This reinforces the need to enhance the connections between the team members, especially between client, therapist, and prescriber. A reduction of side effects may be achieved by reduction of medication and an increase of nutritional methods.

Given all these interactions and the exploration of assessment, food, and nutritional protocols, where do we begin?

Our goal is three-fold:

1. Combine the knowledge we have acquired and analyzed about the client and then apply strategies drawn from psychoeducation, cognitive-behavioral methods with strengths-based methods, motivational interviewing, and coaching.
2. Define an initial mental health nutrition plan that will benefit our clients.
3. Support our clients to engage in and adhere to an increasingly progressive program of self-care; including expanding options for improved diet and supplementation protocols.

To accomplish these goals, we help the client to do the following:
• Identify positive changes that are achievable.
• Incorporate positive behaviors and relinquish negative habits.
• Identify and eliminate addictive foods one at a time.
• Present food and behavior substitutions that are satisfying.
• Choose the option of alternatives to harmful pharmaceuticals.
• Support strengths and work with obstacles.
• Support self-compassion.

NUTRITIONAL CHANGE TAKES TIME

It is natural that we want change to be fast, and we are conditioned to expect this by the promise of fast-acting medications and advertisements. But fast-acting often brings side effects. I advise a client with a chronic illness that it takes time to become ill; the causes have been in place for a while, and it will take time to recover and taking time to recover is worthwhile. Long-term chronic problems often require a period of 1–5 years to resolve, and I advise my clients to expect incremental changes every 3–6 months. I also reinforce that the degree to which they adhere to their program is the degree and rate at which they will recover. This is also not to suggest that false hope is offered. Some people, especially with chronic PTSD, anxiety, TBI, and psychotic disorders may still experience significant symptoms at times, but with this approach we seek a reduction of suffering and overall improvement, not a "cure."

I use the metaphor of the growth of a tree when I talk with clients about the time it takes for nutritional therapies to work. I may guide them through a visualization on this image; a tree grows slowly, but surely, digging roots into the earth for stability as it spreads its branches and leaves to the sky. The roots absorb water from below and the leaves from above. Nourishment comes from many directions. There are many roots and branches and leaves, and over time the tree becomes fuller and stronger. This slow but sure approach promises success so that when a wind blows the tree does not topple over easily but moves with the wind. This is the process of nature and mental health nutrition.

Change takes place by integrating positive activities (habits) first and then eliminating negative habits (activities). Practically, this means a step-by-step approach to identify one positive behavior that will change or replace a negative behavior and by employing the principle of substitutions outlined in this book.

I also focus on the specific actions that will improve well-being. Based on goals we have set together. I ask clients to pay attention and watch for specific changes and suggest how long it will take to observe a change.

I focus on specific changes to watch for, such as the following:

- Reducing caffeine leads to better sleep.
- Eating breakfast and better quality protein will improve energy and mood stability.
- Increasing anti-inflammatory foods will reduce pain.
- Increasing magnesium intake leads to less anxiety and improved sleep.

STARTING OUT

In Chapter 1, I reviewed the spectrum of roles the mental health nutrition clinician might play, including (1) psychoeducation, (2) collaboration, and (3) autonomous practice. The clinician new to nutrition may begin by incorporating aspects of nutrition into treatment. Generally our clients have suffered for many years without knowing why. Psychoeducation provides explanations illustrating the links between nutritional and dietary patterns and mental health. Psychoeducation also includes information about how particular nutritional recommendations are essential to the empowerment process. I explain that B-complex vitamins are used for blood glucose regulation and mood. This can reinforce a better understanding of how a B vitamin every day is important. I will share an herbal tea in the waiting room at each appointment along with a handout of the recipe. The tea is presented with a description of the ingredients and what those ingredients are good for and how to prepare the drink.

As you develop experience and expertise working with a client, you will deepen and broaden a comprehensive plan. When a clinician is just beginning to incorporate nutrition, I suggest first setting aside some time during each appointment to discuss the client's self-care behaviors, focusing on nutrition. This approach provides an opportunity to make recommendations and discuss any obstacles while still carrying out the psychotherapeutic process. Focusing on the information collected in the Food-Mood diary is a good place to begin this process, and this will lead to providing homework that incorporates the results and decisions arising from a discussion about the diary. Providing handouts and resources complements this process. Once this first phase is complete, the next stage involves a more complex analysis and the development of a written report containing dietary and nutritional supplementation protocols.

FIVE STAGES OF CHANGE MODEL

The stages of change model describes five points of readiness and provides a framework for understanding the change process. By identifying where a person is in the change cycle, interventions can be tailored to the individual's "readiness" to progress in the recovery process. Interventions that do not match the person's readiness are less likely to succeed and more likely to hurt rapport, create resistance, and impede change.

The stages of change model, which began in motivational interviewing to treat the addictions, has excellent application in nutritional counseling. Just as we strive to find a method or technique that is isomorphic to the client's belief system, identifying the stage of change of the client promises greater success in aligning intervention and goals.

Providing a Written and Verbal Report

I write a comprehensive written report and analysis for each of my clients. I then allocate time to review it with them while they read along. I suggest recommendations in the report that are tailored to the client's needs along with reference materials.

Based on your client's readiness for change and the degree to which she is willing to make changes in her current nutritional patterns, you may choose to go step by step with small incremental changes, or your client may be ready to implement a comprehensive analysis that points the way to change that will be enacted over the next 6–12 months. Their stage will determine your approach. For example, you may decide to work with a client using the principle of incorporating one healthy behavior while eliminating one unhealthy choice.

Based on the stage of change and motivational interviewing methods I describe next, goals and steps can be divided into 1-, 3-, or 6-month phases that are flexible. This approach allows the client to act immediately and also keep in mind future goals. Following the initial review of the plan, the client will need time to digest the report and ask questions, and it is very likely that when the client returns to the next appointment, more questions and concerns will arise. Subsequent sessions can be designed to continue the conduct of therapy with part of each session assigned to discuss progress, obstacles, and "check in" about the client's progress. Our approach in this work will be colored by our own theoretical orientation, but we must maintain therapeutic rapport and trust regardless of our methods.

During the assessment process you have compiled and integrated information about the client and her narrative and the kinds of strengths and challenges she brings to the change process. At this stage, you will clarify those strengths and identify obstacles and prioritize goals with her. Often too much focus is placed on what clients cannot eat rather than what they can. This can be an emotional trigger. Focus on what they can have, and include foods they enjoy eating. You may discover that your client will benefit from a variety of pills or capsules, but you may also discover that she has difficulty swallowing them. You may want to suggest liquid oils or powdered nutrients. A client may discuss financial obstacles in buying nutrients; part of your emphasis may be to identify how to ensure those nutrients are available through whole food preparation and selected supplement purchases. An example of this approach is exploring whether it might be better to obtain probiotic bacteria by preparing sauerkraut or homemade yogurt at home or by purchasing a (more expensive) supplement.

You may have discovered during the intake that your client is interested in changing her diet, but her family members are not willing or eager to do so. The failure to participate in a whole health program by the family is a sure recipe for failure. You may, therefore, choose at this stage to engage the family in a session or more that informs and educates them about the needs for these changes and that gains their agreement. Finally, as you work with your client, you may find that she will benefit from group support even more than individual counseling, and she can join your food-mood support group.

In the report, I provide narrative sections that include the following:

- Symptoms and complaints
- A list of the goals for change the client named during the intake process
- Three short-term action items of change
- Three medium- and long-term action items of change
- Sample dietary suggestions that are isomorphic to the client
- Basic diet or food guidelines including metabolizer type and ideal range of food ratios
- Suggestions for additional testing
- Nutritional supplement protocol
- Additional resources and handouts including special recipes or suggested reading

Principles of Dietary and Nutrient Recommendations

- Start with where you will observe the fastest and most important changes first.
- Start slowly and build according to adherence capacity.
- Always balance the use of vitamins, minerals, botanicals, and glandulars.
- Review and change the protocol every 3–6 months (or as necessary).
- Combine nutrients where possible to include powders and liquids or reduce the number of pills and capsules required.

Stage of Change 1: Precontemplation

The earliest stage of precontemplation is where clients may not want to change, may be unaware that they need to change, or may feel helpless to change (Herrin & Larkin, 2013, p. 99). Linking the results of the Food-Mood diary is a place to begin as clients start to make connections between mood and food choices and behaviors. This is where I began with Joan the first week as we reviewed her diary. Small incremental changes bring fast results, like a high-protein, low-carbohydrate diet for 7 days to stabilize her blood sugar. The assessment process can also be divided into sections to address relevant symptoms or behaviors so that once the veil of avoidance is lifted your clients do not feel overwhelmed.

The Elicit-Provide-Elicit Technique

At every stage of my consultations with clients, I apply methods that actively engage the client in the change process. The Elicit-Provide-Elicit (E-P-E) technique, presented by Miller and Rollnick (2012) in the motivational interviewing approach, is a way of determining what level of understanding the patient already has regarding the changes she could be making and to clarify misconceptions where needed. It also addresses obstacles to change and allows the practitioner to help the patient find a way to integrate the changes. There are three parts to the E-P-E technique:

Elicit: Asking the patient directly what it is that they already know.

Provide: Clarifying any misconceptions or lack of knowledge they may have.

Elicit: Exploring what this information means to the patient.

Joan's story continues from Chapter 3, Sample Dialogue 2: Food-Mood Diary.

Joan and I discussed her use of poor-quality fats that emerged during the Food-Mood diary and assessment. This is an important first step that can educate her about eliminating the poor-quality fats and substituting them with the good-quality fats, and it identifies a little further the challenges Joan may experience.

Following is an example of how the E-P-E technique worked with Joan to support her use of better quality fats and oils for mental health and elimination of trans fats.

Elicit (Clinician): Joan, I'm curious about what you already know about the effects of fats and oils on depression.

Joan: Well, I heard that some fats are good for you and some are not, but I am not sure which are which.

Provide (Clinician): You are exactly right; there are differences between good fats and bad fats. We now know that good fats improve mood and can help depression, while bad fats can contribute to depression.

Joan: It seems like what they tell us is always changing and it is confusing, so I just don't do anything.

Asking for permission to provide (Clinician): It certainly can be confusing! Would it be helpful if I tried to simplify it a bit for you?

Joan (nods): Yes, please do.

Provide (Clinican): Some things we may have heard about fats in the past, such as butter being bad for you, turn out to be untrue. And now we know that eliminating a lot of fried foods and fast foods is healthy, and eating good quality butter and extra-virgin olive oil and coconut oil is very helpful for the brain and mood.

Joan: That makes sense. But seems like it could be expensive.

Elicit (Clinician): Sounds like you would be willing to make some changes as long as they're not too expensive. We have discussed both eliminating unhealthy foods and adding in some healthy ones. Of the options we discussed, what could you see yourself doing at this point?

Joan: I think if I could do it one thing at a time and find some ways to still enjoy food and treats, then I wouldn't feel deprived. Perhaps if I started with just replacing my processed snacks with those that have these healthier fats.

Provide (Clinician): Joan, I think changing one thing at a time is a great plan and you may be pleasantly surprised that you will still enjoy many of your favorite foods and not feel deprived. And you seem very committed to improving your physical and mental health, so I think you will be successful. What other questions do you have before we end today?

NOTE: Adapted dialogue from Susan Butterworth (2010), Health coaching strategies to improve patient-centered outcomes, *The Journal of the American Osteopathic Association*, 110(4), Suppl. 5, eS12–eS14.

Box 9.1
HAPIfork

The HAPIfork is a biofeedback, electronic fork that helps you monitor and track your eating habits. It also alerts you with the help of indicator lights and gentle vibrations when you are eating too fast. Every time you bring food from your plate to your mouth with your fork, this action is called a "fork serving." The HAPIfork also measures:

- How long it took to eat your meal
- The amount of "fork servings" taken per minute
- Intervals between "fork servings"

Assessing Importance Technique

Another important technique introduced by Miller and Rollnick (2012) involves "Assessing Importance." This provides an opportunity to enhance client motivation to adhere to the nutritional program. This method allows you to score the importance a client assigns to her or his behavior on a scale of 0 to 10, evoke change talk, and then identify what can increase a level of importance for a required change of behavior.

An example of the Assessing Importance technique with Joan is as follows:

Clinician: Joan, we have reviewed some of the changes you can make about the use of good fats versus bad fats. I'd like to hear a little more about where you feel this change fits in to your life currently. Would that be okay?

Joan: (Nods.)

Clinician: On a scale of 0 to 10, with 0 meaning not important at all, and 10 meaning the most important thing in your life, where would you rate the importance of replacing bad fats with good fats in your diet?

Joan: 8.

Clinician: That's pretty high! Why are you an 8 and not a 2 or 3?

Joan: Well, I do like the taste of virgin olive oil, although is can be expensive.

Clinician: Why else?

Joan: It's good to hear that butter isn't all that bad for me, because I've always liked it and it's cheap and easy to use.

Clinician: Why else is this so important to you?

Joan: I'm intrigued by the thought that these changes could actually help my moods. And it's really important for me to feel better in that way.

Clinician: Ok, so although cost is an issue for you, you seem to have a lot of good reasons for making these changes in your diet, especially starting with the butter and olive oil. How confident are you that you could make these changes?

Joan: Oh very confident—it really won't be that hard.

Clinician: So where does this all leave you? What is your next concrete step?

Joan: Well, I'm going to buy butter at the store for sure and check out the cost of olive oil to see where it's cheaper. And I'm going to try to buy some healthier snacks like we talked about as well.

Clinician: I can hear the excitement and commitment in your voice! I look forward to checking in with you next time to see how it all went.

NOTE: Dialogue adapted from Susan Butterworth (2010), Health-coaching strategies to improve patient-centered outcomes, *The Journal of the American Osteopathic Association*, 110 (4), suppl. 5, eS12–eS14.

Stage of Change 2: Contemplation: Acknowledging That There Is a Problem but Struggling with Ambivalence

This is the stage where Joan is positioned and I suspect will return to with each change she contemplates making. In the contemplation stage, Joan considers the positive reasons for change. If I eat less fast food and cook for myself more, for example, I will have more energy and will feel better. On the other hand, it will take a lot more time and energy just to get started. And, of course, there are the obstacles to enacting that change. This is where we work with the ambivalence (Herrin & Larkin, 2013).

The Evoking Change Talk

Evoking change talk is a cornerstone of motivational interviewing and is designed to engage the client to identify reasons to change and elicit a plan of action in at least one area according to the patient's readiness to change. The objective is to evoke the patient's desire, ability, reasons, and need to change in order to strengthen the patient's commitment to the behavior during a session. This "change talk" predicts increased commitment strength to the lifestyle change, which is directly correlated with clinical outcomes.

> **Clinician:** Joan, what might be the top three benefits to you if you changed over to healthy fats?
>
> **Joan:** Well, I think you said it was better for my brain and might prevent memory loss, so that is important to me. I also think my skin would look better, and I believe I might be in a better mood more of the time.
>
> **Clinician:** How would your life be different in 6 months if you were consistently making choices to eat healthy fats?
>
> **Joan:** I have been so moody and fatigued that I would expect in 6 months I would have more energy and not be so depressed. Plus I would feel more in control of my life.
>
> **Clinician:** Wow, that's a pretty powerful statement: feeling more in control of your life. How would that impact you?
>
> **Joan:** It would impact everything—my confidence, my self-esteem, my relationships, my anxiety.

NOTE: Adapted dialogue from Susan Butterworth (2010), Health-coaching strategies to improve patient-centered outcomes, *The Journal of the American Osteo-pathic Association*, 110 (4), suppl. 5, eS12–eS14.

Stage of Change 3: Preparation/Determination

Taking Steps and Getting Ready to Change

The preparation or decision-making stage of change is where action will be undertaken within the next 1–2 months. This is where specific goals and strategies are identified (Herrin & Larkin, 2013). Joan has identified some actions she can take, and these will be reinforced at each of our meetings.

Stage of Change 4: Action/Willpower

This stage of change is about acting on behavioral strategies in specific and practical ways. Joan will engage in menu planning, make new purchases, and may begin to identify who in her life can support her. She may also update her Food-Mood diary that we can review when we meet.

Stage of Change 5: Maintenance

The maintenance stage is still in Joan's future. Her incremental changes with healthy fats may become solidified over the next several months. We will review obstacles to using quality fats, such as eating out or being a guest, and explore how to cope with these challenges while processing any triggers for relapse (Herrin & Larkin, 2013).

COACHING FOR ADHERENCE

There are as many styles of coaching as there are psychotherapeutic styles, and how we coach our clients generally derives from our own approach to counseling. Like therapies, coaching styles should be congruent with the clients' belief systems. Coaching styles can reflect their stage of change, fit their personality, or nudge them gently in a new direction. I prefer an eclectic approach that integrates self-coaching, which supports the client's inner voice or inner coach; is solution focused, which identifies specific actionable changes; and incorporates mindfulness, which supports a compassionate, moment-to-moment approach to self change. Mindfulness balances both goals for change with a "no goals" approach. I also use a little directive coaching when appropriate; when a client's belief in what is possible is flagging, or if the client doubts certain effects, I use a directive approach sparingly, like one adds sea salt to a meal: "If you make the changes I am recommending, you will get better," "I have no doubt that if you do this you will improve," "If you make the commitment, you will see the results." Clients always benefit from unconditional positive regard, but sometimes they also need firm reassurance in spite of their doubts.

Box 9.2 describes simple table designs that support desired behavioral changes.

Box 9.2
Plates and Colors

The size and color of dinnerware affect how much you eat. Smaller plates reduce portion size. Colors that contrast the food on the plate will help you to eat less, and plate colors that match the food will help you to eat more. Tablecloths with a low contrast to plate color will reduce the desire to overeat (Van Ittersum & Wansink, 2012).

Break Down Expected Costs on a Daily or Monthly Basis

Finances are often a concern in making healthful changes. For example, Joan expressed concern that cost was a factor in her decision about changing over to olive oil. It is important to work with your client creatively to reinforce the medicinal benefits of healthy foods and nutrients. Adopting preventive strategies may significantly reduce the costs for health and medicine. Most nutritional products are sold at retail prices that are generally marked up by 100% of the wholesale price. If you coordinate with a nonprofit cooperative purchasing, a wholesale club, or tribal clinics/pharmacies, it is possible to secure the very highest quality nutrients at wholesale prices. This makes them more affordable for your clients with very little markup. Occasionally a physician can prescribe vitamins and oils for diagnoses such as fish oil for major depression, and insurance companies will cover the costs. Many companies will provide product samples that you can share with your clients. Box 9.3 identifies a variety of "tips" to save money while shopping for high-quality foods.

Box 9.3
Money-Saving Shopping and Food-Buying Tips

- Join a CSA or volunteer at a co-op or farm and get reduced prices.
- Day-old bins at the supermarket often have vegetables that make good soups.
- Healthy food is most often on the perimeter of the supermarket.
- Buy in bulk.

- Buy bones and cheap cuts of meat for flavoring and making broths for soups and to sauté.
- Fresh produce is lowest in price when it is in season.
- Shop at ethnic food stores, where they often have less expensive herbs, fresh roots, and low farm-to-store pricing, including Mexican, Asian, Indian stores, and more.
- Buy frozen foods like berries to save money and retain quality.
- Shop so that half of your plate is fruits and vegetables.
- Leafy greens like kale, chard, collards, spinach, and broccoli are some of the most nutritious, least expensive things you can buy.
- Canned salmon, sardines (boneless, skinless), smoked mackerel, and anchovies are inexpensive alternatives to fresh fish.
- If packaged or canned food has more than four ingredients on the label, then avoid it.

Planning meals by writing up a grocery list in advance will save money and time. There are a lot of useful and easy to use apps for the computer or other instruments. Among these is one called "Cooksmarts" that helps with meal planning and recipes.

Some basic principles of meal planning are outlined next.

Meal Planning

1. Create a list of your family's favorite recipes and make sure they are easily accessible, whether these are in cookbooks or bookmarked on your browser.
2. Clean and organize your freezer because you will need to make room for leftovers. Having glass storage containers and glass baking dishes will come in handy for storing leftovers. Plastic freezer bags are also useful.
3. Keep track of items that you are running low on or that you need to restock in your cupboards. A magnetized whiteboard on the fridge can be quite handy for this, or even just a notepad that you keep in the kitchen. Be sure to bring this list with you when you go to the store.
4. Keep track of the meals that you will be cooking for the week using a calendar in the kitchen, a day planner, or a magnetized whiteboard. Use this to make notes about things that may need to be done in advance, like thawing or marinating meat.
5. In addition to planning dinner for each night of the week, it may be useful to also plan the other meals of the day, including snacks.

6. Before going to the store, create your list. Look at your favorite recipes and pick out which ones you want to cook for the week. Write down everything that you will need. Make columns for different parts of the store and list the ingredients that you will need from each one. For instance, use columns for produce, bulk, dairy, meat, and frozen food.

7. During the week save peelings from vegetables in a tub in the fridge so you can add them to your vegetable broth.

A common reason that people do not prepare healthy food is because they do not have enough time to cook. Preparing a large, healthy meal on the weekend and cooking enough so that there are leftovers is one way to ensure that there is healthy food available during busy times. Meals that freeze well include broth-based soups and casseroles. When making a casserole, double the recipe and freeze the extra in small meal-size containers that can be defrosted and warmed on another day.

Plan and Prep a Week at a Time

1. Pick a day of the week to organize food and food prep for the week. For example, many of the basics can be prepared on a Sunday and will last the week.

2. Roast one chicken: eat half on Sunday night and the other half can be boned and prepared as a chicken salad for lunch. Add the leftover bones to the bone broth pot. Make a Crock-Pot chicken soup from the other chicken, adding vegetables, onions, and garlic, then strain the broth and use as a base for preparing rice or as a soup later in the week, and bone the chicken and store for later in the week or as a snack.

3. Integrate the family in cooking or plan a potluck or food exchange with friends. If you are making soup, make a double batch and trade it with a friend who is making another soup or casserole.

4. When beginning to cook a meal, think ahead for the next few meals and take any preparation methods into account, such as soaking legumes or nuts, or marinating meat.

5. Wash and prepare your vegetables for the week to have them ready for easy use in cooking or for snacking. Include carrots, celery, broccoli, lettuce, bell peppers, mushrooms, zucchini, and so on.

6. Gather all the vegetables you want for salads and prepare raw salads in jars for 3–4 days at a time.

7. Make a vegetable broth rich in potassium by placing all the stems and ends of vegetables in a Crock-Pot.

8. Peel large amounts of garlic, place whole bulbs in the oven, and bake at 300 degrees Fahrenheit until the individual cloves open. Remove from oven and pull apart individual cloves.

9. Use a Crock-Pot in which you place all your meat bones for bone broth.

10. Fill a baking tray of sweet potatoes and bake; store in the fridge. They can be sliced and eaten cold, made into a custard as a dessert, reheated and topped with butter, or sliced and pan-fried quickly in butter and balsamic vinegar.

11. Steam beets and store in the fridge; you can add yogurt and eat as a snack, or eat sliced over salad.

12. Prepare 2–3 salad dressings, choosing from among the recipes in the appendices, and store in bottles in the fridge (see Appendix Y for Salad Dressings).

13. Prepare several cups of brown rice or another grain, which can be reheated and added to soups or stir-fried as needed throughout the week.

14. Soak almonds and raisins—cover almonds and raisins with water and place in Tupperware. Let it sit overnight. Use as needed.

15. Place a cheese slice and a hard-boiled egg together in a Tupperware for an easy protein snack.

16. Put bone broth in a thermos to have it available throughout the day.

Traveling With Cooler Bags and Thermoses

Having cooler bags with you when you travel allows you to buy healthy foods that are easy to eat on the road, rather than relying on fast food and restaurants for your meals. Fill baggies with water and freeze, and then use these as freezer packs to keep things cool. Good travel foods include hard-boiled eggs; dried fruit and nuts; fresh fruit and raw vegetables; aged hard cheeses; gluten-free or whole grain crackers; canned Pacific wild salmon, sardines, or anchovies; water in glass bottles; olive oil and vinegar to add to salads; a Tupperware filled with fresh greens; Kombucha or herbal beverages in glass bottles; and almond butter.

Tips for Traveling and Eating While on Vacation

1. Avoid high-carbohydrate foods at breakfast and opt for simple protein foods like fried eggs and bacon (note that at hotels and buffets most scrambled

eggs come from a premade egg mix and sausage meat has additives, so choose the fruit and hard-boiled eggs when possible and avoid the pastries).

2. Order salad with grilled meat for lunch and ask for simple dressings like olive oil and vinegar/lemon. They usually have it in the kitchen.

3. Choose proteins that are less likely to be mass produced, like venison, bison, or lamb, and choose wild-caught fish (preferably from Alaska).

4. Avoid soups in restaurants as they are usually made with broths high in wheat and MSG.

5. Travel with a small supply of energy bars, almonds, rice cakes, almond butter, hard-boiled eggs, and canned sardines until you can get to a store.

6. If staying with family, you can buy groceries to contribute healthy options to meals.

COOKING METHODS

The relationship between whole foods, slow or minimal processing, freshness, and good nutrition is unquestionable. But many people do not know where to begin. For many foods, the least amount of processing (raw) ensures the maximum nutrition and healthful benefits while for others a long slow cook or a quick steam is best. Slow cooking in water, boiling, salting, broiling, pickling, roasting, baking, drying, steaming, fermenting, and smoking are the preferable processing methods that ensure maximum nutrition. Frying, deep-fat frying, high-temperature cooking, and preserving with nitrates and nitrites are the most injurious methods and contribute to poor mental health.

Eliminating Microwave Use

Microwaves alter the molecular structure of food and hence its nutritional benefits; therefore, microwave ovens should never be used to prepare food. Microwaves produce unnatural molecules in food and transform other molecules and amino acids into toxic and carcinogenic forms. The "lazy Susan" plate inside the microwave is ideal for the storage of spice and herb bottles.

Crock-Pot

If you have only one appliance in the kitchen, it should be the versatile Crock-Pot. Crock-Pot cooking is one of the best ways to introduce cooking to someone who does not cook or who does not have a lot of time to cook. Using a Crock-Pot is inexpensive, and slow-cooking foods, especially bones, meats, and legumes at low temperatures is the best way to retain nutrients. Always use unsalted butter and sea salt when cooking with the Crock-Pot, and be sure to put meat juices back into sauces and stews—they are rich in "happiness" amino acids.

Blenders

Blenders are the next appliance to buy for making smoothies, sauces, and dressings. High-speed blenders are the best option, as the typical household blenders do not have the ability to process hard foods like nuts and seeds, and will not produce as smooth of a liquid.

PROVIDE RESOURCES

In our work with clients we also may take on the role as advocates for social change and food security. Thus, knowing local resources and referral points for clients will be essential. Guiding them with forms such as their flexible spending accounts and health savings accounts can often cover some of their expenses for nutritional supplements. Certain diagnostic categories also can bring the cost down; for example, a diagnosis of "obesity" will provide support for health club membership.

Community-Supported Agriculture and Home Gardens

Many regions have community-supported agriculture programs (CSAs.) These are local food production farms that also have a centralized area of distribution in urban settings. Volunteering on a farm during the summer brings cost down, and many of these farms also engage in humane animal husbandry, which can supply quality animal-based proteins. Encouraging home gardens, an herbal kitchen with culinary herbs, or just the exploration of the use of herbal roots and leaves is an important start for clients making changes.

COUPLES AND FAMILIES

Mindful eating extends to couples, families, and group activity as well. Even the simple though often forgotten act of eating together as a family and sharing news of the day leads to reduction of weight gain compared to families who watch TV (Wansink & Van Kleef, 2013). How do we get children to participate in healthy nutritional and behavioral changes?

Beginning at age 8, children are at a good point to start helping in the kitchen.

Cooking together is fun and involves skill building, including learning math and measurements, geography, chemistry, and nutrition along with patience and teamwork. If your child is studying something in school, why not plan a theme dinner around that geographic location and include ethnic cuisine and invite one of her or his friends, or their family, to participate. The skill of cooking is becoming a lost art and equipping your child to cook is a lasting healthy gift. For example, we have tamale-making night; in addition to the fun group effort, it is an opportunity to talk about tamales and where corn is from, where salsas and chilies are from, as well as coconut and chocolate. Younger children can learn to count by measuring and practice their reading skills by reading recipes.

Cooking With Kids

- Take children shopping so they can help pick ingredients.
- Have healthy snacks in easy-to-reach places for kids to encourage healthy eating.
- Make it fun and exciting to encourage them—play music, have a conversation.
- Make a list of activities for children to help with in the kitchen.
- Make yogurt.
- Make sprouts and watch them grow.
- Plant wheat berries and watch them grow into wheatgrass.
- Make healthy cupcakes.
- Measure ingredients.
- Make Healthy Chocolate Almond Coconut treats.
- Make smoothies.
- Make sauerkraut and then put it on hot dogs.
- Make gluten-free pizza dough and then have a pizza party.
- Use a spiralizer; they are a lot of fun.

Psychoeducation Nutrition Groups

Developing a mental health nutrition group focused on food/mood can be effective for all clients, including those with eating disorders, those in sexual abuse recovery or addiction recovery, and for people with depression or schizophrenia. These groups can also be organized for children with a diagnosis of ADHD and for the elderly.

I have worked with many of these diagnostic specific groups and the basics are the same: Engage people to be more compassionate with themselves; consider the role of food and eating behaviors in their lives; engage a more social psychoeducational approach infused with mindfulness exercises; educate about the second brain; review myths about foods; and reframe food as medicine and share recipes, tips, and support.

This psychoeducational program combines experiential methods of mindful eating with nutrition education and psychotherapeutic exchange and sharing among participants. The groups are limited to 6–8 people and may run from 90 to 120 minutes over a renewable, 12-week series.

A 12-Week Food/Mood Psychoeducational Group Format

- Week 1: Introductions and compassionate goal setting; introduction to mindfulness.
- Week 2: Mindfulness practice; introduction of food/mood diary; further reflection on goals and obstacles
- Week 3: Sharing about the meaning of food and one's relationship with food; the mindfulness raisin exercise.
- Week 4: Foods in the family of origin/current family; the chewing mindfulness exercise.
- Week 5: Food and the addictions: How do we use food to self-medicate? What are the healthy alternatives to sugar and refined foods?
- Week 6: Food and body image: How do we make decisions about what we eat?
- Week 7: The second brain: Food and digestion. How do we feel when we eat? From mouth to elimination: What foods and nutrients enhance digestion?
- Week 8: Fear of fats; fear of fat.
- Week 9: Making healthy foods; smoothies.
- Week 10: Overcoming obstacles; making a list for support.
- Week 11: Identifying strengths and next steps; plan for final gathering.
- Week 12: Final "party" where each person brings a healthy dish with a copy of the recipe and shares its benefits for mental well-being.

Integrating nutrition into mental health practice is both feasible and essential. It is the missing piece in our work as mental health clinicians. The approaches outlined in this book promise improvement—ranging from the most basic level of stabilizing mood by managing blood glucose levels along with more advanced approaches of medication withdrawal and comprehensive nutrient schedules for the prevention and treatment of chronic illness. Every clinician can make the steps necessary to integrate the approaches I have presented. To do so requires exploring these methods first for oneself, and then initiating the process step by step with willing clients. If the clinician offers these services, people will respond positively. To do this effectively may require collaboration with various other clinicians or more training. A resource list for options is provided in Appendix Z. This, in turn, will lead to a thriving practice in any setting that will enhance treatment efficacy for people of all cultures and ages.

Essential Next Steps

- Work with the client to identify first steps for change.
- Incorporate motivational interviewing into nutritional changes.
- Coach for adherence.
- Provide a written nutritional report and review it with the client.
- Provide specific resources and handouts to support success.
- Consider the role of group support and develop your Food/Mood group.
- Enjoy a healthy meal with family and friends.

To access a multitude of bonus recipes, downloadable sample forms, and other supplementary resources, visit http://nutitionessentialsformentalhealth.com

APPENDIX A

General Guidelines for a Hypoglycemic Diet

- Eat six small meals a day, or three meals with snacks in between.
- Always mix proteins and carbohydrates.
- No refined sugar or flour.
- Eat 2–3 ounces of food every 2–3 hours depending on need.
- Don't allow yourself to get hungry.
- Never eat carbohydrates alone—always include protein.
- Eat a little before exercise and after.
- Drink plenty of water.

An Example of a Hypoglycemic Meal Plan

Time	Snack	Meal
6 a.m.		1 egg and 1 piece of whole grain (or gluten-free bread), with some herbal tea
8 a.m.	2 oz of protein with whole grains, or oatmeal with nuts	
10 a.m.	1 apple, or 1 oz of dried fruit (such as organic dried apricots) and 10 almonds	
12 p.m.		4–6 oz of protein (animal) with 1 sweet potato and 1 cup of raw vegetables with olive oil and vinegar or lemon salad dressing
2 p.m.	1 tablespoon nut butter (rice cake optional)	
4 p.m.	Hard-boiled egg (whole grain, gluten-free bread optional)	
6 p.m.		4–6 oz protein (beans or animal protein) with 1 cup greens (salad or steamed) with vegetables, and 1 cup of whole grains
Before bed	2 crackers (gluten-free optional) and 1 oz. of cheese; or 1 oz turkey or tuna	

Client Intake Form

Client Name _____ Date _____

Client Information

Address _____

City _____State _____ Zip _____

Phone (Home) _____Work _____

Cell _____

E-mail _____

Date of Birth _____ Gender: M F

Employer_____ Occupation_____

Marital Status: Single   Married   Partnership   Divorced   Separated   Widowed

Spouse/Partner Name _____# of Children_____

Emergency Contact _____

Contact Phone:

Home _____Work _____C ell _____

Primary Health Care Provider

Name _____

Address _____

City/State/Zip _____

Phone _____ Fax _____

I give my therapist permission to consult with my health care provider regarding my health and treatment.

Comments _____

Initials _____ Date _____

1. Current Health Information

Height _____ Weight _____

List Health Concerns

Primary _____

_____

_____

o Mild   o Moderate   o Disabling   o Constant   o Intermittent

o Symptoms □ w/activity

o Symptoms □ w/activity

o Getting worse   o getting better   o no change

Treatment received _____

_____

Secondary _____

_____

o Mild   o Moderate   o Disabling   o Constant   o Intermittent

o Symptoms □ w/activity

o Symptoms □ w/activity

o Getting worse   o getting better   o no change

Treatment received_____

_____

Have you ever received Energy Therapy before?

o Y   o N   Frequency? _____

Have you ever received Manual Therapy before?

o Y   o N   Frequency? _____

Have you ever received Psychotherapy before?

o Y   o N   Frequency? _____

What kinds of practitioners (formal/informal) have you worked with around food/diet/nutrition (example: Dietician, Health Coach, or Nutritional Therapist)?

_____

_____

List all conditions currently monitored by a Health Care Provider.

_____

_____

List Daily Activities

Work _____

Work Hours and Schedule _____

Do you now or have you ever worked the night shift?   o Y   o N

If so, please explain _____

If currently, what are your hours? _____

Home/Family _____

Social/Recreational _____

Circle the above activities affected by your condition.

       o all of the above

Check other activities affected:

      o sleep   o washing   o dressing   o fitness

How do you reduce stress? _____

Pain?_____

What are your goals for receiving therapy? _____

2. Health History

List & include dates & treatments. Add pages if necessary.

Surgeries _____

_____

Accidents (physical-psychological) _____

_____

Major Illnesses _____

_____

Women

Last Pap _____ First day of last menstrual period _____

Marital/Partner History (Years Married) _____ Number of Children _____

Ages of Children _____ Number of pregnancies _____

Complications _____

Use of Contraceptive   o Y   o N

What type? _____

Abortions/Miscarriages? _____

4. Family Medical History

Please give age, lists of any illness, or if deceased. If deceased, list cause of death and age of death.

Mother:

Father:

Siblings:

Mother's parents:

Father's parents:

5. Current Dietary Habits

Please list any specific diets that you are currently following, for example, vegan diet (no dairy, meat, fish or eggs), vegetarian, Atkins, paleo, DASH, raw, GAPS, etc.:_____

_____

Eating Behaviors

Briefly describe your mealtime and snack patterns:

_____

_____

_____

Food Allergies and Sensitivities

o Wheat allergy   o Wheat sensitivity

o Dairy allergy   o Dairy sensitivity

Please list any other known or suspected food allergies and sensitivities: _____

Are there foods you could not give up? If so, which ones? _____

Current Food Preparation Methods

Who's doing the shopping?   o You   o Family member   o Friend   o Other

Do you eat with people or alone   o People   o Alone

Do you eat out?   o Yes   o No

If so, how often?   o Once monthly   o Twice monthly   o Weekly   o Daily

What kinds of places do you eat out?_____

Do you prepare your own food?   o Yes   o No

Do you enjoy cooking?   o Yes   o No

How do you feel about food preparation and cooking? _____

_____

How much time do you spend preparing food each day?

o Never   o 1 hour   o 2 hours   o 3 hours

Food Symptoms

Please circle any of the following food symptoms that you experience on a regular basis:

Stomachaches	Burping	Itching
Sinus	Flatulence	Flushing
Fatigue	Bloating	

6. Diet History

Were you breastfed, and if so, until what age?   o Yes   o No   Until age: _____

Were you fed formula as a baby?   o Yes   o No

Did you experience ear infections as a child?   o Yes   o No

Use of antibiotics as a child/adult?   o Yes   o No

Please list any other childhood illnesses and the age at which they occurred: _____

_____

Please list any digestive complaints you recall having as a child (for example, stomach pains, diarrhea, constipation, gas, etc.) _____

_____

Please list any other physical complaints you recall as a child (for example, fatigue, headaches, pain):

_____

Acne as an adolescent?   o None   o Mild   o Moderate   o Severe

History of fasting?   o Yes   o No

Did you experience any eating disorders during adolescence?   o Yes   o No

If so, please describe: _____

_____

Briefly describe your family's eating habits and meal times (Did you eat as a family? Did you eat at the table or in front of the television? Did you fend for yourself? Were foods prepared from packages? Was there fighting at meal-time?): _____

_____

_____

_____

_____

7. Medications (Current and Past Use)

In the table below, please list any medications, including pharmaceuticals and antibiotics that you are currently or have previously taken.

Medication	Prescribed For	Dosage	Frequency	Dates/Duration
E.g., Wellbutrin	Depression	100 mg	2/day	2010 – present

8. Use of Non-Pharmaceutical Substances

CURRENT	PAST	TIMES PER WEEK / COMMENTS
o	o	tobacco _____
o	o	alcohol/drugs _____
o	o	coffee/soda _____
o	o	other _____

Are you a recovering alcoholic?　　o Yes　　o No

History of drug or alcohol abuse?　　o Yes　　o No

Long term use of prescription/recreational drugs?   o Yes   o No

If yes, how often and in what form? _____

Do you use Nutrasweet (aspartame)?   o Yes   o No

9. Use of Nutritional Supplements / Herbs / Minerals

In the table below, please list any supplements, including vitamins, minerals, herbs, amino acids, and hormones that you are currently or have previously taken.

Supplements	Manufacturer	Dosage	Frequency	Dates/Duration
E.g., Vitamin C	Biotics Research	500 mg	2/day	2012—4 months

10. Detoxification

If you are currently or have previously done any detoxification methods, please indicate which ones by filling in the table below. If you have done a detoxification method that is not listed in the table, write the name of it in the row marked "other."

Method	How Often	When	Dates/Duration	Desired/Perceived Benefits
E.g., Skin Brushing	1–2 times / day	Before bathing	2013–present	Strengthen immunity
Skin Brushing				
Coffee Enema				
Liver Flush				
Juice Fast				
Colon Cleanser				
Epsom Salt Bath Soak (magnesium sulfate)				

Salt and Baking Soda Bath				
Vinegar Bath				
Sweats/ Saunas				
Castor Oil Packs				
Master Cleanse				
Other				

11. Pain / Discomfort

Mark areas of pain/discomfort:

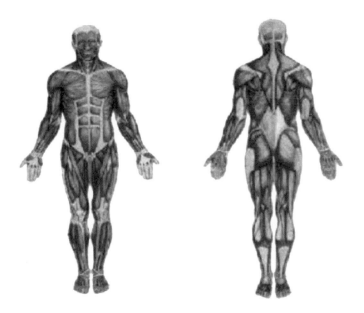

Please describe the location and experience of pain:

_____

_____

_____

_____

Rate your stress level as of today

1 ——————————————————————— 10

Low   **High**

12. Check all Current and Previous Conditions (please explain)

General

CURRENT	PAST	COMMENTS
o	o	headaches_____
o	o	pain _____
o	o	sleep disturbances _____
o	o	fatigue _____
o	o	infections in the ears _____
o	o	fever _____
o	o	sinus _____
o	o	other _____

Skin Conditions

CURRENT	PAST	COMMENTS
o	o	rashes_____
o	o	athelete's foot, warts _____
o	o	other _____

Allergies

CURRENT	PAST	COMMENTS
o	o	scents, oils, lotions _____
o	o	detergents _____
o	o	other _____

Muscles and Joints

CURRENT	PAST	COMMENTS
o	o	rheumatoid arthritis _____
o	o	osteoarthritis _____
o	o	scoliosis _____
o	o	broken bones_____
o	o	spinal problems_____
o	o	disk problems_____
o	o	lupus_____
o	o	TMJ, jaw pain _____
o	o	spasms, cramps_____
o	o	sprains, strains _____
o	o	tendonitis, bursitis_____
o	o	stiff or painful joints_____
o	o	weak or sore muscles_____
o	o	neck, shoulder, arm pain_____
o	o	low back, hip, leg pain _____
o	o	other _____

Nervous System

CURRENT	PAST	COMMENTS
o	o	head injuries, concussions _____
o	o	dizziness, ringing in the ears _____
o	o	loss of memory, confusion _____
o	o	numbness, tingling _____
o	o	sciatica, shooting pain_____
o	o	chronic pain _____
o	o	depression _____
o	o	other _____

Respiratory, Cardiovascular

CURRENT	PAST	COMMENTS
o	o	heart disease_____
o	o	blood clots_____
o	o	stroke_____
o	o	lymphadema_____
o	o	high, low blood pressure _____
o	o	irregular heart beat _____
o	o	poor circulation _____
o	o	swollen ankles_____
o	o	varicose veins _____
o	o	other _____
o	o	pregnancy _____
o	o	chest pain, shortness of breath _____
o	o	asthma _____
o	o	palpable heartbeat in abdomen _____

Digestive/Elimination System

CURRENT	PAST	COMMENTS
o	o	bowel dysfunction _____
o	o	gas, bloating _____
o	o	bladder/kidney dysfunction _____
o	o	abdominal pain _____
o	o	ulcers, colitis _____
o	o	belching/gas within 1 hour after eating _____
o	o	heartburn/acid reflux_____
o	o	bloating within 1 hour after eating _____

o	o	bad breath (halitosis)_____
o	o	sweat has strong odor_____
o	o	feel like skipping breakfast _____
o	o	feel better if you don't eat _____
o	o	sleepy after meals_____
o	o	stomach pains/cramps_____
o	o	diarrhea _____
o	o	undigested food in stool _____
o	o	pain between shoulder blades _____
o	o	stomach upset by greasy foods _____
o	o	nausea _____
o	o	light or clay colored stools _____
o	o	gallbladder attacks _____
o	o	gallbladder removed _____
o	o	hemorrhoids or varicose veins _____
o	o	chronic fatigue / fibromyalgia _____
o	o	pulse speeds after eating _____
o	o	airborne allergies, hives _____
o	o	sinus congestion, "stuffy head" _____
o	o	crave bread or noodles_____
o	o	alternating constipation/diarrhea ____
o	o	crohn's disease _____
o	o	asthma_____
o	o	sinus infections _____
o	o	use over-the-counter pain medica-tions _____

o	o	anus itches_____
o	o	history of antibiotic use _____
o	o	fungus or yeast infections _____
o	o	irritable bowel/colitis_____
o	o	other _____

Endocrine System

CURRENT	PAST	COMMENTS
o	o	thyroid dysfunction _____
o	o	HIV/AIDS_____
o	o	diabetes _____
o	o	other _____

Reproductive System

CURRENT	PAST	COMMENTS
o	o	pregnancy _____
o	o	reproductive problems _____
o	o	painful, emotional menses _____
o	o	fibrotic cysts _____

Cancer/Tumors

CURRENT	PAST	COMMENTS
o	o	benign _____
o	o	malignant_____

13. Meaning of Food

Please describe in a few sentences what food means to you. There may be both positive and negative associations. There is no right or wrong to this answer. For example, is food important to you? Are you preoccupied with it? Does it feel nourishing? Does food cause fear or discomfort?

_____

_____

_____

_____

14. Motivation for Nutritional Change

Identify 3 reasons to improve your diet:

1. _____

2. _____

3. _____

Identify 3 obstacles to improving your diet:

1. _____

2. _____

3. _____

Identify 3 goals to improve your diet:

3 month goal: _____

6 month goal: _____

12 month goal: _____

Identify 3 goals to improving your food preparation:

3 month goal: _____

6 month goal: _____

12 month goal: _____

Food-Mood Diary and Clinician Checklist

Food/Mood Diary

Name: _____ Date: (dd/mm/yy)_____

Write down everything you eat and drink for three days, including all snacks, beverages, and water. Please include approximate amounts. Describe energy, mood or digestive responses associated with a meal/snack, and record it in the right-hand column. Use an up arrow (↑) for an increase in energy/mood, down arrow (↓) for a decrease in energy/mood, and an equal sign (=) if energy/mood is unchanged.

Time of waking:_____a.m. / p.m.

Meal	Beverages	Energy Level (↑, ↓, or =)	Mood (↑, ↓, or =)	Digestive Response (gas, bloating, gurgling, elimination, etc.)
Breakfast (Time:_____)				
Snacks (Time:_____)				
Lunch (Time:_____)				
Snacks (Time:_____)				
Dinner (Time:_____)				
Snacks (Time:_____)				

Clinician Checklist for the Food-Mood Diary		
Question	**Answer**	**Goals and Recommendations**
1. How much time passed between when the client awakens and when they eat breakfast? Is the client eating breakfast?		One should always eat breakfast, containing at least 3–4 ounces of protein within 30 minutes of waking for proper energy and blood sugar balancing.
2. How much water/broth is the client drinking throughout the day?		Water intake should be about 50 percent of body weight every day in ounces (example: if a person weighs 160 lb, they should be drinking 80 ounces of water daily).
3. How often is the client eating? How many hours between each meal or snack?		Food should be eaten every 3–4 hours to prevent mood swings, and the client should have at least 3 meals/day and 2 snacks.
4. How many servings of vegetables is the client eating per day?		At least 3 servings of vegetables should be eaten every day. A serving equals from ½ to 1 cup.
5. Is the client eating raw vegetables and fruits?		At least 1–3 servings of raw fruit or vegetables should be eaten every day.
6. Is the client eating enough protein? Note if lack of protein corresponds to drops in mood.		Proteins help to stabilize energy and balance mood and should be emphasized during the daytime hours.
7. Is the client eating enough fats? Note if lack of fats corresponds to mood shifts.		Fats help to stabilize energy and balance mood and should be emphasized during the daytime hours.
8. How many servings of starchy carbohydrates is the client eating and at what times of day?		During the day carbohydrates are best when combined with protein, and carbohydrates should be emphasized in the evening for relaxation.
9. What is the quality of the food the client is eating (freshly prepared vs. canned or prepackaged foods)?		Recommend whole, fresh, organic foods over packaged and canned foods.
10. Is the client eating enough soluble fiber?		Soluble fiber is found in foods like oat bran, nuts, beans, lentils, psyllium husk, peas, chia seeds, barley, and some fruits and vegetables. Men should be eating about 38 grams/day, and women 25 grams/day.
11. Is the client eating enough insoluble fiber?		Insoluble fiber is found in wheat bran, corn, whole grains, oat bran, seeds and nuts, brown rice, flaxseed, and the skins of many fruits and vegetables.

Crockpot Recipes

▆ Sweet Vegetable and Meat Stew

These three recipes are my "go-to recipes" for making easy, nourishing, and rich-tasting meals. The recipes can be modified as you wish and still taste good. The Sweet Vegetable and Meat Stew is a variation on the traditional Jewish Passover stew called Tzimmes. Because each of these recipes has its own version of sweet—from dried fruit, to balsamic vinegar, to white wine or sherry—they are ideal for coming off sweets, carbohydrates, and alcohol addiction.

Ingredients

2 pounds stew meat or inexpensive fatty meat

3 medium carrots, peeled and sliced into ¼ inch coins

2 bay leaves

½ lemon, including peel, pitted and chopped into ½ inch pieces

½ juice orange, including peel, pitted and chopped into ½ inch pieces

¼ tsp. cinnamon

½ cup mixed dried fruit* (prunes, pears, apricots, and apples), chopped into 1-inch pieces

2 cups water

Directions:

1. Cut the meat and carrots into 2-inch pieces and place in the crockpot with 2 cups of water. Cook for 2 hours on high.
2. Add the rest of the ingredients and cook on low for 2 more hours.
3. Serve in bowls.

* Use organic fruit with no sulfites. Make sure you purchase dried fruits without preservatives because the preservatives can be allergenic or exacerbate asthma or breathing difficulties.

▆ Lamb With Balsamic-Glazed Vegetables

Ingredients

1 teaspoon salt

1 teaspoon freshly ground black pepper

1 teaspoon ground coriander

2 teaspoon dried rosemary leaves

1 teaspoon dried mint

1 teaspoon dried thyme

1 teaspoon ground fennel

3 lb lamb roast, deboned and well-trimmed of fat

1 large red onion, cut into eighths

1 large parsnip

2 medium new potatoes, quartered

3 tablespoon balsamic vinegar

Directions

1. Combine the salt, pepper, coriander, rosemary, mint, thyme, and fennel in a small bowl. Rub the seasonings all over the lamb roast.

2. Place the onion in the bottom of the slow cooker and add the lamb roast. Add the remaining vegetables. Drizzle the balsamic vinegar over the vegetables.

3. Cover and cook on high for 1 hour, then turn to low for 10–12 hours.

Lemon Chicken

Ingredients

1 whole chicken

4 stalks celery

8 small red potatoes

1 onion or sliced leeks

¼ cup sherry or dry white wine

2 lemons

1 teaspoon of lemon zest

Directions

1. Wash chicken and place whole in the crockpot along with vegetables, fluids, and only 1 lemon.

2. Cook for 8–10 hours on low.

3. Add the juice from the second lemon and lemon zest before serving.

Gluten-Containing Foods

Foods That Often Contain Gluten		
Beer	Emergen-C in raspberry and	Oats (see section on
Blue cheese—	mixed berry flavors only, the	oats below)
check with the company;	other flavors are fine.	Pastas
many are fine but not all	Flour or cereal products	Pastries
Bouillon cubes	Flour tortillas	Processed meats
Bran	Fried foods	Rice Dream—processed
Bread, breading, bread crumbs	Gravy	w/ barley
Broth	Hot dogs	Roux—a sauce base
Brown rice syrup	Hydrolyzed vegetable protein	Salad dressings
(frequently made from barley)	(HVP), vegetable protein,	Sauces
Cakes	hydrolyzed plant protein	Sausages (some)
Candies	(HPP), hydrolyzed soy pro-	Seitan
Caramel color (infrequently	tein, or textured vegetable	Seasoned chips and other
made from barley)	protein (TVP)—label will say	seasoned snack foods
Cereal	"wheat"	Seasoned rice and
Coating mixes	Imitation bacon	pasta mixes
Communion wafers	Imitation seafood	Self-basting poultry
Cookies	Lunch meats	Soup bases
Couscous	Malt or malt flavoring (usually	Soy-based veggie burgers
Crab cakes	made from barley)	Soy sauce or soy sauce solids—
Crackers	Malt vinegar	wheat-free is available
Croutons	Marinades	Starch—label will say
Dextrin (usually corn	Matzo	"wheat"Stuffing
but may be derived	Meatballs	Tamari
from wheat)	Meat loaf	Textured vegetable pro-
Dressings	Meat substitutes (Tofurky and	tein—label will say
Dry roasted nuts—	others)	"wheat"Thickeners
processing agents may con-	Modified food starch—	Vital wheat gluten found in
tain wheat	label will say "wheat"	imitation meats
	Monosodium glutamate	Ricola cough drops
	Muffins	

Gluten and Gluten-Free Alternatives

Contains Gluten		Gluten-Free	
Barley	Triticale	Amaranth	Beans
Bulgur	Oats*	Rice	Flax
Couscous	Oat bran*	Corn	Garfava
Durum wheat	Oat fiber*	Soy	Sorghum
Farina	Rye	Potato	Millet
Graham flour	Wheat	Quinoa	Buckwheat
Kamut	Wheat bran	Tapioca	Arrowroot
Matzo	Wheat germ	Teff	Nut flours
Seitan	Wheat grass		
Semolina	White flour		
Spelt	Whole wheat flour		

Pineapple-Coconut Cognitive Smoothie

This recipe is easy to make and satisfying for people of all ages who want to support cognitive function by feeding the brain nutrients and fats it can readily use for fuel.

Ingredients

1 cup frozen or fresh pineapple

½ cup coconut milk

1 cup coconut cream

1 tablespoon coconut oil

10 drops stevia liquid

Directions

1. Blend all ingredients and serve cold.
2. Add specific nutrients from the cognitive protocol to the smoothie.

Variations

Frozen mango or blueberries also go well with pineapple and can be substituted. For example, using ½ cup of pineapple and 1 cup of mango or ½ cup blueberries. Another option is to substitute 2 heaping tablespoons of pure cocoa for the fruit. If you want to gain weight, you can add 1 heaping scoop of whey protein.

Practitioners Working in the Field of Nutrition

The following practitioners can serve as resources and referrals for collaboration and for prescribing nutritional programs. Following the descriptions is a table that includes the credentials, training, and approach for each profession. Share the table with a client who wants to explore her or his options.

NUTRITIONAL COUNSELORS/THERAPISTS

These include certified clinical nutritionists, certified nutritional consultants, certified nutritionists, and board-certified physician nutrition specialists (medical professionals with specialized training in nutrition).

Nutritional counselors work with people to assess their nutritional needs and make recommendations for dietary changes to improve health and well-being. A nutritionist has specific nutritional training but is not a registered dietitian (RD). Regulation of the terms "nutritionist" and "nutritional counselor" varies from state to state.

The Nutritional Therapy Association (NTA) offers a program that trains nutritional therapy practitioners (NTPs) and nutritional therapy consultants (NTCs) with a holistic approach and the philosophy that poor nutrition is behind many of today's health problems, and that each individual has unique dietary needs.

> Nutritional Therapy Association
> Website: http://nutritionaltherapy.com/
> The National Association of Nutrition Professionals provides a list of a range of continuing education and graduate degree programs.
> Website: http://nanp.org/

REGISTERED DIETITIANS

Registered dieticians (RDs) can help to manage and prevent chronic illness, provide sports nutrition and culinary education, assist with presurgery and postsurgery nutrition, help with eating disorders, lead community efforts to improve food resources, provide guidance with prenatal and perinatal nutrition, and assist with healthy food and nutrition for the elderly. RDs administer medical nutrition therapy in which they review a person's eating habits, review the individual's nutritional health, and create a nutritional treatment plan that is personalized for the individual. Often, though not always, the course of study promotes conventional nutritional guidelines rather than more progressive ones, and thus one should explore the approach taken by the dietician.

RDs are required to have a bachelor's degree with courses on the disease process, food chemistry, food service systems management, physiology, sociology, and biology.

The coursework must be approved by the Academy Accreditation Council for Education in Nutrition and Dietetics. Many RDs also have advanced degrees. RDs are also required to complete an internship and pass a national exam with the Commission on Dietetic Registration. They are also required to receive continuing education. RDs have limits on what they can do, but they often work in health care facilities, hospitals, and private practice facilities, or HMOs as part of a medical team. Physicians often refer patients to RDs for nutritional therapy. To find a RD in your area, go to the website for the Academy of Nutrition and Dietetics at http://www.eatright.org, then click on "Find a Registered Dietitian."

NATUROPATHIC PHYSICIANS

Naturopathy is a holistic medical system that is guided by the major principle: The Healing Power of Nature (Vis Medicatrix Naturae). It is a blend of natural medicine and allopathic (allopathic) medicine. Naturopathic doctors (NDs) are licensed as primary care physicians in some states (see below) in the United States. Naturopathic practice includes the following diagnostic and therapeutic modalities: clinical and laboratory diagnostic testing, nutritional medicine, botanical medicine, physical medicine (including manipulative therapy), counseling, minor surgery, homeopathy, acupuncture, prescription medication, and obstetrics (natural childbirth).

There are five Naturopathic Medical Schools in the United States; each school provides a low-cost clinic in which physicians complete their training as interns and residents. Some insurance will pay for naturopathic services. NDs are licensed to diagnose and prescribe medicine. Unless they specialize in mental health, they generally have basic training in mental illness medications as well. Their training is a minimum of a four-year program that includes the first two years of basic sciences of a medical (MD) education with the last two years focused on natural, alternative, and preventative medicine. They are required to take board certification exams to obtain state licenses.

Collaborate with an ND to prescribe dietary changes that also include the use of nutrients, glandulars, and reducing or eliminating pharmaceutical drugs. The certifying body is the American Association of Naturopathic Physicians and can be a source of referrals. The following states license NDs: Alaska, Arizona, California, Colorado, Connecticut, District of Columbia, Hawaii, Kansas, Maine, Maryland, Minnesota, Montana, New Hampshire, North Dakota, Oregon, Utah, Vermont, Washington, and territories: Puerto Rico and Virgin Islands. The following states are pending: Illinois, Iowa, Massachusetts, New York, North Carolina, Pennsylvania, and Wisconsin.

Please note that licensed naturopathic physicians should not be confused with naturopath, naprapath, or unlicensed naturopathic practitioners who also practice naturopathic methods but are not licensed by the state.

American Association of Naturopathic Physicians
Website: www.naturopathic.org

FUNCTIONAL MEDICINE PRACTITIONERS

Functional medicine uses a systems-oriented and patient-centered approach, addressing the patient as a whole person. Practitioners of functional medicine take extensive patient histories and take time to understand an individual's unique health needs. They draw from Western and complementary/alternative medicine focusing on science-based prevention and treatments for body, mind, spirit, lifestyle, family, career, and the environment. To become a functional medicine practitioner, you must already have graduated from an accredited osteopathic, medical, chiropractic, nursing, physician assistant, dentistry, naturopathic, dietetics, pharmacy, acupuncture, or nutrition program; have completed a series of courses in Functional Medicine; and passed written examinations.

Institute for Functional Medicine
Website: www.functionalmedicine.org

INTEGRATIVE MEDICAL PRACTITIONERS

Integrative medicine draws on both allopathic and complementary/alternative medical practices. It is often evidence-based and takes into account the patient as a whole person, the relationship between the practitioner and the patient, and uses all available therapies that may help in the treatment of a client.

The American Board of Physician Specialties certifies integrative medical doctors once they have successfully passed the Integrative Medicine board certification exam. To take the exam, you must be an MD or DO and have received training specifically in integrative medicine, acupuncture, naturopathy, or chiropractic education.

> The American Board of Integrative Holistic Medicine (ABIHM)
> Website: http://www.abihm.org
>
> The National Center for Complementary and Integrative Health
> Website: https://nccih.nih.gov/

HEALTH COACHES

A health coach supports, educates, mentors, and serves as a role model to motivate individuals, couples, families, and communities to explore and enact positive health choices. A variety of health coach training and certification programs exist and training credentials can vary.

The Institute for Integrative Nutrition combines motivational interviewing–type strategies with nutritional education.

> Website: http://www.integrativenutrition.com/career/healthcoaching
> Duke University has a program in Integrative Health Coaching
> Website: http://www.dukeintegrativemedicine.org/patient-care/
>   integrative-health-coaching

OSTEOPATHIC DOCTORS

Osteopathy is a comprehensive medical system that focuses on disease prevention while using the technology of modern medicine to diagnose and treat illness. It is holistic, looking at the patient as a whole person and not just treating isolated symptoms. Osteopathic physicians (DOs) are fully trained physicians like MDs, who are able to perform surgery and work with prescription drugs. They also emphasize nutritional therapies and manipulative therapies such as cranial osteopathy. They are also trained in a specialty such as surgery, psychiatry, or pediatrics. Examinations to receive state licenses are required for DOs to practice. DOs are more likely to practice primary care specialties and also receive additional training on the musculoskeletal system and osteopathic manipulative medicine, so they use their hands and palpation skills to aid in their diagnoses and treatments.

American Osteopathic Association
Website: http://www.osteopathic.org

TRADITIONAL CHINESE MEDICINE AND ACUPUNCTURISTS

Traditional Chinese medical practitioners and acupuncturists prescribe individualized diets for the whole person. They take a comprehensive history and conduct a thorough assessment that includes pulse taking, tongue reading, and facial diagnosis. The Chinese nutritional approach is based on having a balance of the five tastes (spicy, sour, bitter, sweet, and salty) and six food groups (meats, dairy, fruit, vegetables, grains, and herbs and spices). Chinese medicine also incorporates the concepts of yin and yang to nutrition and recommends different foods for different times of year. For example, the summer is a more active, or yang, time of year, and so to create balance one would eat more grounding, yin foods. Foods are recommended based on their ability to balance conditions of heat, dampness, coldness, dryness, moistness, or an excess or deficiency of yin or yang.

Acupuncture is a traditional Chinese medicine (TCM) approach to healing. Oriental medical practitioners and acupuncturists receive at least master's-level training in an accredited 3- to 4-year program and must pass certification examinations. Other health care practitioners may also receive abbreviated training (in some states) in acupuncture detoxification protocols that trains them to treat a limited number of points on the body for the treatment of the addictions.

American Association of Oriental Medicine
Website: http://aaom.org

National Association of Detoxification Acupuncture
Website: http://www.acudetox.com/

TRADITIONAL MEDICINE HEALERS/PRACTITIONERS

Traditional medicine involves ways of healing that are passed on from one generation to the next, among families and healers, and is based on indigenous, practical, and observational arts and science. Medicinal plants, animals, foods, the elements, rituals, spirit ways, and touch are all part of the earth's gifts that make up traditional medicine. Traditional medicine is the property of the communities and nations that it originates from, and it emphasizes restoration of balance and prevention of causes, and requires the vital preservation of the culture and natural resources of its origin. Traditional medicine exists in every culture and is based on the knowledge acquired over many thousands of generations of observation and learning. Traditional medicine contributes many methods to what is now called complementary and alternative medicine.

Center for Traditional Medicine
Website: http://centerfortraditionalmedicine.org/

Center for World Indigenous Studies
Website: http://cwis.org/

World Health Organization
Website: http://www.who.int/en/

Spectrum of Practitioners			
Practitioner	**What They Do**	**Approach**	**Education**
Functional medicine practitioner	Patient histories Individual health needs Prevention	Western and alternative medicine Systems oriented Patient centered Practitioner–patient relationship Science based	Graduation from an accredited program Completion of Functional Medicine courses Examinations
Integrative medicine practitioner	Practitioner–patient relationship Use of all available therapies	Evidence based Holistic Allopathic and alternative medicine	Certification exam Could be an MD or DO, RN/ARNP, or PA and have received specific training
Naturopathic physician	Holistic Primary care Diagnosis Prescriptions Testing Nutrition Botanicals Physical medicine Counseling Minor surgery Homeopathy Acupuncture Intravenous and injection therapy Naturopathic obstetrics (natural childbirth)	Holistic The healing power of nature Natural and allopathic medicine	Four-year program Two years of basic sciences of a medical (MD) Two years natural, alternative, and preventative medicine Board certification exams required to obtain state licenses Basic training in mental illness medications
Nutritional counselors/therapists	Nutritional assessment Dietary recommendations Health coaching Meal planning Cooking instruction	Holistic Philosophy: poor nutrition is behind many of today's health problems Each individual has unique dietary needs	Nutritional therapy consultant (NTC): 9 months of training Nutritional therapy practitioner (NTP): 9 months of training, hands-on functional evaluation training
Osteopathic doctors	Nutritional therapies Manipulative therapies such as cranial osteopathy Psychiatry Pediatrics Prescriptions Surgery	Comprehensive medical system Disease prevention Modern medicine Holistic	Fully trained physicians Examinations to receive state licenses are required

Spectrum of Practitioners			
Practitioner	**What They Do**	**Approach**	**Education**
Registered dietitians	Nutritional therapy Personalized nutritional treatment plan Manage and prevent chronic illness Sports nutrition Culinary education Presurgery and postsurgery nutrition Eating disorders Community efforts Prenatal and perinatal nutrition Nutrition for the elderly	Medical nutrition Sometimes hospital/institutional base Some people who begin as RDs expand into holistic approaches	Bachelor's degree in a related subject required Coursework approved by the Academy Accreditation Council for Education in Nutrition and Dietetics Internship required Must pass a national exam with the Commission on Dietetic Registration Continuing education required
Traditional Chinese medicine and acupuncturists	Individualized diets Comprehensive history Assessment includes pulse taking, tongue reading, and facial diagnosis Acupuncture Herbal therapies	Holistic Alternative medicine	Master's-level training in an accredited 3- to 4-year program required Certification examinations
Traditional medicine healers/practitioners	Medicinal plants Medicinal foods Rituals Spirit ways Touch	Complementary and alternative medicine Indigenous, practical, and observational arts and science Emphasizes restoration of balance and prevention of causes	Knowledge acquired over many thousands of generations of observation and learning Passed on from one generation to the next

Measuring Basal Body Temperature for Thyroid Function

There are several methods used to assess thyroid function.

BLOOD TESTS

A blood test can be conducted to determine the level of thyroid-stimulating hormone (TSH) released by the pituitary.

ACHILLES REFLEX

A delayed Achilles return reflex is a classic sign of hypothyroidism along with the other noted symptoms.

AN IODINE SKIN TEST

A 2% solution of iodine is painted onto the skin and watched to see how quickly the body absorbs the available iodine. The quicker the iodine fades, the greater the hypothyroid deficiency can be assumed.

THE BARNES THYROID TEMPERATURE TEST

This test may be conducted at home every morning for 5 days using a thermometer. It will measure functional hypothyroidism, which is not always identified by blood tests.

Barne's Thyroid Test Instructions

Shake down the thermometer the night before and place on your night table. First thing in the morning before getting out of bed tuck the thermometer in your armpit and lay very still for 10 minutes.

Indicate the first day of your menstrual period by circling the temperature on the chart for that day. Indicate the last day of your menstrual period by making an "X" through the temperature on the chart.

If the thyroid is overactive, (or you have a fever) your temperature will show 1–2 degrees above normal. If the thyroid is underactive, your temperature will show 1–2 degrees below normal.

The normal underarm temperature is between 36.6 and 36.8 degrees Celsius. If your temperature is consistently below this level, blood tests for evaluating thyroid function are indicated. However, be aware that these tests are often normal even if the thyroid gland is malfunctioning. That is because the tests show only how much thyroid hormone is circulating in the blood and tell nothing of how well the hormones are functioning on a cellular level. Additionally, the loss of up to 70% of thyroid function may occur before blood tests become abnormal.

This test was developed by Broda O. Barnes, MD, PhD, a practicing physician in the state of Colorado. It is Dr. Barnes's opinion that this test is superior to standard blood studies for evaluation of thyroid function. Blood tests measure only pituitary (TSH) and T3 hormone blood levels, while temperature readings measure how much energy is actually being generated in cells.

Foods Containing Lactose

Foods That Often Contain (Hidden) Lactose	
Bread and other baked goods	Prescription drugs (birth control pills, thyroid medication, gastrointestinal medications)
Breakfast cereals	
Breakfast drinks	Processed breakfast foods (frozen waffles and pancakes, doughnuts)
Candies	
Chips (potato, corn, and other)	Processed meats (bacon, sausage, hot dogs, and lunch meats)
Liquid and powdered milk-based meal replacements	
Nondairy liquid and powdered coffee creamers	Protein powders and bars
Nondairy whipped toppings	Salad dressings
Instant potatoes	Waffles, pancakes, biscuits, cookies, and mixes to make them
Instant soups	
Margarine	Vitamins (many kinds)

Casein and Dairy Charts

Foods and Ingredients That Contain Casein	
Butter, butter flavoring, butter fat	Lactalbumin, lactoalbumin phosphate, lactaglobulin, lactose
Calcium casein, casein hydrolysate, magnesium casein, potassium casein, rennet casein, sodium casein	Margarine
Cheese flavoring	Milk chocolate
Custard	Nondairy creamers
Dairy products like cheese, yogurt, milk, kefir, ice cream, sour cream, half & half, and cream	Powdered milk
	Protein powder
	Pudding
	Sherbert
	Whey, whey hydrolysate

Casein-Free Dairy and Nondairy Foods	
Coconut butter	Pareve/parve creams and creamers
Coconut milk	Proteins like meat and fish (read labels if processed or packaged)
Foods certified as kosher nondairy or pareve/parve	Rice, soy, nut, oat, or potato-based milks
ghee (look for casein-free guaranteed)	Sorbet (read label)
Fruits and vegetables	Soy, rice, and coconut ice cream (not all flavors)
Italian ices	Whole grains in their natural state

Dairy Foods and Their Alternatives	
Dairy Foods	**Substitutes**
Cheese	Nondairy cheeses (made from nuts, hemp, soy,* and rice—look out for "casein" or "caseinate," a milk protein used in cheese substitutes if you have a milk allergy as opposed to a lactose intolerance) Goat or sheep cheese (if tolerated) Nutritional yeast
Milk	Nondairy milks such as soy,* oat, coconut, hazelnut, almond, rice, and hemp milk Goat milk (if tolerated)
Kefir	Nondairy kefir products
Butter and margarine	Vegan butter,* ghee (usually casein/lactose free), goat butter (if tolerated), coconut oil
Nondairy coffee creamer (contains casein)	Try coconut or soy* coffee creamers
Ice cream	Rice, soy,* hemp, coconut, or almond ice cream
Sour cream	Nondairy sour cream*
Yogurt	Coconut, soy,* or rice yogurt with live cultures

* Soy is often found in dairy substitutes, but it has been linked to some serious negative health effects. Unfermented soy contains antinutrients, such as saponins, soyatoxin, phytates, trypsin inhibitors, goitrogens, and phytoestrogens. Phytic acid, found in high amounts in soy, suppresses digestive enzymes; it also depresses thyroid function (Fallon & Enig, 1999) and is high in protease inhibitors, which suppress pancreatic enzymes. Soybeans also contain hemagglutinin, which causes red blood cells to clump. Soy should be avoided (Fallon & Enig, 1999) except in the form of fermented soy products such as miso, shoyu, and tempeh, and then only in very small quantities and on rare occasions. The antinutrients are destroyed during the fermentation process, so fermented soy products are more easily tolerated and can provide many health benefits. Another reason to avoid soy is that nonorganic soy is heavily sprayed with pesticides, and it is almost always genetically modified unless specifically labeled otherwise.

Grain Recipes

SOAKING AND COOKING GRAINS

Soaking grains before cooking them shortens the cooking time, releases nutrients, and increases their digestibility.

1. Wash grains.
2. Place grains in a bowl and cover with warm water.
3. For each cup of grain, add 1 tablespoon apple cider vinegar or lemon juice.
4. Soak at room temperature for 8 to 12 hours.
5. Drain the water from the grains, place them in a cooking pot, and fill with fresh water according to specific grain to water ratios. Add about a ¼ teaspoon of sea salt per cup of grain, or use seaweed.
6. Bring the water to a boil, reduce heat to low, cover, and cook according to specific grain cooking times. Cooking time may be reduced by as much as half after soaking, so check the grains halfway through.

Black Rice Breakfast Pudding With Coconut and Fruit

Adapted from Sarah Britton, *My New Roots* (Retrieved from http://www.mynewroots.org/site/2014/01/coconut-black-rice-breakfast-pudding/

Serves 3–4

Ingredients

1 cup black rice, soaked overnight
1 can coconut milk (full-fat)
¼ teaspoon fine grain sea salt
½ vanilla bean, seeds and pod (optional)

½ cup water

1 tablespoon maple syrup, raw honey, or raw agave

1/3 cup coconut flakes, lightly toasted

Mango, raspberries, blueberries, pomegranate, banana, kiwi, pineapple, or other fruit of your preference

Directions

1. Cover the rice with water and soak overnight or for up to 8 hours. Drain and rinse.
2. Combine the rice in a pot with the coconut milk, salt, vanilla bean, and the ½ cup of water. Bring to a boil, reduce to a simmer, and cover. Cook, stirring frequently, until the rice is tender and most of the liquid has been absorbed (you still want a little liquid), about 25–30 minutes.
3. While the rice is cooking, prepare all the fruit that you would like to accompany the pudding.
4. When the rice is done cooking, remove from the heat and gently stir in the maple syrup, honey, or agave.
5. Serve the black rice in bowls and top with the fruit and toasted coconut.

Congee

A traditional Chinese recipe, congee is a rice porridge cooked with lots of water for a long amount of time. It is a real comfort food that promotes strong digestion and is easily assimilated, in addition to being easy and affordable to make. It can be adapted to increase its medicinal properties by adding other beneficial vegetables, grains, legumes, medicinal or culinary herbs, or even animal proteins. These other ingredients will also be more easily digested and assimilated by cooking with the rice and water.

Ingredients

1 cup grain (usually white or brown rice)

5 to 6 cups liquid (usually water, but homemade broths like Dashi are excellent)

Pinch of sea salt

Directions

1. If you are using a crock-pot, add the ingredients and set to low, leaving it on overnight.
2. If you are using the stovetop, add the ingredients to a stockpot, cover, and bring to a boil. Reduce heat to very low and simmer for four to six hours.
3. Too much water is better than too little, and the longer the congee cooks, the better it gets.

Additions

Try adding carrot to aid with digestion and to reduce gas, or ginger for its warming effects and to improve digestion.

Khichadi

Khichadi (also called kitcheree, khichdi, khicari, and khichri, etc.) means "mixture," and it refers to an Ayurvedic dish combining basmati rice, mung beans, and nutritional spices. It is a comforting gluten-free and vegetarian dish that is easy to digest and has many nutrients. It is also high in protein, calcium, iron, fiber, vitamin C, magnesium, phosphorus, and potassium. Its nutritional benefits are amplified when cooked with turmeric and black pepper, and served with ghee. Khichadi is detoxifying, increases immunity and energy, and stimulates digestive enzymes. This light and satisfying dish is good for those with digestive problems and good during times of illness or upset stomach. The dish uses split yellow mung beans, which are easier to digest than other beans and do not produce as much gas. Khichadi can be eaten for three meals a day as a cleansing food, as it provides adequate protein to balance blood sugar, which can become easily out of balance during water, juice, or other restrictive fasts. If using it to cleanse, use less ghee or omit it altogether. However, ghee should always be used when eating khichadi as a regular meal. White rice is better than brown if using khichadi to cleanse—digestion is weakened during a cleanse and brown rice too hard to digest.

Recipe adapted from John Douillard (2013), What's So Amazing About Kitchari?
Retrieved from http://lifespa.com/whats-so-amazing-about-khichadi/

Ingredients

1 cup split yellow mung dahl beans
¼ – ½ cup long grain white or white basmati rice
1 tablespoon fresh ginger root, grated
1 teaspoon each: black mustard seeds, cumin, and turmeric powder
½ teaspoon each: coriander powder, fennel, and fenugreek seeds
3 cloves
3 bay leaves
7–10 cups water
½ teaspoon sea salt
1 small handful cilantro leaves, chopped

2 scallions, thinly sliced

Directions

1. Soak beans overnight and then drain.
2. Place split yellow mung beans and rice together in a pot and rinse with water, using your hands to swish the rice and beans around. When the water becomes cloudy, drain it, add fresh water, and rinse again. Continue this process until water runs clear. Then strain the rice and beans.
3. Preheat a large pot on the stove. When it is ready, dry-roast all the spices (except the bay leaves) on medium heat for a few minutes to enhance their flavors.
4. Add the bean and rice mixture, and mix well.
5. Add water and bay leaves and bring to a boil. Boil for 10 minutes.
6. Reduce the heat to low, cover, and continue simmering about 30–40 minutes, or until the rice and beans are soft.
7. Just before serving, top with the cilantro leaves, scallions, and sea salt to taste.

NOTES: When not cleansing, or if more blood sugar support is needed during a cleanse, steamed vegetables or lean meat can be added. Be sure to get split yellow mung beans, also called "moong dal." Do not use whole mung beans (they are green) or yellow split peas.

Mushroom Risotto

I love all risotto recipes because they require patience. It can become a meditation to gather and prepare everything that goes into the risotto, and then the stirring; the gentle, rhythmic, mindful stirring is in itself relaxing. Invite friends over to share because there will be enough for several plates. Then the treat is sitting down to eat the comforting richness of a smooth risotto that warms the heart and belly. Pair this with a green salad in which some bitter greens are added to help digest the brain-healing fats. Enjoy a meal made with love.

NOTE: If alcohol is contraindicated, just leave it out.

Ingredients

5–6 cups chicken stock

2 tablespoons butter

2 cups of shitake and oyster mushrooms, cleaned, trimmed, and cut into half inch to inch pieces

1/3 cup finely chopped sweet onion

1¾ cups arborio rice

2/3 cup brandy or dry white wine

1/3 cup freshly grated Parmesan cheese

Sea salt and freshly ground black pepper, to taste

2 tablespoons chopped fresh parsley

Directions

1. Bring stock to a simmer in a saucepan.
2. Melt the butter in a deep, heavy, medium-sized saucepan over medium-high heat. Add mushrooms and onions and sauté about 5 minutes. Add the rice and stir to combine.
3. Add brandy, bring to a boil, and reduce liquid by half, about 3–4 minutes. Add simmering stock, ½ cup at a time, stirring enough to keep the rice from sticking to the edges of the pan. Stir the rice almost constantly—stirring sloughs off the starch from the rice, making the creamy sauce you are looking for in a risotto. Wait until the stock is almost completely absorbed before adding the next ½ cup. This process will take about 25 minutes. The rice should be just cooked and slightly chewy.
4. Stir in the Parmesan cheese and season to taste with salt and pepper. Garnish with chopped fresh parsley or chives.

Oatmeal

Ingredients

1 part steel-cut oats

3 or 4 parts water (more water makes it creamier, less keeps the oats more intact)

1/8 teaspoon salt

Options include topping with raw walnuts, dried fruit, and whole cream or almond milk.

Directions

1. Boil the water and add the oats and salt, reduce the heat, and simmer 20–30 minutes until tender.

Overnight Oatmeal

Ingredients

1 part rolled oats

1 part water or milk (soy, rice, almond, or coconut milk)

Agave miel or honey to taste (Optional)

Dried fruit and nuts (Optional)

Directions

1. Place all ingredients in a bowl and mix well.
2. Pour into a glass container and store in the refrigerator overnight.
3. In the morning it will be ready, and you can top with other fresh ingredients if desired.

Granola

I like to make granola with more nuts and fruit than the traditional oats-dominant recipes. It makes a wonderful breakfast or snack for school or travel, and it allows you to control the contents of your cereal and make it protein rich. If you are gluten sensitive, make sure that you purchase oats called gluten-free oats. While oats themselves are gluten-free, they are often processed alongside wheat or other gluten grains. It is essential to purchase organic and raw products, and dried fruit should not be sweetened or have preservatives, which can be neurotoxic. After you make your first batch, experiment with adding different dried fruit, nut, and seed options. Add a little almond, coconut, hemp, or rice milk, or a goat yogurt with a banana, and you have a perfect brain food meal, rich in coconut and healthy sweeteners for brain energy, protein-rich nuts and seeds providing amino acids, and a good dose of fiber from the oats, which aids the colon and induces relaxation.

Ingredients

Use all raw organic items:

5 cups oats

1 cup pumpkin seeds

1 cup sunflower seeds

1 cup almonds

1 cup pecans

1 cup cashews

½ cup sesame seeds

½ cup chia seeds

1 cup grated coconut

¼ – ½ cup coconut oil

½ cup raw honey, raw organic maple syrup, or dark agave syrup

1 cup raisins

Dried cranberries or blueberries, chopped dates, black mission figs, and hemp seeds (Optional)

Directions

1. Mix all the ingredients in a large mixing bowl except the grated coconut, coconut oil, sweetener of choice (honey/maple/agave), raisins, and other dried fruit.

2. Gently melt the coconut oil and the sweetener in a pot over a light heat.

3. Pour coconut oil/sweetener mixture into the bowl of ingredients, mixing well so the ingredients are coated.

4. Option 1: Heat a cast-iron skillet over low heat. Place a layer of oat mixture (2 inches thick) in the pan, stirring constantly until lightly toasted.

5. Option 2. Place a layer of parchment paper on a large cookie sheet and cover it with 2 inches of the granola mixture. Place in an oven at 350 degrees. Set the timer for 15 minutes and stir the mixture at 15 minutes, making sure the edges are not getting too brown, and then place in the oven for another 10 minutes or so. The goal is to gently brown but not overcook the ingredients, so watch them well.

6. Note that once out of the cast-iron pan or the oven that the granola mixture will continue to cook.

7. As each batch is finished, put in a large glass or ceramic bowl. Add the grated coconut, organic raw raisins, and other dried fruit. Mix well and let cool before adding to quart-size bottles or plastic bags.

Curried Quinoa

Ingredients

1½ cups water

¾ cup quinoa

2 tablespoons coconut oil

½ cup coarsely chopped sweet onion

¼ cup red bell peppers, chopped

½ cup frozen peas

¾ cup chopped Fuji apple

½ cup pecans, coarsely chopped

1 tablespoon freshly grated ginger

1 tablespoon curry powder

¼ teaspoon salt

Directions

1. Bring the water to a boil. Add the quinoa, reduce the heat to a low simmer, cover and cook for 15–20 minutes.
2. While the quinoa is cooking, heat the coconut oil in a medium skillet and sauté the onions on low until lightly browned.
3. Add the chopped bell peppers and cook for two minutes.
4. Add the peas, apple, pecans, and ginger to the pan and cook for another 2 minutes.
5. When the quinoa is finished cooking, add to the onion mixture. Add the curry and salt, and stir to combine.

Cooking Millet

Ingredients

1 cup raw millet

2 cups water (or broth)

¼ teaspoon salt, optional

1 tablespoon unsalted butter or coconut oil

Directions

1. In a large, dry saucepan, toast the raw millet over medium heat for 4–5 minutes or until it turns a rich golden brown and the grains become fragrant. Do not burn.
2. Add the water and salt to the pan and stir. Bring to a boil; then turn the heat to low. Add the butter and cover the pot. Simmer until the grains absorb most of the water, about 15 minutes.
3. Remove from the heat and allow it to sit, covered and removed from heat, for 10 minutes.
4. Fluff the millet with a fork and add additional salt, if desired. Millet does not keep well and is best served warm.

Variations

To make millet porridge, increase the liquid to 3 cups and stir every few minutes as the millet simmers.

Corn-Containing Foods

Products and Ingredients Commonly Containing Corn		
Beverages	yogurt to salad dressings)	products
Cereals	Hydrolized corn	Sorbitol (derived from corn,
Candies	Hydrolized corn protein	used in toothpaste, gum)
Canned fruits	Iodized salt (dextrose)	Syrups
Citric acid (organic applesauce)	Jams	Tea bags (corn is used to
Corn alcohol	Maize	adhere the teabags together)
Corn extract	Malt syrup from corn	Toothpaste
Corn gluten	Maltitol (derived from corn,	Vanilla extract
Corn meal	used in gum)	Vegetable oils
Corn solids	Modified cornstarch	Vitamin D (in fortified milk)
Cornstarch	Monosodium glutamate	Vitamin E
Corn sweetener	Mineral-enhanced water	Wax used on vegetables
Corn syrup	Natural flavors	(cucumbers)
Corn flour	Perfume	Yeast packets (as ascorbic acid)
Corn/vegetable oil	Prepared meats like hot dogs	Zea mays
Dextrose	and deli meats	Zein
Envelopes (the gum that is	Popcorn	
usually licked to seal an	Sauces	
envelope)	Shampoo	
High fructose corn syrup (used	Snack foods	
to sweeten everything from	Soaking pads for fresh meat	

Corn Foods and Their Alternatives	
Corn Foods	**Substitutes**
Baking Powder	Corn-free baking powder
Corn tortillas	Wheat, spelt, brown rice, teff, or coconut flour tortillas
Corn flour	Wheat, spelt, rice, oat, coconut, amaranth, or potato flour
Corn starch	Tapioca starch, arrowroot powder, potato starch
Corn oil	Olive oil, coconut oil, safflower oil, sesame oil
Corn syrup/sweeteners	Stevia, honey, maple syrup, brown rice syrup, agave syrup, cane sugar
Vanilla extract	Corn-free vanilla extract

Foods Containing Histamines

Alcohol Artificial food colors and preservatives Chocolate, cocoa, and cola drinks Citrus fruits (oranges, grapefruit, lemons, lime) Eggs Dried fruit Fermented foods: sauerkraut, kombucha, pickles, relishes, fermented soy products, etc. Fermented milk products, including most cheeses Leftover meat (after meat is cooked, the histamine levels increase due to microbial action as the meat sits) Most berries	Processed, cured, smoked, and fermented meats such as lunch meat, bacon, sausage, salami, pepperoni Seafood: shellfish or fin fish, fresh, frozen, smoked, or canned Spices: cinnamon, chili powder, cloves, anise, nutmeg, curry powder, cayenne pepper Spinach Tea (herbal or regular) Tomatoes and tomato products like ketchup and tomato sauces Vinegar and foods containing vinegar such as pickles, relishes, ketchup, and prepared mustard Yogurt, buttermilk, kefir

Foods Containing Salicylates

Foods High in Salicylates

Fruits: all dried fruits, apples, apricots, avocados, blackberries, blackcurrants, blueberries, boysenberries, cherries, cranberries, currants, dates, figs, grapefruit, grapes, guava, kiwi fruit, oranges, peaches, raspberries, pineapple, plums, strawberries, cherries, prunes, raspberries, red currants, tangelos, tangerines, tomatoes

Vegetables: alfalfa, artichokes, broad beans, broccoli, canned olives, cauliflower, chicory, cucumbers, eggplant, hot peppers, mushrooms, okra, peppers, radishes, spinach, tomatoes, zucchini, water chestnut, watercress

Herbs, spices, and condiments: dry spices, dried herbs, powders, tomato pastes and sauces, vinegar, soy sauce, jams, and jellies

Beverages: apple cider, beer, coffee, liquor, orange juice, port, regular and herbal tea, rum, sherry, wine

Nuts: almonds, Brazil nuts, macadamia nuts, pine nuts, peanuts, pistachios, water chestnuts

Sweets: fruit flavors, gelatin, honey, ice cream, jam, licorice, mint-flavored gum and breath mints, peppermints

Products That May Contain Salicylates

Fragrances and perfumes
Shampoos and conditioners
Herbal remedies
Cosmetics such as lipsticks, lotions, and skin cleansers

Mouthwash and mint-flavored toothpaste
Shaving cream
Sunscreens or tanning lotions
Muscle pain creams
Alka Seltzer

Ingredients That Contain Salicylates

Aspirin
Acetylsalicylic acid
Artificial food coloring and flavoring
Benzoates
Beta-hydroxy acid
Magnesium salicylate
Menthol

Mint
Salicylic acid
Peppermint
Phenylethyl salicylate
Sodium salicylate
Spearmint

Foods Containing Sulfites

Foods Containing Sulfites	
Apple cider	Maraschino cherries
Baked goods	Molasses
Beer (most do not contain sulfites)	Pickled foods
Bottled lemon juice and lime juice	Potato chips
Canned vegetables	Shrimp (sometimes treated with sulfites)
Condiments (many)	Soup mixes
Dehydrated, precut or peeled potatoes	Sparkling grape juice
Dried fruit	Tea
Gravies	Trail mix
Guacamole	Vegetable juices
Jams	Wine

APPENDIX P

Papaya Barbeque Sauce

Papaya Barbeque Sauce

This is an exotic and healthy alternative to traditional barbeque sauce. If you want to make an anti-inflammatory, nightshade-free version, just leave out the crushed red chili pepper.

Ingredients

1 tablespoon organic extra-virgin coconut oil
1 medium onion, chopped
2 cloves garlic, minced
1 teaspoon crushed red chili pepper
½ teaspoon cumin powder
1 teaspoon oregano
1 cup dark brown sugar
5 drops of stevia liquid
1 lime (zest and juice)
½ cup apple cider vinegar, to taste
2 lbs papaya, diced
½ teaspoon sea salt
3-4 drops liquid smoke

Directions

1. Cook and stir onions and garlic in oil until onions are translucent. Add the chilies, cumin, and oregano.
2. Add sugar, stevia, lime, and apple cider vinegar. Bring to a boil.
3. Add liquid smoke, papaya and salt. Return to a boil and simmer 15 minutes.
4. Remove mixture from the heat and allow it to cool. Puree in a blender until smooth.

Elimination Diet

Guide to Foods on the Elimination Diet		
Foods to Include in the Diet	**Foods to Eliminate From the Diet**	
Buckwheat	Alcohol	Hydrogenated oils
Coconut oil	Beans (all beans—soybeans, tofu,	Margarine
Cold-pressed olive oil	tempeh, peas, lentils)	Mayonnaise
Fish	Caffeine (coffee, black tea, green	Meats (beef, chicken, pork, cold
Flaxseed oil	tea, yerba mate, soda)	cuts, bacon, hot dogs, sausage)
Fresh water	Canned meat and fish products	Meat substitutes (made from soy
Fruits (fresh)	Chocolate	or gluten)
Herbal teas	Citrus fruits	Nightshade vegetables (tomatoes,
Herbs and spices	Condiments (ketchup, mustard,	eggplant, potatoes, bell peppers,
Lamb	soy sauce, vinegar, relish, chut-	chili peppers, paprika)
Rice	ney, barbeque sauce)	Nuts
Rice or coconut milk—	Corn	Seeds
unsweetened	Dairy—milk, cream, cheese,	Shellfish
Sea salt	yogurt, butter, cottage cheese,	Sweeteners (honey, sugar, maple
Stevia	kefir, ice cream, nondairy	syrup, corn syrup)
Sweet potatoes or yams	creamer	
Turkey	Eggs	
Vegetables (raw, steamed,	Gluten—wheat, barley, spelt,	
sautéed, or roasted)	kamut, rye, oats (unless gluten-	
Wild game	free), and any other products	
	containing gluten	

Guide to the Modified Elimination Diet

Foods to Include on the Diet	Foods to Avoid on the Diet
Chicken, lamb, cold-water fish (salmon, mackerel, halibut) All legumes Unsweetened live yogurt Nut and rice milks Vegetables Baked goods and cereal products made from gluten-free flours like buckwheat, corn, potato, coconut, tapioca, rice, teff (see section on gluten for more acceptable foods) Unsweetened juices from fruits and vegetables, water, noncitrus herbal teas Fresh fruits except for citrus fruits and strawberries Cold/expeller-pressed, unrefined oils like ghee, flax, olive, coconut, sesame	Red meat and processed meats Eggs Milk, cheese, ice cream, cream, nondairy creamers Gluten and all foods containing gluten (see section on gluten for a full list of foods to avoid) Coffee, tea, soda, cocoa, sweetened beverages, decaffeinated coffee, herbal coffee Citrus juices, fruit drinks Alcohol Strawberries, citrus fruits, dried fruits Margarine, shortening, butter, refined oils, peanut oil, peanuts, salad dressings, spreads

Cruciferous Vegetable Recipes

Raw Cultured Vegetables

The fermentation process goes through two phases; the first phase is when the salty brine kills off harmful bacteria. The second phase is when the good Lactobacillus bacteria convert sugars into lactic acid, which gives it that distinctly tangy flavor, and also acts as a preservative.

Ingredients

4 cups of vegetables, using a mixture of 3 parts cabbage and 1 part kale or other vegetable, chopped (Use organic vegetables that have been washed and dried)

Water, as needed

Starter culture

3–5 cabbage leaves, whole

Directions

1. Chop the vegetables by hand and mix in a bowl.
2. Take several cups of the mixture and blend with water to make a brine (should be a thick liquid). Add the starter cultures to the brine.
3. Use an air-tight container, either glass or steel, with a rubber or plastic seal and a lid that clamps down. Add the remaining chopped veggies and brine to this jar, packing them in snuggly, leaving 2 inches at the top. Take the additional cabbage leaves, roll them up and lay them across the top of the jar to fill this 2-inch space.
4. Let the jar sit for a minimum of three days at room temperature. It's best to let them sit for a week or more. The culture should be kept at around 70 degrees F. Warmer temperatures will speed up the culturing, so the vegetables will be ready in about half the time, but if it's too warm it's possible for the vegetables to spoil. When it's colder it may be necessary to insulate the container to keep it from getting too cold.
5. When the vegetables are done (you can taste them throughout the fermentation period to get a sense of this), place them in the refrigerator. They will stay good for up to 8 months.

Coleslaw With Yogurt

Adapted from Jeffrey Goettemoeller (1998), *Stevia Sweet recipes: Sugar-Free— Naturally!* (Garden City Park, NY: Square One Publishers).

Ingredients

2 cups shredded cabbage

½ cup chopped cauliflower

¾ cup shredded carrots

¼ cup toasted pecans

1/3 cup currants or raisins

1/8 teaspoon stevia extract powder

2 teaspoons fresh lemon juice

Few drops vanilla extract

½ cup plain yogurt

Directions

1. Combine the cabbage, cauliflower, carrots, pecans, and currants in a large bowl.
2. In a smaller bowl, whisk together the remaining ingredients and pour over the cabbage mixture, stirring well to combine.

Asian Slaw

Serves 4–5

Ingredients

5 cups shredded cabbage and carrots, mixed

4 tablespoons brown rice vinegar

4 tablespoons Bragg's liquid aminos

1 tablespoon maple syrup

1 tablespoon dark toasted sesame oil

1 tablespoon olive oil

2 teaspoons black pepper

Directions

1. Mix all ingredients together in a large bowl. Refrigerate for at least 1 hour prior to serving.

Pineapple-Cabbage Slaw With Chile-Coconut Dressing

Serves 4

Ingredients

Roasted Chile-Coconut Dressing/Sauce:

½ cup organic extra-virgin coconut oil

4 generous teaspoons coarsely ground Aleppo chile or other flavorful medium-hot to hot ground chile

4 large garlic cloves, finely chopped

11/3 cups full-fat coconut milk

2–2½ tablespoons Asian fish sauce

¼ teaspoon liquid stevia

¼ –1/3 teaspoon pink or gray sea salt

Juice of 1 to 1½ large limes (optional)

Salad:

3–4 cups mixed greens

8 leaves Napa cabbage, thinly sliced

4 whole scallions, thinly sliced

1½ cups fresh pineapple, cut into bite-sized pieces

½ cup dry-roasted and salted broken cashews

1½ to 2 cups cooked and diced tempeh, chicken, or seafood

½ cup fresh mint, coriander, or basil leaves, torn

Sea salt and fresh ground black pepper

Directions

1. To make the dressing, heat the coconut oil in a large sauté pan over medium heat. Add the chile and garlic and heat slowly for about 2 minutes, stirring often until the garlic is fragrant and sizzling, but not browned.

2. Add the coconut milk and increase heat, bringing the mixture to a boil. Allow it to boil for 30 seconds while stirring. Add 2 tablespoons of the fish sauce, the stevia, and the salt. Boil for 30 seconds, or until it is thickened, bubbly, and a rich caramel color.

3. Immediately transfer the sauce to a bowl. The sauce can be refrigerated for several days.

4. To make the salad, mix all the greens and cabbage in a bowl, then divide between four plates. Divide the remaining ingredients between each plate, tossing them over the greens. Season with salt and pepper.

5. If the sauce was made in advance, simply reheat it on the stove until bubbly, and then drizzle it over each salad. Squeeze fresh lime juice over the salads and serve.

Coconut Turmeric Cauliflower

Adapted from Mikaela Reuben (2014), Mind body green. Retrieved from http://www.mindbodygreen.com/0-13198/anti-inflammatory-coconut-turmeric-cauliflower-vegan.html

Ingredients

1 head cauliflower, stem removed, and cut into

1- to 2-inch florets

1 stalk lemon grass

2½ tablespoons coconut oil

1 shallot, chopped

1-inch piece of ginger, peeled and chopped

6 kaffir lime leaves

1 tablespoon turmeric powder

1 pinch sea salt

Directions

1. Turn the oven on to broil.

2. Peel the outer leaf of the lemon grass off. Bruise the lemon grass by pounding or pressing the inside with a wooden spoon. Chop into ½-inch pieces.

3. Add 1½ tablespoons of the coconut oil to a medium-sized pot and put on medium heat. Add shallot and ginger. Cook until softened. Add lemon grass and kaffir lime leaf. Reduce to low and simmer for at least 30 minutes.

4. Toss the cauliflower and remaining 1 tablespoon coconut oil together in a bowl with a little sea salt. Place on a baking pan and put in the oven, watching closely as it will cook quickly. Broil until it is lightly browned and then take it out of the oven.

5. Strain the lemon grass mixture and drizzle the sauce over the cauliflower. Add sea salt and turmeric, tossing until the cauliflower is thoroughly coated and a lovely yellow color.

Stuffed Cabbage

Ingredients

For the sauce:

3 tablespoons extra-virgin olive oil

1½ cups chopped onion (2 onions)

2 (28-oz) cans crushed tomatoes with juice

¼ cup red wine vinegar

2 tablespoons raw honey

½ cup raisins

1½ teaspoons sea salt

¾ teaspoon freshly ground black pepper

1 large head Savoy or green cabbage, including outer leaves, core removed

For the filling:

2½ pounds ground chuck

3 extra-large eggs, lightly beaten

½ cup finely chopped onion

½ cup brown rice (or other grain of choice)

1 teaspoon minced fresh thyme leaves

1½ teaspoons sea salt

½ teaspoon freshly ground black pepper

Directions

1. To make the sauce, heat the olive oil over medium-low heat and cook the onions until translucent, 5–10 minutes. Add the tomatoes with their juice, vinegar, honey, raisins, salt, and pepper. Turn the heat up and bring to a boil, then return to low heat and simmer 30 minutes, uncovered. Stir occasionally. Set aside.
2. While the sauce is cooking, bring a large pot of water to a boil.
3. Immerse the head of cabbage in the boiling water for a few minutes, peeling off each leaf with tongs as soon as they are soft. Set the leaves to the side.
4. For the filling, in a large bowl, combine the ground chuck, eggs, onion, brown rice, thyme, salt, and pepper. Add 1 cup of the sauce to the meat mixture.
5. Preheat the oven to 350 degrees F.
6. To assemble, cut out the hard triangular rib from the base of each cabbage leaf with a small paring knife. Spread 1 cup of the sauce in the bottom of a large Dutch oven or glass

baking dish. Place 1/3 to ½ cup of filling in an oval shape near the rib edge of each leaf and roll up toward the outer edge, tucking the sides in as you roll. Place half the cabbage rolls, seam sides down, over the sauce. Add more sauce and more cabbage rolls until all the cabbage rolls are in the pot, and cover with the remaining sauce. Cover the dish tightly with the lid (or aluminum foil) and bake for 1 hour or until the meat is cooked and the rice is tender. Serve hot.

Soaking Legumes and Nuts

Legumes

1. Place the legumes in a bowl and cover with warm water.
2. For each cup of beans, add 1 tablespoon apple cider vinegar or lemon juice (do not add vinegar or lemon juice to lentils and split peas). For smaller beans, use twice as much vinegar or lemon juice.
3. Soak at room temperature for a minimum of 7 hours. Larger beans should be soaked for 24 hours, being sure to change the water if they begin to ferment.
4. After soaking, drain and cook according to how they are normally cooked.

Nuts

1. To soak nuts, simply cover in warm water and soak for 7 hours.
2. Drain the nuts and let sit at room temperature to dry out.

Root Vegetable Recipes

Honey and Chipotle Roasted Sweet Potato Spears

Adapted from Diane Morgan (2012), *Roots: The Definitive Compendium With More Than 225 Recipes* (San Francisco, CA: Chronicle Books).

Ingredients

4 lb medium sweet potatoes or yams, peeled, halved crosswise, and sliced into ½-inch wedges

1 tablespoon plus ½ cup unsalted organic butter, at room temperature

1 teaspoon chipotle chile powder

½ cup honey

1/3 cup fresh lime juice

1 teaspoon fine sea salt

Directions

1. Position a rack in the center of the oven and preheat to 400 degrees F. Put the sweet potatoes in a large bowl. Coat a large rimmed baking sheet with 1 tablespoon of butter.
2. In a small saucepan, melt the remaining ½ cup butter over medium heat. Whisk in the chile powder and then add the honey, lime juice, and salt. Bring to a simmer, stirring constantly, and simmer for 3 minutes to meld the glaze.
3. Pour the glaze over the sweet potatoes and toss until well coated. Spread the sweet potatoes in a single layer on the prepared baking sheet, making sure to scrape all of the glaze from the bowl onto them. Cover the pan tightly with aluminum foil.
4. Roast the sweet potatoes for 40 minutes. Remove the foil and baste the sweet potatoes with the pan glaze. Continue to bake, basting every 10 minutes, until the sweet potatoes are tender, nicely browned, and caramelized at the edges, about 20 minutes longer. Serve immediately, or keep warm in a low oven for up to 30 minutes and then baste again just before serving.

Honeyed Carrots

By Rudolph C. Ryser

Ingredients

1 pound carrots

2 tablespoons unsalted butter

¼ teaspoon dried French tarragon

4 drops stevia liquid

2 tablespoons raw honey

Directions

1. Peel the carrots and cut into halves and quarters of equal size.
2. Heat a cast-iron pan on medium and slowly melt butter.
3. Place cut and quartered carrots in the pan and sauté for 5 to 10 minutes or until tender.
4. Add tarragon, stevia, and honey to the carrots and stir lightly. When all ingredients are fully integrated, turn out onto a serving dish and serve immediately.

Yucca Fries With Cilantro-Lime Dipping Sauce

Recipe adapted from Diane Morgan (2012), *Roots: The Definitive Compendium With More Than 225 Recipes* (San Francisco, CA: Chronicle Books)

Cilantro is a powerful detoxifier of heavy metals.

Ingredients

Dipping Sauce

½ cup sour cream

½ cup fresh cilantro, finely chopped

2 tsp fresh lime juice

¼ tsp fine sea salt

Fries

1½ lb yucca

8 cups water

Fine sea salt

3 small dried red chiles such as chile de árbol

About 5 cups peanut, grapeseed, or vegetable oil for

deep frying

Directions

1. Begin by making the dipping sauce. Combine all dipping sauce ingredients in a blender and purée until smooth. Transfer to a bowl, cover, and refrigerate until ready to serve.

2. Trim the ends off of the yucca and peel off the skin. Cut the yucca in half and remove the fibrous core in the center.

3. Bring the water to a boil in a large pot, add 2 tbsp of salt and the chiles, and then add the yucca. Simmer, uncovered, until tender (but not mushy) when pierced with a wooden skewer or fork, about 20 minutes. The yucca may cook at different rates, so check often for tenderness and remove the tender ones. Drain the yucca in a colander, and then transfer to a bowl of ice water. When it has cooled down, drain and pat dry with paper towels. Slice the yucca into thick fries about ¾ inch thick.

4. Line two baking sheets with two layers of paper towels. Have ready a slotted spoon or wire mesh skimmer. Pour the oil in a deep, heavy pot or wok so it is about 3 inches deep, heat to 360 degrees F (use a deep-frying thermometer). Fry the yucca in small batches. Add a handful of fries to the hot oil and fry, and cook until they are golden brown, stirring once or twice, 2 ½ to 3 minutes (test a fry to make sure it is crispy on the outside and soft inside). Use the slotted spoon/skimmer to remove the fries from the oil and place them on the paper towels to absorb the oil. Sprinkle with salt. Continue cooking small batches of fries, rechecking the oil temperature to make sure it stays at 360 degrees F.

5. Serve hot with the dipping sauce.

Fermented Foods

Kimchi

Ingredients

2 heads of Napa cabbage (or another Chinese cabbage variety), shredded in a food processor

5–10 scallions, finely chopped

2–3 cloves garlic, crushed

1 teaspoon fresh ginger, crushed

2 jalapeños, finely minced

2 tablespoons crushed fresh red chili pepper

Half an onion, chopped (Optional)

Filtered or distilled water, as needed

½ teaspoon Celtic sea salt or Himalayan pink salt

2 tablespoons of raw honey

Directions

1. Mix together all ingredients (except salt and honey) in a bowl.
2. Add several cups of the mixture to a blender with filtered or distilled water, the sea salt, and the honey and blend to make a brine (should be a thick liquid). Starter cultures can be added to the brine if desired.
3. Add chopped vegetables and brine to a 1½ quart glass or stainless steel jar, packing them in snuggly, leaving 2 inches at the top. Take several cabbage leaves, roll them up and place them at the top to fill this 2-inch space.
4. Let the jar sit for a minimum of three days at room temperature. It is best to let them sit for a week or more. The culture should be kept at around 70 degrees F.

Homemade Yogurt

You will need a starter culture to begin. You can purchase it as a specific product or you can buy any live-culture yogurt available at the store. Make sure it says "contains live-cultures." Once you have finished your first batch, you can reserve a little bit as the starter culture for the next batch.

Basic Steps

1. Heat the milk.
2. Cool the milk.
3. Add a cup of store-bought yogurt.
4. Pour mixture into sterilized mason jars.
5. Let the jars sit in a cooler with warm water for several hours.

Ingredients

1 gallon of milk
1 cup yogurt starter (use a small cup of plain yogurt, or a cup from your previous batch)
Four quart-size glass canning jars with four lids and four screw tops
A cooler that will fit the four glass jars
1 gallon of water

Directions

1. Sterilize your glass jars, lids, and screw tops by placing them in a large pot. Fill with an inch of water; cover with lid and heat to boiling. Boil for 10 minutes. Leave the lid on the pot and move it off the heat until you are ready to use the jars.

2. Pour the milk into a large, heavy-bottomed stockpot or Dutch oven. Heat the milk to 185–190 degrees Fahrenheit (90–90 Celsius).

3. Cool the milk by placing the pot in a sink filled with cold water. Let it sit until the temperature goes down to 120 degrees Fahrenheit (50–55 degrees Celsius).

4. Add the yogurt starter to the cooled milk and mix with a whisk, stirring well to distribute the starter throughout the milk.

5. Pour the milk into the jars, and put the lids and screw tops on. Place them into a cooler.

6. Heat the gallon of water to 120 degrees F (50–55 degrees C) and pour into the cooler around the sealed yogurt jars. Close the cooler lid and let it sit for 3 hours.

7. After 3 hours, remove the yogurt jars from the cooler and place in the refrigerator.

Garlic and Yogurt Salad Dressing

Adapted from Jeffrey Goettemoeller (1998), *Stevia Sweet Recipes: Sugar-Free—Naturally!* (Garden City Park, NY: Square One Publishers).

Ingredients

¾ cup plain yogurt

1 small garlic clove, minced

¼ teaspoon dried basil

½ tablespoon apple cider vinegar

1/16 teaspoon green stevia powder

1 teaspoon chopped fresh parsley

4 tablespoons mayonnaise

Directions

1. Whisk all ingredients together in a bowl and serve.

Homemade Kefir

Ingredients

Whole cow milk, goat milk, sheep milk, coconut milk, or raw milk

Starter culture

Directions

1. Gently heat the milk to about 90 degrees. Remove from the heat.
2. Add the starter culture, mix it up, cover, and let sit at room temperature for 24 hours.
3. It will thicken up enough for a toothpick to stand up in it. When it is ready, it will be thick but still pourable. Shake the kefir and place in the refrigerator.
4. A second batch of kefir can be made by simply adding a few spoonfuls of the first batch to warmed milk.

Miso Soup With Natto

Ingredients

¼ cup dried wakame seaweed

| 2 cups dashi* |
| 4–5 shiitake mushrooms, sliced |
| 2 tablespoons of natto, or to taste |
| 2 tablespoons brown miso |
| 2 tablespoons sweet white miso, such as Saikkyo |
| 2 scallions, sliced (for garnish) |

Directions

1. Soak the seaweed in warm water for 30 minutes prior to cooking.

2. Bring the dashi to a simmer in a soup pot and add the mushrooms and the seaweed. Simmer for 10 minutes. Reduce the heat to low.

3. In a separate bowl, mix together the natto, brown miso, and sweet white miso, adding as much of the broth as it takes to make a smooth creamy paste. Place this mixture into the soup pot and let it heat through for 1 minute while stirring to dissolve the paste.

4. Serve immediately. Garnish with scallions.

*Dashi is a type of stock used in Japanese soups and other recipes. Dashi is usually made from dried bonito (fish) flakes and/or kombu seaweed. It can also be made using store-bought dashi powder or granules, but homemade dashi is higher quality, more nutritious, and better tasting. See the recipe below for how to make your own.

Dashi

This basic Japanese soup stock is a key ingredient to many Japanese dishes, like Miso Soup and Congee (see recipes). It is made from kelp (kombu) and dried bonito flakes (fish flakes), and it only takes about thirty minutes to make. The stock ingredients are strained to make "first dashi," a light broth with a milder flavor. "Second dashi" is made by taking the kombu and bonito from the first dashi and cooking it again to make a stronger, darker broth than first dashi.

Ingredients:

| 5 cups cold water |
| 1 ounce dried kombu (about 5" x 5") |
| 3 cups loosely packed bonito flakes ("katsuobushi") |

Directions

1. Gently wipe the kombu with a damp cloth or paper towel, removing some of the powdery excess but not all of it.

2. Place the kelp in a pot with the cold water. (If making ahead of time, soak the kombu for several hours to bring out its flavor).

3. Put the water on medium heat and slowly bring to near boiling. Once the water is trembling and you see bubbles forming in the pot, just before boiling, remove the kelp (reserve for second dashi¾see Note).

4. Add the bonito flakes and bring the stock to a full boil. Turn off the heat and let it sit for 5 minutes while the bonito flakes sink to the bottom of the pot.

5. Using a fine strainer or sieve, strain and separate the bonito flakes from the broth. Reserve the bonito flakes for use in second dashi. The broth, or first dashi, can be used immediately in recipes (see Miso Soup with Natto recipe) or it may be refrigerated 3-7 days or stored in the freezer for 3 weeks.

6. If you're making second dashi, add the reserved kombu and bonito flakes to a medium pot with 5 cups of water. Simmer over low heat for 10 minutes. Do not boil.

7. Strain the stock through a fine strainer or sieve. Discard the bonito. The kombu can be discarded or eaten with sesame oil and sesame seeds and salt, or added to other soups or stews.

8. Second dashi can be stored in the refrigerator for 3-7 days or frozen for 3 weeks.

Kicking the Coffee (Caffeine) Addiction

A PROTOCOL FOR WITHDRAWAL

Coffee is a drug, not a beverage. So use it wisely.

Coffee, a favorite beverage in our culture, enhances mood, stimulates alertness, and increases mental performance. However, it contains hundreds of chemicals, including the powerful and well-known caffeine, an addictive chemical that is known to cause a number of negative health effects. It should be used in moderation, if at all. Not only does the coffee bean itself contain naturally occurring chemicals, but nonorganic coffee may also contain traces of pesticides, herbicides, and other harmful chemicals that can harm your body, as well as the environment and communities where it is grown. Decaffeinated coffee, although nearly caffeine-free, still contains the naturally occurring chemicals as well as harmful chemicals such as methylene chloride used in the decaffeination process. Although there are some proven health benefits to drinking organic coffee, it should be consumed in moderation (1–2 cups a day) due to its addictive qualities and potential for negative effects on health. Espresso has less caffeine than drip coffee. People with anxiety or panic should avoid coffee; however, people who are depressed, have ADHD, or need cognitive support may benefit.

Short-Term Negative Effects
- Restlessness, anxiety, and nervousness
- Increased blood pressure
- Sleep disturbances
- Increased heart rate
- Irregular heartbeat
- Nausea and headache
- Muscle tension
- Increased acidity
- Adrenal fatigue (see below)
- Frequent urination

- Jitteriness
- Lightheadedness
- Diarrhea
- Upset stomach
- Irregular breathing
- Heartburn

Adrenal Fatigue

Caffeine raises the body's adrenaline levels and can lead to adrenal exhaustion. The adrenal glands regulate stress response, but when the adrenals are exhausted it may be difficult to respond to stress because they cannot efficiently produce the necessary hormones. Imagine driving a car with your foot on the accelerator while the car is in neutral. Eventually this will cause the engine to burn out. Your adrenal glands are like your body's engine, ready to pump out hormones in response to stresses in your environment. When the adrenal glands are repeatedly overstimulated, which can occur with regular coffee drinking (and stress), they become less efficient.

Long-Term Negative Health Effects of Caffeine
- Heartburn
- Ulcers
- Fibrocystic breast disease
- Heart problems
- Heart disease

Caffeine Withdrawal Symptoms
- Headache
- Fatigue
- Anxiety
- Nausea and vomiting
- Loss of appetite
- Intense desire for coffee
- Irritability
- Intensified premenstrual symptoms
- Muscular tension
- Constipation
- Lack of concentration
- Disorientation
- Forgetfulness

Caffeine Content Chart

	Serving Size (oz)	Caffeine Content (mg)
Coffee (brewed)	8	102–200
Black tea	8	23–110
Yerba mate*	8	110
Soft drinks	12	23–71
Green tea	8	20–30
White tea	8	15
Cocoa beverage	8	3–32
Dark chocolate	1	5–35

Note: Prescription and over-the-counter drugs also contain caffeine. Mixing caffeine with other drug ingredients like phenylpropanolamine (ephedrine) can cause severe hypertension, stroke and myocardial infarction.

Coffee Substitutes

Beverage	Caffeinated?	Ingredients
Inka	No	Roasted barley, rye, chicory and beet roots
Roastaroma	No	Roasted barley, roasted chicory, roasted carob, cinnamon, all-spice, and Chinese star anise. *Contains gluten
Teeccino	No	Carob, barley, chicory, almonds, dates, figs, coffee flavor
Roasted dandelion root	No	Roasted dandelion root
Dark roast yerba mate	Yes*	Roasted yerba mate
Chai	Yes	Black tea, cardamom, cloves, cinnamon, ginger
Genmaicha	Yes	Green tea and roasted brown rice

*The caffeine content of yerba mate is currently being debated. Some say that the stimulant in yerba mate is caffeine, but that the nutritional benefits of mate (vitamins, minerals, amino acids, and antioxidants) act to balance out the negative effects of the caffeine. Other research indicates that yerba mate's stimulating factor is not caffeine at all, but a compound called "mateine," which is similar to caffeine. In either case, many individuals report that drinking yerba mate does not have the same negative side effects as drinking coffee or other caffeinated beverages.

Health Benefits of Drinking Coffee

Although there are many studies showing coffee's negative effects, there are also a number of studies indicating that coffee, if moderately consumed, may actually be beneficial. The following is a list of some potentially beneficial effects of moderate coffee consumption:

- Reduced risk of gallstone development
- Reduction in colon cancer risk
- Improved cognitive function
- Reduced risk for Parkinson's disease
- Improvement in physical endurance
- Reduced risk of liver damage
- Treatment for headaches, asthma, and mood enhancement

Three Methods to Kick the Caffeine Habit

Here are a few methods to transition from coffee addiction to a more balanced, healthy lifestyle. These methods will help you avoid the common withdrawal symptoms of quitting coffee.

Decaf Coffee Method

- Week 1: Using all organic coffee, brew ¾ regular coffee to ¼ decaf coffee.
- Week 2: The following week reduce the ratio to ½ regular coffee and ½ decaf.
- Week 3: Now brew just ¼ regular coffee and ¾ decaf.
- Finally, transition to completely decaf coffee and you are caffeine-free!

Lowered Caffeine Method

- Week 1: Instead of coffee, brew yourself some caffeinated coffee substitute (these will all have less caffeine than coffee and will help in the transition).
- Week 2: Replace ½ of your caffeinated coffee with a caffeine-free coffee substitute or herbal tea.
- Week 3: Completely replace your caffeinated coffee substitute with a caffeine-free choice and thank yourself for overcoming the addiction!

Quick and Easy Method

- Week 1: Replace ½ of your coffee with herbal tea or a caffeine-free coffee substitute.

- Week 2: Brew just a ¼ of your original coffee intake and replace the rest with a caffeine-free choice.
- Week 3: Drink only caffeine-free coffee substitutes or herbal tea and be free of caffeine!

And If You're Still Needing an Energy Boost . . .

Here is a list of naturally energizing and stimulating herbs and plants that can easily be incorporated into your diet:

Licorice root: Sweet, energizing, and detoxifying. Used in cases of adrenal gland insufficiency.

Rhodiola: Reduces fatigue; improves physical and mental performance. Adaptogenic (increases the body's resistance to stress).

Ginseng: Adaptogenic and stimulating root. Improves memory, concentration, and focus.

Schizandra: Adaptogenic and mood enhancing. Improves learning ability, memory, and mental function.

Cacao: Increases blood circulation and improves mood. Contains magnesium, sulphur, and antioxidants.

Maca: Adaptogenic, energizing, and increases endurance. Helps with fatigue, sexual function, anxiety, and stress.

Cold-Brewed Coffee

To reduce the acidity of your coffee by about 70%, a cold-brewing method can be used. It can be used for hot or iced coffee.

1. Start with coarsely ground, organic coffee. If you are grinding your beans at the store, use the "French Press" setting.
2. Combine grounds with water in a glass container. Use 1/3 cup of grounds with 1½ cups of water at room temperature. Stir well.
3. Cover the container and let steep in a cool, dark place for 12–16 hours.
4. Strain the mixture using a coffee filter. This is a concentrated coffee extract and should be mixed with water to taste.
5. To make iced coffee, mix equal parts coffee extract with cold water and add ice.
6. To make hot coffee, use equal parts coffee extract (at room temperature) and boiling water. These ratios can be adjusted depending on how strong you like your coffee.
7. Use the coffee concentrate within 1–2 weeks.

Smoothie Recipes

Fruity Turmeric Smoothie

Ingredients

½ cup frozen pineapple or mango

1 fresh banana

1 cup milk (hemp or coconut milk)

1 tablespoon coconut oil, melted

½ teaspoon turmeric, fresh

½ teaspoon cinnamon

½ teaspoon ginger, fresh

¼ teaspoon ground black pepper

1 teaspoon chia seeds

1 teaspoon green tea powder (optional)

¼ cup goat yogurt (optional)

1 teaspoon raw honey or 10 drops of liquid stevia (optional)

Directions

1. Add ingredients to a blender in the following order: frozen fruit, banana, milk, oil, spices, and remaining ingredients.
2. Blend until smooth.

Cashew-Apple Smoothie

By Marlene Bremner

Ingredients

2 tablespoons raw organic cashews

¼ of a sweet apple, coarsely chopped

½ of a banana

2 tablespoons organic full-fat coconut milk

¼ cup coconut yogurt, dairy yogurt, or kefir

½ cup milk of choice (hazelnut, almond, rice, etc.)

1 tablespoon ground flax seeds

1 tablespoon chia seeds

Directions

Add all ingredients to a blender in the order they are listed in, and blend until smooth.

Avocado-Coconut Smoothie

Makes 2 servings

Ingredients

1 avocado

1 banana (fresh or frozen)

1 cup coconut milk (full fat)

½ cup orange juice

2 tablespoons freshly squeezed lime juice

1 pinch salt

1 teaspoon honey or 1–2 drops liquid stevia extract (Optional)

Directions

1. Peel the avocado and remove the pit. Cut it into chunks and place in a blender.
2. Peel the banana, break in two, and place in the blender.
3. Add the remaining ingredients (and honey or stevia, if using) to the blender and blend until smooth, or about 1 minute.
4. Pour into two large glasses and serve.

Onion-Garlic Soup

Onion-Garlic Soup

Onion soup with garlic is medicine. It makes for an inexpensive meal that is rich in sulfur compounds. Garlic and onions should be eaten daily, but this soup can be made on special occasions, especially to boost mood and enjoy a rich dinner on a cool evening. Sulfur compounds support glutathione synthesis as well, making this a powerful detoxification meal. It is also an ideal meal if you have sinus congestion or during a cold.

Ingredients

6 large red or yellow onions (about 3 pounds), peeled and thinly sliced

2 tablespoons olive oil

½ teaspoon honey (Optional)

1 teaspoon sea salt

4 cloves garlic, minced

½ cup dry white wine

8 cups fresh beef/bone broth, chicken stock, vegetable stock, or a combination

2 bay leaves

¼ teaspoon dried thyme

Sea salt and pepper to taste

3 tablespoons brandy (Optional)

Optional: French bread (or gluten-free bread) and 1½ cups grated Swiss Gruyere, goat cheddar, or Parmesan cheese (Optional)

Directions

1. In a 5- to 6-quart, thick-bottomed pot, heat the olive oil on medium heat. Add the onions and toss to coat with the olive oil. Cook the onions, stirring often, until they have softened, about 15 to 20 minutes. Increase the heat to medium high and cook, stirring often, until they start

to brown, about 15 more minutes. Then sprinkle with the honey and 1 teaspoon of salt and continue to cook until the onions are well browned, about 10 to 15 more minutes.

2. Add the minced garlic and cook for a minute more. Add the wine to the pot and scrape up the browned bits on the bottom and sides of the pot, deglazing the pot as you go.

3. Add the stock, bay leaves, and thyme. Bring to a simmer, cover the pot, and lower the heat to maintain a low simmer. Cook for about 30 minutes. Season to taste with more salt and with freshly ground black pepper. Discard the bay leaves and add brandy.

4. You can prepare bread (or gluten-free bread) to place on the soup when it is done. First, slice and toast the bread. Then transfer the soup to overproof serving bowls, place a piece of bread on the top of the soup, and sprinkle some cheese on top. Place the bowls under the broiler for a few minutes until bubbling and brown.

Salad Dressings

Vinaigrette Salad Dressing

The best salad dressings are those you make yourself. They are healthy, medicinal, and taste good. Vinaigrettes are especially good for decreasing fatigue and apple cider vinegar increases energy, reduces depression, and improves mood.

Make this dressing and keep it in a glass bottle in the fridge for up to 2 weeks, or use with the Salad Jars recipe.

Makes 4 cups

Ingredients

½ cup of cold-pressed, extra-virgin olive oil

1/2 cup organic flax seed oil

2 cups of organic apple cider vinegar

1 fresh lime or lemon (optional)

2 cloves of fresh garlic, crushed

½ teaspoon of your favorite herb (dill, basil, oregano, caraway seed, etc.)

Directions

Combine all ingredients in a glass bottle, shake, and refrigerate. Use 1 tablespoon over your salad each day.

Addition

Add some cranberries! Use fresh berries that are cooked and strained, cranberry concentrate, or soaked dried cranberries that have no sugar or added preservatives.

Creamy Ginger Vinaigrette

Ingredients

½ cup olive oil

1 cup white wine vinegar

10 drops of stevia or 1 tablespoon honey

2 teaspoons fresh grated ginger

Pinch of cayenne pepper

1/3 teaspoon freshly ground black pepper

Directions

1. Combine all ingredients in a jar with a tight fitting lid. Shake well.
2. Store in refrigerator and use within 2 weeks.

Creamy Dill Dressing

Avocado is rich in fats for the brain and skin. In Mexico, it is called "poor man's butter." Dill is a carminative, which means it helps digestion and reduces gas. Cayenne pepper also stimulates digestion and brings blood and oxygen to the stomach lining. This dressing may be used over any type of raw vegetable salad, or leave out the water and use it as a vegetable dip.

Makes 1½ cups

Ingredients

1 avocado

½ cup–1 cup water for desired consistency

2 tablespoons olive oil

2–3 tablespoons fresh dill

1–2 tablespoons lemon juice

½ teaspoon Celtic salt

2 tablespoons fresh chives, minced (Optional)

Dash of cayenne (Optional)

Directions

In a blender, process all ingredients until smooth and creamy.

Lemon Tahini Dressing

Makes 1 cup

Ingredients

¼ cup flax oil

¼ cup olive oil

½ cup lemon juice

1 tablespoon raw tahini

2 teaspoons dill

½ teaspoon sea salt

Freshly ground black pepper, to taste

Dash of cayenne pepper (Optional)

Directions

In a blender, process all ingredients until smooth and creamy.

NOTE: You may like this dressing thinner or thicker—add water as needed.

Resources

DATABASES

Drug–Nutrient Interactions Virtual Database

Use this database to enter a drug or supplement; receive a full interaction report that includes notice of potential interactions. Mailing address: Integrative Therapeutics, LLC, 825 Challenger Drive Green Bay, WI 54311; Phone: 800-931-1709; Fax: 800-380-8189. Website: http://www.integrativepro.com/Resources/Professional-Resources/Drug-Nutrient-Interaction-Checker?utm_medium=email&utm_source=2014-08-07-newsletter&utm_campaign=drug-nutrient-interactions&utm_content=sub-feature

Book: Stargrove, M. B., Treasure, J., & McKee, D. L. (2007). *Herb, nutrient, and drug interactions: Clinical implications and therapeutic strategies. Maryland Heights, MI: Mosby.*

Nutrition Data

Detailed nutrition information, plus unique analysis tools that tell you more about how foods affect your health and make it easier to choose healthy foods.
Website: http://nutritiondata.self.com/

RxISK

RxISK is a free and independent website where patients, doctors, and pharmacists can research prescription drugs and easily report a drug side effect. Website: https://www.rxisk.org/Default.aspx

ASSESSMENTS, TESTING, AND LAB WORK

Diagnos-Techs

Provides saliva testing for evaluating stress, hormone-related disease, food allergies, gastrointestinal health, 24 hr Cortisol Test to evaluate HPA axis function, and other health conditions. Website: http://www.diagnostechs.com/Pages/Intro.aspx

Eating Attitudes Test 26

This test can be used for education and screening. A score of 20 or greater implies the need for further assessment. Website: http://www.eat-26.com/

Gluten and Food Allergy/Food Sensitivity Testing

Cyrex™ specializes in testing for autoimmune conditions. Website: https://www.cyrexlabs.com/; Tests: https://www.cyrexlabs.com/CyrexTestsArrays/tabid/136/Default.aspx

Great Plains Laboratory

Provides specialized testing, including Organic Acids test, Gluten/Casein, Vitamin D, amino acid levels testing (urinary and blood), urinary/serum peptide tests, and zinc taste test.

Website: http://www.greatplainslaboratory.com/home/eng/; Tests: http://www.greatplainslaboratory.com/home/eng/peptide.asp

Life Extension

Provides requisitions for client-ordered blood tests for a variety of markers, including inflammatory markers, homocysteine, high-sensitivity C-reactive protein (CRP), fibrinogen, and micronutrient tests (blood). Website: http://www.lef.org/Vitamins-Supplements/Blood-Tests

The Mediator Release Test

Tests for food- and food-chemical-induced inflammation. Website: http://nowleap.com/mediator-release-testing/the-patented-mediator-release-test-mrt/

SpectraCell

Provides nutritional testing, including MTHFR, telomere testing, micronutrient tests (blood), and nutrient status for physicians and their clients. SpectraCell Labs also conducts telomere testing via blood sample submission. Website: http://www.spectracell.com/

Standard Process

NutrSync: DNA test for 45 variables that affect nutritional status. Website: https://www.standardprocess.com/Standard-Process/NutriSync#.VSQkwmahY29

Trace Elements

Provides hair tissue mineral analysis for metabolic type, mineral ratios, and heavy metals. **Website:** http://www.traceelements.com/

HIGH-QUALITY NUTRITIONAL SUPPLEMENTS SOURCES

Life Extension

Provides nutritional information, products, and services. Website: http://www.lef.org/

Life Extension Magazine

A monthly publication of the Life Extension Foundation on topics of nutrition, hormones, and antiaging supplements. Website: http://www.lef.org/magazine/index.htm

Thorne Metabolic Nutrition

Quality nutritional supplements. Website: https://shop.thorne.com/products/thorne-metabolic-nutrition

HIGH-QUALITY NUTRIENT BRANDS

Allergy Research Group

Excellent source of vitamins, minerals, and glandulars.
Website: http://www.allergyresearchgroup.com/

Biotics Research Corp

Address: PO Box 7027, Olympia, WA 98507; Phone: (360) 438-3600;
    Excellent source of vitamins, minerals, and glandulars, as well as De-Stress and Liquid Zinc.
    Toll-free: (800) 636-6913; Website: http://bioticsnw.com/

Carlson Labs

Excellent source for vitamin E and fish oil.
Website: http://www.carlsonlabs.com/

Fungi Perfecti

Provides medicinal mushroom supplements and products. Address: Fungi Perfecti LLC, PO Box 7634, Olympia, WA 98507; Phone (toll-free in US & Canada): 800-780-9126; Phone (local): 360-426-9292; E-mail: info@fungi.com

Green Pastures

High-quality fermented cod liver oil and butter-oil blend.
Website: http://www.greenpasture.org/public/Home/index.cfm

Integrative Therapeutics

Website: http://www.integrativepro.com/

Nordic Naturals

Website: https://www.nordicnaturals.com/
High-quality fish oil combinations for all ages.

Standard Process

Excellent source of chlorophyll and glandulars.
Website: http://www.standardprocess.com/home

DISTRIBUTORS OF HIGH-QUALITY SUPPLEMENTS

These companies will establish accounts for professionals and provide wholesale pricing for most quality brands, and they ship nationally. Clinicians may make arrangements for client purchase at small discounts.

Emerson Ecologics

Quality nutritional supplements. Website: https://emersonecologics.com/

Natural Partners

Quality nutritional supplements. Website: http://www.naturalpartners.com/

SPECIFIC SUPPLEMENTS

Prevagen

Prevagen® (apoaequorin) is clinically shown to help with mild memory problems associated with aging. Address: Quincy Bioscience, 301 S. Westfield Rd, Suite 200, Madison, WI 53716; Phone: 888-565-5385; E-mail: customerservice@prevagen.com; Website: https://www.prevagen.com/

Sonic Cholesterol

A purified cholesterol supplement to support healthy cholesterol levels. Address: New Beginnings Nutritionals, 7797 Quivira Road, Lenexa, KS 66216; Phone: (913) 754-0458; Toll-free: (877) 575-2467; Fax: (913) 248-7609; E-mail: info@nbnus.com; Website: http://www.nbnus.net/shopexd.asp?id=399

FOODS AND FOOD-RELATED TECHNOLOGIES

Bragg's Apple Cider Vinegar

Organic raw apple cider vinegar. Phone (toll-free): 800-446-1990; Fax: 805-968-1001; E-mail: General information: info@bragg.com; Website: http://www.bragg.com/

Find Real Food App

An app that lists of over 13,000 researched foods and brands highest in nutrient density, without additives and processing. Website: https://itunes.apple.com/us/app/find-real-food/id716877330?mt=8&ign-mpt=uo%3D4

HAPIfork

The HAPIfork is an electronic fork that helps you monitor and track your eating habits. Website: http://www.hapi.com/

COOKING SKILLS

Cooking Matters

Helps families to shop for and cook healthy meals on a budget. Address: 1030 15th Street NW, Suite 1100, Washington DC, 20005; Website: http://cookingmatters.org/

Food Scores App

Produced by Environmental Working Group, this app rates the quality of the food/brand name and produces an overall score between 1 and 10. Website: http://www.ewg.org/foodscores?inlist=Y&sdf=1

Knife Skill Video Techniques—HD

This HD video series teaches the basics of how to work with knives and also has tutorials on how to sharpen your knife, and butchery. Website: http://www.stellaculinary.com/knife-skill-video-techniques-hd

Rouxbe Online Cooking School

Rouxbe (ROO-bee) is a members-only, online cooking school delivering culinary and wellness instruction to home cooks, schools, restaurants, and professional culinary academies. Phone (toll-free): 1-800-677-0131; Phone (international): 1-604-677-6000; E-mail: pr@rouxbe.com; Website: http://rouxbe.com/

COOKBOOKS/BLOGS

These two resources are among the best food cookbooks and blogs. Watch out for use of some ingredients like sugar that you will want to avoid. Just make a substitution.

Canal Street Cooking

Website: http://thecanalhouse.com/buythebook.html

Food52

Website: http://food52.com/

DVDS

Microwarriors: The Power of Probiotics, Special Edition

DVD Documentary Narrated by Leonard Nimoy about probiotics, including their history, production, scientific research, and more. Address: Health Point Productions, 4335 Van Nuys Blvd., Sherman Oaks, CA 91403; Phone: (818) 788-2040;

E-mail: microwarriorsmovie@sbcglobal.net; Website: http://www.microwarrior-smovie.com/index.html

Beyond Fish Oil Nutritional and Complementary Therapies With Dr. Leslie Korn

This 7-hour continuing education course for clinicians provides a comprehensive overview of nutritional therapies for mental health and their integration with other modalities. Website: http://shop.pesi.com/product/beyondfishoilcomplementary andnutritionaltreatmentsformentalhealthdisorders%287436%29

KITCHEN APPLIANCES

Blenders

Brands to look for include Vitamix, K-Tec Blender, Juiceman Smoothies, and Tribest Blender.

Juicer

Champion Juicer is a very high-quality juicer. Website: http://championjuicer.com/

Dehydrator

The Excalibur is a good choice, as it has temperature control, it is fan-operated, and it is easy to clean. Website: http://www.excaliburdehydrator.com/

NUTRITIONAL THERAPIES TRAINING

Bastyr University Nutrition Programs

Bastyr University offers undergraduate and graduate nutrition degree programs, as well as nondegree programs that encompass a "whole food" approach. Address: Bastyr University, 14500 Juanita Drive N.E., Kenmore, WA 98028-4966; Phone: (425) 602-3000; Fax: (425) 823-6222 (fax); Website: http://www.bastyr.edu/academics/areas-study/study-nutrition

Health Coach Training Program

Integrative Nutrition's Health Coach Training Program is online, with lectures by leading health experts. Phone (US): (877) 730-5444; Phone (International): +1 (212) 730-5433; Website: http://www.integrativenutrition.com/

National Association of Nutrition Professionals (NANP)

This webpage lists training programs that have been reviewed and approved as meeting NANP's educational standards. These programs qualify their graduates for professional membership and to sit for the holistic nutrition national board exam. Website: http://nanp.org/schools

Nutritional Therapy Practitioner Program (NTP)

This distance-learning program provides students with 9 months of distance training with the flexibility of self-paced study, teleconference calls, and three separate multiple-day, instructor-led workshops during the 15-module course. Website: http://nutritionaltherapy.com/ntt-programs/ntp-classes/

ORGANIZATIONS

Center for Nutrition Advocacy

The Center for Nutrition Advocacy tracks nutritional practice regulation for each state. Website: http://nutritionadvocacy.org/laws-state

International Network of Integrative Mental Health, Inc. (NIMH)

Provides education, research, networking, and advocacy. Website: http://www.inimh.org/

Weston-Price Foundation

Provides education, research, and activism for restoring nutrient-dense foods to the human diet. Website: http://www.westonaprice.org/

References

Abumaria, N., Yin, B., Zhang, L., Li, X-Y., Chen, T., Descalzi, G., ... Liu, G. (2011). Effects of elevation of brain magnesium on fear conditioning, fear extinction, and synaptic plasticity in the infralimbic prefrontal cortex and lateral amygdala. *Journal of Neuroscience, 31*(42), 14871–14881.

Abumaria, N., Yin, B., Zhang, L., Zhao, L., & Liu, G. (2009, October 20). *Enhancement of cognitive control of emotions by elevated brain magnesium leads to anti-depressants like effect.* Poster presentation #549, Society for Neuroscience 2009 Meeting, Chicago, IL.

Abu-Taweela, G. M., Zyadah, M. A., Ajarem, J. S., & Ahmad, M. (2014). Cognitive and biochemical effects of monosodium glutamate and aspartame, administered individually and in combination in male albino mice. *Neurotoxicology and Teratology, 42*(2014), 60–67.

Agarwal, S., Reider, C., Brooks, J. R., & Fulgoni, V. L. (2015, January 7). Comparison of prevalence of inadequate nutrient intake based on body weight status of adults in the United States: An analysis of NHANES 2001–2008. *Journal of the American College of Nutrition.* Retrieved May 2015, from http://www.tandfonline.com/doi/full/10.1080/07315724.2014.901196#.VLhghsa2828

Alcock, J., Maley, C. C., & Aktipis, C. A. (2014). Is eating behavior manipulated by the gastrointestinal microbiota? Evolutionary pressures and potential mechanisms. *BioEssays, 36*(10), 940–949.

Aleppo, G., Nicoletti, F., Sortino, M. A., Casabona, G., Scapagnini, U., & Canonico, P. L. (1994). Chronic L-alpha-glyceryl-phosphoryl-choline increases inositol phosphate formation in brain slices and neuronal cultures. *Journal of Pharmacology and Toxicology, 74*(2), 95–100.

Alhamoruni, A., Wright, K. L., Larvin, M., & O'Sullivan, S. E. (2012). Cannabinoids mediate opposing effects on inflammation-induced intestinal permeability. *British Journal of Pharmacology, 165*(8), 2598–2610. doi: 10.1111/j.1476-5381.2011.01589.x.

Allison, K. C., Engel, S. G., Crosby, R. D., de Zwaan, M., O'Reardon, J. P., Wonderlich, S. A., Stunkard, A. J. (2008). Evaluation of diagnostic criteria for night eating syndrome using item response theory analysis. *Eating Behaviors, 9*(4), 398–407.

Aneja, A., & Tierney E. (2008). Autism: The role of cholesterol in treatment. *International Review of Psychiatry, 20*(2), 165–170. doi: 10.1080/09540260801889062.

Arafat, E. S., Hargrove, J. T., Maxson, W. S., Desiderio, D. M., Wentz, A. C., & Andersen, R. N. (1988). Sedative and hypnotic effects of oral administration of micronized progesterone may be mediated through its metabolites. *American Journal of Obstetrics and Gynecology, 159*(5), 1203–1209.

Ashton, H. (2002). *Benzodiazepines: How they work and how to withdraw.* Retrieved May 2015, from http://www.benzo.org.uk/manual/

Bachhuber, M. A., Saloner, B., Cunningham, C. O., & Barry, C. L. (2014). Medical cannabis laws and opioid analgesic overdose mortality in the United States, 1999-2010. *JAMA Internal Medicine, 174*(10), 1668–1673. doi:10.1001/jamainternmed.2014.4005.

Bakulski, K. M., Rozek, L. S., Dolinoy, D. C., Paulson, H. L., & Hu, H. (2012). Alzheimer's disease and environmental exposure to lead: The epidemiologic evidence and potential role of epigenetics. *Current Alzheimer Research, 9*(5), 563–573.

Bal, B. S., Finelli, F. C., & Koch, T. R. (2011). Origins of and recognition of micronutrient deficiencies after gastric bypass surgery. *Current Diabetes Reports, 11*(2), 136–141. doi: 10.1007/s11892-010-0169-4.

Baldi, I., Filleul, L., Mohammed-Brahim, B., Fabrigoule, C., Dartigues, J. F., Schwall, S., ... Brochard, P. (2001). Neuropsychologic effects of long-term exposure to pesticides: Results from the French phytoner study. *Environmental Health Perspectives, 109*(8), 839–844.

Balerio, G. N., Aso, E., Berrendero, F., Murtra, P., & Maldonado, R. (2004). Delta9-tetrahydrocannabinol decreases somatic and motivational manifestations of nicotine withdrawal in mice. *European Journal of Neuroscience, 20*(10), 2737–2748.

Bambico, F. R., Katz, N., Debonnel, G., & Gobbi, G. (2007). Cannabinoids elicit antidepressant-like behavior and activate serotonergic neurons through the medial prefrontal cortex. *Journal of Neuroscience, 27*(43), 11700–11711.

Bara, A. C., & Arber, S. (2009). Working shifts and mental health: Findings from the British Household Panel Survey (1995–2005). *Scandinavian Journal of Work, Environment, and Health, 35*(5), 361–367. doi:10.5271/sjweh.1344

Baughman, F. (2006). There is no such thing as a psychiatric disorder/disease/chemical imbalance. *PLoS Medicine, 3*(7), e318.

Baum, J. I., Layman, D. K., Freund, G. G., Rahn, K. A., Nakamura, M. T., & Yudell, B. E. (2006). A reduced carbohydrate, increased protein diet stabilizes glycemic control and minimizes adipose tissue glucose disposal in rats. *Journal of Nutrition, 136*(7), 1855–1861.

Bell, J. G., MacKinlay, E. E., Dick, J. R., MacDonald, D. J., Boyle, R. M., & Glen, A. C. A. (2004). Essential fatty acids and phospholipase A2 in autistic spectrum disorders. *Prostaglandins, Leukotrienes and Essential Fatty Acids, 71*(4), 201–204.

Bello, N. T., & Hajnal, A. (2010). Dopamine and binge eating behaviors. *Pharmacology Biochemistry and Behavior, 97*(1), 25–33.

Bercik, P., Park, A. J., Sinclair, D., Khoshdel, A., Lu, J., Huang, X., ... Verdu, E. F. (2011). The anxiolytic effect of bifidobacterium longum NCC3001 involves vagal pathways for gut–brain communication. *Neurogastroenterology and Motility, 23*(12), 1132–1139. doi: 10.1111/j.1365-2982.2011.01796.x.

Bested, A. C., Logan, A. C., & Selhub, E. M. (2013). Intestinal microbiota, probiotics and mental health: From Metchnikoff to modern advances: Part III – convergence toward clinical trials. *Gut Pathogens, 5*(1), 4. doi:10.1186/1757-4749-5-4.

Bhattacharjee, S., Zhao, Y., Hill, J. M., Percy, M. E., & Lukiw, W. J. (2014). Aluminum and its potential contribution to Alzheimer's disease (AD). *Frontiers in Aging Neuroscience, 6*, 62.

Bland, J. (1980, July). Glandular based food supplements: Helping to separate fact from fiction, 1979-80. *Nutritional Perspectives*, 15–39.

Bland, J. S. (2004). *Clinical nutrition: A functional approach.* Gig Harbor, WA: Institute for Functional Medicine.

Bravo, J. A., Forsythe, P., Chew, M. V., Escaravage, E., Savignac, H. M., Dinan, T. G., ... Cryan, J. F. (2011). Ingestion of lactobacillus strain regulates emotional behavior and central GABA receptor expression in a mouse via the vagus nerve. *Proceedings of the National Academy of Sciences USA, 108*(38), 16050–16055. doi: 10.1073/pnas.1102999108.

Bredesen, D. E. (2014). Reversal of cognitive decline: A novel therapeutic program. *Aging, 6*(9), 707–717.

Breggin, P. R. (2013). *Psychiatric drug withdrawal: A guide for prescribers, therapists, patients, and their families.* New York: Springer.

Brinkworth, G. D., Noakes, M., Buckley, J. D., Keogh, J. B., & Clifton, P. M. (2009). Long-term effects of a very-low-carbohydrate weight loss diet compared with an isocaloric low-fat diet after 12 mo. *American Journal of Clinical Nutrition, 90*(1), 23–32. doi: 10.3945/ajcn.2008.27326.

Brown, R. P., Gerbarg, P. L., & Bottiglieri, T. (2000). S-adenosylmethionine in the clinical practice of psychiatry, neurology, and internal medicine. *Clinical Practice of Alternative Medicine, 1*(4), 230–241.

Brownley, K. A., Von Holle, A., Hamer, R. M., La Via, M., & Bulik, C. M. (2013). A double-blind, randomized pilot trial of chromium picolinate for binge eating disorder: Results of the Binge Eating and Chromium (BEACh) study. *Journal of Psychosomatic Research, 75*(1), 36–42. doi: 10.1016/j.jpsychores.2013.03.092.

Buang, Y., Wang, Y. M., Cha, J. Y., Nagao, K., & Yanagita, T. (2005). Dietary phosphatidylcholine alleviates fatty liver induced by orotic acid. *Nutrition, 21*(7–8), 867–873.

Burke, N. J., Hellman, J. L., Scott, B. G., Weems, C. F., & Carrion, V. G. (2011). The impact of adverse childhood experiences on an urban pediatric population. *Child Abuse and Neglect, 35*(6), 408–413.

Butterworth, S. (2010). Health-coaching strategies to improve patient-centered outcomes. *Journal of the American Osteopathic Association, 110*(4), eS12–eS14.

Buydens-Branchey, L., & Branchey, M. (2003). Association between low plasma levels of cholesterol and relapse in cocaine addicts. *Psychosomatic Medicine, 65*(1), 86–91.

Buysse, D. J., Reynolds, C. F., Monk, T. H., Berman, S. R., & Kupfer, D. J. (1989). The Pittsburgh Sleep Quality Index (PSQI): A new instrument for psychiatric research and practice. *Psychiatry Research, 28*(2), 193–213.

Capasso, A., Petrella, C., & Milano, W. (2010). Pharmacological profile of SSRIs and SNRIs in the treatment of eating disorders. *Current Clinical Pharmacology, 4*(1), 78–83.

Careaga, M., Hansen, R. L., Hertz-Piccotto, I., Van de Water, J., & Ashwood, P. (2013). Increased anti-phospholipid antibodies in autism spectrum disorders. *Mediators of Inflammation, 2013*(2013), 935608.

Cascella, N. G., Kryszak, D., Bhatti, B., Gregory, P., Kelly, D. L., McEvoy, J. P., ... Eaton, W. W. (2011). Prevalence of celiac disease and gluten sensitivity in the United States clinical antipsychotic trials of intervention effectiveness study population. *Schizophrenia Bulletin, 37*(1), 94–100.

Center for Nutrition Advocacy. (2014). *State laws.* Retrieved May 2015, from http://www.nutritionadvocacy.org/laws-state

Chauhan, A., Essa, M. M. M., Muthaiyah, B., Chauhan, V., Kaur, K., & Lee M. (2010). Walnuts-rich diet improves memory deficits and learning skills in transgenic mouse model of Alzheimer's disease. *Alzheimer's and Dementia, 6*(4, Suppl), S69.

Chedid, V., Dhalla, S., Clarke, J. O., Roland, B. C., Dunbar, K. B., Koh, J., ... Mullin, G. E. (2014). Herbal therapy is equivalent to rifaximin for the treatment of small intestinal bacterial overgrowth. *Global Advances in Health and Medicine, 3*(3), 16–24. doi: 10.7453/gahmj.2014.019.

Chen, M-H., Su, T-P., Chen, Y-S., Hsu, J-W., Huang, K-L., Chang, W-H., ... Bai, Y-M. (2013). Association between psychiatric disorders and iron deficiency anemia among children and adolescents: A nationwide population-based study. *BMC Psychiatry, 13*, 161.

Chen, X., Redline, S., Shields, A. E., Williams, D. R., & Williams, M. A. (2014). Associations of allostatic load with sleep apnea, insomnia, short sleep duration, and other sleep disturbances: Findings from the National Health and Nutrition Examination Survey. *Annals of Epidemiology, 24*(8), 612–619.

Cheney, G. (1952). Vitamin U therapy of peptic ulcer. *California Medicine, 77*(4), 248–252.

Chouinard, G., Beauclair, L., Geiser, R., & Etienne, P. (1990). A pilot study of magnesium aspartate hydrochloride (Magnesiocard) as a mood stabilizer for rapid cycling bipolar affective disorder patients. *Progress in Neuro-Psychopharmacology and Biological Psychiatry, 14*(2), 171–180.

Clare, D. A., & Swaisgood, H. E. (2000). Bioactive milk peptides: A prospectus. *Journal of Dairy Science, 83*(6), 1187–1195.

Clark, M. M., Hanna, B. K., Mai, J. L., Graszer, K. M., Krochta, J. G., McAlpine, D. E., … Sarr, M. G. (2007). Sexual abuse survivors and psychiatric hospitalization after bariatric surgery. *Obesity Surgery, 17*(4), 465–469.

Cohen, J. S. (2001). Peripheral neuropathy associated with fluoroquinolones. *Annals of Pharmacotherapy, 35*(12), 1540–1547.

Concas, A., Sogliano, C., Porcu, P., Marra, C., Brundu, A., & Biggio, G. (2006). Neurosteroids in nicotine and morphine dependence. *Psychopharmacology (Berl), 186*(3), 281–292.

Cope, E. C., Morris, D. R., & Levenson, C. W. (2012). Improving treatments and outcomes: An emerging role for zinc in traumatic brain injury. *Nutrition Review, 70*(7), 410–413.

Crumpacker, D. W. (2008). Suicidality and antidepressants in the elderly. *Proceedings (Baylor University Medical Center), 21*(4), 373–377.

Curi, R., Alvarez, M., Bazotte, R. B., Botion, L. M., Godoy, J. L., & Bracht, A. (1986). Effect of Stevia rebaudiana on glucose tolerance in normal adult humans. *Brazilian Journal of Medical and Biological Research, 19*(6), 771–774.

Czapp, K. (2009). The good Scots diet. *Weston A. Price Foundation.* Retrieved May 2015, from http://www.westonaprice.org/health-topics/the-good-scots-diet/

Dean, O., Giorlando, F., & Berk, M. (2011). N-acetylcysteine in psychiatry: Current therapeutic evidence and potential mechanisms of action. *Journal of Psychiatry and Neuroscience, 36*(2), 78–86. doi: 10.1503/jpn.100057.

DebMandal, M., & Mandal, S. (2011). Coconut (Cocos nucifera L.: Arecaceae): In health promotion and disease prevention. *Asian Pacific Journal of Tropical Medicine, 4*(3), 241–247.

de la Monte, S. M., & Wands, J. R. (2008). Alzheimer's disease is type 3 diabetes: Evidence reviewed. *Journal of Diabetes Science and Technology, 2*(6), 1101–1113.

Delini-Stula, A., & Holsboer-Trachsler, E. (2009). Treatment strategies in anxiety disorders: An update. *Therapeutische Umschau, 66*(6), 425–431.

de Saint-Hilaire, Z., Messaoudi, M., Desor, D., & Kobayashi, T. (2009). Effects of a bovine alpha S1-casein tryptic hydrosylate (CTH) on sleep disorder in Japanese general population. *Open Sleep Journal, 2,* 26–32.

Dickerson, F., Stallings, C., Origoni, A., Vaughan, C., Khushalani, S., Alaedini, A., & Yolken, R. (2011). Markers of gluten sensitivity and celiac disease in bipolar disorder. *Bipolar Disorders, 13*(1), 52–58. doi: 10.1111/j.1399-5618.2011.00894.x.

Dickerson, F., Stallings, C., Origoni, A., Vaughan, C., Khushalani, S., & Yolken, R. (2012). Markers of gluten sensitivity in acute mania: A longitudinal study. *Psychiatry Research, 196*(1), 68–71. doi: 10.1016/j.psychres.2011.11.007.

Dinan, T. G., Stanton, C., & Cryan, J. F. (2013). Psychobiotics: A novel class of psychotropic. *Biological Psychiatry, 74*(10), 720–726. doi: 10.1016/j.biopsych.2013.05.001.

Diniz, B. S., Machado-Vieira, R., & Forlenza, O. V. (2013). Lithium and neuroprotection: Translational evidence and implications for the treatment of neuropsychiatric disorders. *Journal of Neuropsychiatric Disease and Treatment, 9,* 493–500. doi: 10.2147/NDT.S33086.

Dohan, F. C. (1996). Cereals and schizophrenia data and hypothesis. *Acta Psychiatrica Scandinavica, 42*(2), 125–152.

Donini, L. M., Marsili, D., Graziani, M. P., Imbriale, M., & Cannella, C. (2004). Orthorexia nervosa: A preliminary study with a proposal for diagnosis and an attempt to measure the dimension of the phenomenon. *Eating and Weight Disorders, 9*(2), 151–157.

Dorman, T., Bernard, L., Glaze, P., Hogan, J., Skinner, R., Nelson, D., … Head, D. (1995). The effectiveness of stabilium on reducing anxiety in college students. *Journal of Advancement in Medicine, 8*(3), 193–200.

Drum, R. (2013). *Medicinal uses of seaweeds.* Retrieved May 2013, from http://www.ryandrum.com/seaweeds.htm

Eggers, A. E. (2012). Extending David Horrobin's membrane phospholipid theory of schizophrenia: Overactivity of cytosolic phospholipase A(2) in the brain is caused by overdrive of coupled serotonergic 5HT(2A/2C) receptors in response to stress. *Medical Hypotheses, 79*(6), 740–743. doi: 10.1016/j.mehy.2012.08.016.

Elias, P. K., Elias, M. F., D'Agostino, R. B., Sullivan, L. M., & Wolf, P. A. (2005). Serum cholesterol and cognitive performance in the Framingham Heart Study. *Psychosomatic Medicine, 67*(1), 24–30.

Eliaz, I., Weil, E., & Wilk, B. (2007). Integrative medicine and the role of modified citrus pectin/alginates in heavy metal chelation and detoxification: Five case reports. *Forschende Komplementärmedizin, 14*(6), 358–364.

Enig, M. G. (2000). *Know your fats: The complete primer for understanding the nutrition of fats, oils, and cholesterol.* Silver Spring, MD: Bethesda Press.

Epling, W. F., & Pierce, W. D. (Eds.). (1996). *Activity anorexia: Theory, research, and treatment.* Mahwah, NJ: Erlbaum.

Eubanks, L. M., Rogers, C. J., Beuscher IV, A. E., Koob, G. F., Olson, A. J., Dickerson, T. J., & Janda, K. D. (2006). A molecular link between the active component of marijuana and Alzheimer's disease pathology. *Molecular Pharmacology, 3*(6), 773–777. doi: 10.1021/mp060066m

Exley, C. (2014). Why industry propaganda and political interference cannot disguise the inevitable role played by human exposure to aluminium in neurodegenerative diseases, including Alzheimer's disease. *Frontiers in Neurology, 5,* 212. doi: 10.3389/fneur.2014.00212

Fallon, S., & Enig, M. (1999). *Nourishing traditions: The cookbook that challenges politically correct nutrition and the diet dictocrats.* Washington, DC: Newtrends Publishing.

Fasano, A. (2011). Zonulin and its regulation of intestinal barrier function: The biological door to inflammation, autoimmunity, and cancer. *Physiology Review, 91*(1), 151–75. doi: 10.1152/physrev.00003.2008.

Felton, C. V., Crook, D., Davies, M. J., & Oliver, M. F. (1994). Dietary polyunsaturated fatty acids and composition of human aortic plaques. *Lancet, 344*(8931), 1195–1196.

Forlenza, O. V., Diniz, B. S., Radanovic M, Santos, F. S., Talib, L. L., & Gattaz, W. F. (2011). Disease-modifying properties of long-term lithium treatment for amnestic mild cognitive impairment: Randomised controlled trial. *British Journal of Psychiatry, 198*(5), 351–356.

Fournier, J. C., DeRubeis, R. J., Hollon, S. D., Dimidjian, S., Amsterdam, J. D., Shelton, R. C., & Fawcett, J. (2010). Antidepressant drug effects and depression severity: A patient-level meta-analysis. *Journal of the American Medical Association, 303*(1), 47–53.

Frazier, E. A., Fristad, M. A., & Arnold, L. E. (2012). Feasibility of a nutritional supplement as treatment for pediatric bipolar spectrum disorders *Journal of Alternative and Complementary Medicine, 18*(7), 678–685. doi:10.1089/acm.2011.0270.

Frost, G., Sleeth, M. L., Sahuri-Arisoylu, M., Lizarbe, B., Cerdan, S., Brody, L., … Bell, J. D. (2014). The short-chain fatty acid acetate reduces appetite via a central homeostatic mechanism. *Nature Communications, 5,* 3611.

Gaby, A. R. (2002). Intravenous nutrient therapy: The "Myers' cocktail". *Alternative Medicine Review, 7*(5), 389–403.

Gates, D. (2011). *The body ecology diet: Recovering your health and rebuilding your immunity.* Carlsbad, CA: Hay House.

Gelber, D., Levine, J., & Belmaker, R. H. (2001). Effect of inositol on bulimia nervosa and binge eating. *Interntaional Journal of Eating Disorders, 29*(3), 345–348.

George, M. S., Guidotti, A., Rubinow, D., Pan, B., Mikalauskas, K., & Post, R. M. (1994). CSF neuroactive steroids in affective disorders: Pregnenolone, progesterone, and DBI. *Biological Psychiatry, 35*(10), 775–780.

Gershon, M. (1998). *The second brain: The scientific basis of gut instinct and a groundbreaking new understanding of nervous disorders of the stomach and intestines.* New York: HarperCollins.

Gershuny, B. S., Keuthen, N. J., Gentes, E. L., Russo, A. R., Emmott, E. C., Jameson, M., … Jenike, M. A. (2006). Current posttraumatic stress disorder and history of trauma in trichotillomania. *Journal of Clinical Psychology, 62*(12), 1521–1529.

Gilbert, P. (2009). Introducing compassion-focused therapy. *Advances in Psychiatric Treatment, 15*, 199–208.

Gimpl, G., & Fahrenholz, F. (2002). Cholesterol as stabilizer of the oxytocin receptor. *Biochimica et Biophysica Acta, 1564*(2), 384–392.

Grant, J. E., Odlaug, B. L., & Kim, S. W. (2009). N-acetylcysteine, a glutamate modulator, in the treatment of trichotillomania: A double-blind, placebo-controlled study. *Archives of General Psychiatry, 66*(7), 756–763. doi: 10.1001/archgenpsychiatry.2009.60.

Greenblatt, J. (2013). Don't suffer with OCD. *Bottom Line Health.* Retrieved May 2015, from http://www.bottomlinepublications.com/content/article/health-a-healing/don-t-suffer-with-ocd

Guo, X., Park, Y., Freedman, N. D., Sinha, R., Hollenbeck, A. R., Blair, A., & Chen, H. (2014). Sweetened beverages, coffee, and tea and depression risk among older US adults. *PLoS One, 9*(4), e94715. doi: 10.1371/journal.pone.0094715

Gupta, M. A., & Gupta, A. K. (1998). Depression and suicidal ideation in dermatology patients with acne, alopecia areata, atopic dermatitis and psoriasis. *British Journal of Dermatology, 139*(5), 846–850.

Hadhazy, A. (2010, February 12). Think twice: How the gut's "second brain" influences mood and well-being. *Scientific American.* Retrieved May 2015, from http://www.scientificamerican.com/article/gut-second-brain/

Hamlin, J. C., Pauly, M., Melnyk, S., Pavliv, O., Starrett, W., Crook, T. A., & James, S. J. (2013). Dietary intake and plasma levels of choline and betaine in children with autism spectrum disorders. *Autism Research and Treatment, 2013*, 578429.

Harris, C. B., Chowanadisai, W., Mishchuk, D. O., Satre, M. A., Slupsky, C. M., & Rucker, R. B. (2013). Dietary pyrroloquinoline quinone (PQQ) alters indicators of inflammation and mitochondrial-related metabolism in human subjects. *Journal of Nutritional Biochemistry, 24*(12), 2076–2084.

Hatoum, I. J., Greenawalt, D. M., Cotsapas, C., Daly, M. J., Reitman, M. L., & Kaplan, L. M. (2013). Weight loss after gastric bypass is associated with a variant at 15q26.1. *American Journal of Human Genetics, 92*(5), 827–834.

Hausenblas, H. A., Saha, D., Dubyak, P. J., & Anton, S. D. (2013). Saffron (Crocus sativus L.) and major depressive disorder: A meta-analysis of randomized clinical trials. *Journal of Integrative Medicine, 11*(6), 377–383. doi: 10.3736/jintegrmed2013056.

Heinberg, L. J., Ashton, K., & Windover A. (2010). Moving beyond dichotomous psychological evaluation: The Cleveland clinic behavioral rating system for weight loss surgery. *Surgery for Obesity and Related Diseases, 6*(2), 185–190. doi: 10.1016/j.soard.2009.10.004.

Herbert, M. R., & Buckley, J. A. (2013). Autism and dietary therapy: Case report and review of the literature. *Journal of Child Neurology, 28*(8), 975–982. doi: 10.1177/0883073813488668.

Heresco-Levy, U., Javitt, D. C., Ermilov, M., Mordel, C., Silipo, G., & Lichtenstein, M. (1999). Efficacy of high-dose glycine in the treatment of enduring negative symptoms of schizophrenia. *Archives of General Psychiatry, 56*, 29–36.

Herrin, M., & Larkin, M. (2013). *Nutrition counseling in the treatment of eating disorders.* New York: Routledge.

Higdon, J. (2003). *Iodine.* Retrieved May 2015, from http://lpi.oregonstate.edu/infocenter/minerals/iodine/

Higdon, J. (2004). *Potassium.* Retrieved May 2015, from http://lpi.oregonstate.edu/infocenter/minerals/potassium/

Hoffer, A. (1962). *Niacin therapy in psychiatry (American lecture series).* Springfield, IL: Thomas.

Hoffer, L. J. (2008). Vitamin therapy in schizophrenia. *Israeli Journal of Psychiatry and Related Sciences, 45*(1), 3–10.

Holick, M. (2003). Vitamin D deficiency: What a pain it is. *Mayo Clinic Proceedings, 78*(12), 1457–1459.

Horrobin, D. F. (2001). Phospholipid metabolism and depression: The possible roles of phospholipase A2 and coenzyme A-independent transacylase. *Human Psychopharmacology: Clinical and Experimental, 16*(1), 45–52.

Howatson, G., Bell, P. G., Tallent, J., Middleton, B., McHugh, M. P., & Ellis, J. (2012). Effect of tart cherry juice (Prunus cerasus) on melatonin levels and enhanced sleep quality. *European Journal of Nutrition, 51*(8), 909–916.

Hsu, R-L., Lee, K-T., Wang, J-H., Lee, L. Y-L., & Chen, R. P-Y. (2009). Amyloid-degrading ability of nattokinase from bacillus subtilis natto. *Journal of Agricultural and Food Chemistry, 57*(2), 503–508.

Hyung, S. J., DeToma, A. S., Brender, J. R., Lee, S., Vivekanandan, S., Kochi, A., … Lim, M. H. (2013). Insights into antiamyloidogenic properties of the green tea extract (-)-epigallocatechin-3-gallate toward metal-associated amyloid- species. *Proceedings of the National Academy of Sciences USA, 110*(10), 3743–3748. doi: 10.1073/pnas.1220326110.

Igna, C. V., Julkunen, J., & Vanhanen, H. (2011). Vital exhaustion, depressive symptoms and serum triglyceride levels in high-risk middle-aged men. *Psychiatry Research, 187*(3), 363–369.

Iliades, C. (2014). How stress affects digestion. *Everyday Health.* Retrieved May 2015, from http://www.everydayhealth.com/health-report/better-digestion/how-stress-affects-digestion.aspx

Imhoff, L. R., Liwanag, L., & Varma, M. (2012). Exacerbation of symptom severity of pelvic floor disorders in women who report a history of sexual abuse. *Archives of Surgery, 147*(12), 1123–1129. doi:10.1001/archsurg.2012.1144.

Ingenbleek, Y., & McCully, K. S. (2012). Vegetarianism produces subclinical malnutrition, hyperhomocysteinemia and atherogenesis. *Nutrition, 28*(2), 148–153. doi: 10.1016/j.nut.2011.04.009.

Insel, T. (2013, August 28). Director's blog: Antipsychotics: Taking the long view. *National Institute of Mental Health.* Retrieved May 2015, from http://www.nimh.nih.gov/about/director/2013/antipsychotics-taking-the-long-view.shtml

Jackson, J. R., Eaton, W. W., Cascella, N. G., Fasano, A., & Kelly, D. L. (2012). Neurologic and psychiatric manifestations of celiac disease and gluten sensitivity. *Psychiatric Quarterly, 83*(1), 91–102.

James, S. J., Cutler, P., Melnyk, S., Jernigan, S., Janak, L., Gaylor, D. W., & Neubrander, J. A. (2004). Metabolic biomarkers of increased oxidative stress and impaired methylation capacity in children with autism. *American Journal of Clinical Nutrition, 80*(6), 1611–1617.

Jaminet, P., & Jaminet, S-C. (2013). *Perfect health diet: Regain health and lose weight by eating the way you were meant to eat.* New York: Scribner.

Jefferson, T., Jones, M. A., Doshi, P., Del Mar, C. B., Hama, R., Thompson, M. J., ... Heneghan, C. J. (2014). Neuraminidase inhibitors for preventing and treating influenza in healthy adults and children. *Cochrane Database of Systemic Reviews, 10*(4), CD008965. doi: 10.1002/14651858. CD008965.pub4.

Johnson, E. J. (2012). A possible role for lutein and zeaxanthin in cognitive function in the elderly. *American Journal of Clinical Nutrition, 96*(suppl), 1161S–1165S.

Jou, S-H., Chiu, N-Y., & Liu, C-S. (2009). Mitochondrial dysfunction and psychiatric disorders. *Chang Gung Medical Journal, 32*(4), 370–379.

Jung, I. H., Jung, M. A., Kim, E. J., Han, M. J., & Kim, D. H. (2012). Lactobacillus pentosus var. plantarum C29 protects scopolamine-induced memory deficit in mice. *Journal of Applied Microbiology, 113*(6), 1498–1506.

Kang, J. E., Lim, M. M., Bateman, R. J., Lee, J. J., Smyth, L. P., Cirrito, J. R., ... Holtzman, D. M. (2009). Amyloid-ꞵ dynamics are regulated by orexin and the sleep-wake cycle. *Science, 326*(5955), 1005–1007.

Katzman, M., & Logan, A. C. (2007). Acne vulgaris: Nutritional factors may be influencing psychological sequelae. *Medical Hypotheses, 69*(5), 1080–1084.

Kelly, A. C., Carter, J. C., & Borairi, S. (2014). Are improvements in shame and self-compassion early in eating disorders treatment associated with better patient outcomes? *International Journal of Eating Disorders, 47*(1), 54–64. doi: 10.1002/eat.22196.

Khantzian, E. J. (1997). The self-medication hypothesis of substance use disorders: A reconsideration and recent applications. *Harvard Review of Psychiatry, 4*(5), 231–244.

Kharrazian, D. (2013). *Why isn't my brain working: A revolutionary understanding of brain decline and effective strategies to recover your brain's health?* Carlsbad, CA: Elephant Press, LP.

Kidd, P. M. (2000). Attention deficit/hyperactivity disorder (ADHD) in children: rationale for its integrative management. *Alternative Medicine Review, 5*(5), 402–428.

Kikkert, M. J., Schene, A. H., Koeter, M. W. J., Robson, D., Born, A., Helm, H., ... Gray, R. J. (2006). Medication adherence in schizophrenia: Exploring patients', carers' and professionals' views. *Schizophrenia Bulletin, 32*(4), 786–794.

Kim, J. H., Desor, D., Kim, Y. T., Yoon, W. J., Kim, K. S., Jun, J. S., ... Shim, I. (2007). Efficacy of alphas1-casein hydrolysate on stress-related symptoms in women. *European Journal of Clinical Nutrition, 61*(4), 536–541.

Kirsch, I. (2010). *The emperor's new drugs: Exploding the antidepressant myth.* New York: Basic Books.

Kirsch, I., Deacon, B. J., Huedo-Medina, T. B., Scoboria, A., Moore, T. J., & Johnson, B. T. (2008). Initial severity and antidepressant benefits: A meta-analysis of data submitted to the Food and Drug Administration. *PLoS Medicine, 5*(2), e45.

Knuchel, F. (1979). Double blind study in patients with alcohol-toxic fatty liver. *Die Medizinische Welt, 30*, 411–416.

Konturek, P. C., Brzozowski, T., & Konturek, S. J. (2011). Stress and the gut: Pathophysiology, clinical consequences, diagnostic approach and treatment options. *Journal of Physiology and Pharmacology, 62*(6), 591–599.

Korn, L. (2013). *Rhythms of recovery: Trauma, nature, and the body.* New York: Routledge.

Korn, L., & Rÿser, R. (2009). *Preventing and treating diabetes naturally: The native way.* Olympia, WA: DayKeeper Press.

Kubik, J. F., Gill, R. S., Laffin, M., & Karmali, S. (2013). The impact of bariatric surgery on psychological health. *Journal of Obesity, 2013*(2013), 1–5.

Lake, J. (2006). *Textbook of integrative mental health care.* New York: Thieme.

Lakhan, S. E., & Kirchgessner, A. (2010). Gut inflammation in chronic fatigue syndrome. *Nutrition and Metabolism, 7*(79), 1–10.

Lakhan, S. E., & Vieira, K. F. (2008). Nutritional therapies for mental disorders. *Nutrition Journal*, *21*(7), 2.

Lam, J. R., Schneider, J. L., Zhao, W., & Corley, D. A. (2013). Proton pump inhibitor and histamine 2 receptor antagonist use and vitamin B12 deficiency. *Journal of the American Medical Association*, *310*(22), 2435–2442. doi:10.1001/jama.2013.280490.

Lapin, I. (2001). Phenibut (beta-phenyl-GABA): A tranquilizer and nootropic drug. *CNS Drug Reviews*, *7*(4), 471–481.

Landolt, H. P., Dijk, D. J., Gaus, S. E., & Borbely, A. A. (1995). Caffeine reduces low- frequency delta activity in the human sleep EEG. *Neuropsychopharmacology*, *12*(3), 229–238.

Lardner, A. L. (2014). Neurobiological effects of the green tea constituent theanine and its potential role in the treatment of psychiatric and neurodegenerative disorders. *Nutritional Neuroscience*, *17*(4), 145–155.

Lemer, P. (2014). *Outsmarting autism*. Tarentum, PA: Word Association Publishers.

Leung, C. W., Laraia, B. A., Needham, B. L., Rehkopf, D. H., Adler, N. E., Lin, J., … Epel, E. S. (2014). Soda and cell aging: Associations between sugar-sweetened beverage consumption and leukocyte telomere length in healthy adults from the national health and nutrition examination surveys. *American Journal of Public Health*, *104*(12), 2425–2431. doi:10.2105/AJPH.2014.302151

Levenson, C. W. (2006). Zinc: The new antidepressant? *Nutrition Reviews*, *64*(1), 39–42.

Levine, J. (1997). Controlled trials of inositol in psychiatry. *European Neuropsychopharmacology*, *7*(2), 147–155.

Lewis, M., Ghassemi, P., & Hibbeln, J. (2013). Therapeutic use of omega-3 fatty acids in severe head trauma. *American Journal of Emergency Medicine*, *31*(1), 273.e5–273.e8.

Leyse-Wallace, R. (2008). *Linking nutrition to mental health: A scientific exploration*. New York: iUniverse.

Liechti, M. E., & Vollenweider, F. X. (2001). Which neuroreceptors mediate the subjective effects of MDMA in humans? A summary of mechanistic studies *Human Psychopharmacology*, *16*(8), 589–598.

Lindseth, G. N., Coolahan, S. E., Petros, T. V., & Lindseth, P. D. (2014). Neurobehavioral effects of aspartame consumption. *Research in Nursing and Health*, *37*(3), 185–193.

Loflin, M., & Earleywine, M. (2014). A new method of cannabis ingestion: The dangers of dabs? *Addictive Behaviors*, *39*(10), 1430–1433.

Logan, A. C., & Katzman, M. (2005). Major depressive disorder: Probiotics may be an adjuvant therapy. *Medical Hypotheses*, *64*(3), 533–538.

Luyer, M. D., Greve, J. W. M., Hadfoune, M., Jacobs, J. A., Dejong, C. H., & Buurman, W. A. (2005). Nutritional stimulation of cholecystokinin receptors inhibits inflammation via the vagus nerve. *Journal of Experimental Medicine*, *202*(8), 1023–1029.

Lyoo, I. K., Demopulos, C. M., Hirashima, F., Ahn, K. H., & Renshaw P. F. (2003). Oral choline decreases brain purine levels in lithium-treated subjects with rapid-cycling bipolar disorder: A double-blind trial using proton and lithium magnetic resonance spectroscopy. *Bipolar Disorders*, *5*(4), 300–306.

Maczurek, A., Hagera, K., Kenkliesa, M., Sharmand, M., Martinsd, R., Engele, J., … Münchc, G. (2008). Lipoic acid as an anti-inflammatory and neuroprotective treatment for Alzheimer's disease. *Advanced Drug Delivery Reviews*, *60*(13–14), 1463–1470.

Maggio, M., Corsonello, A., Ceda, G. P., Cattabiani, C., Lauretani, F., Buttò, V., … Lattanzio, F. (2013). Proton pump inhibitors and risk of 1-year mortality and rehospitalization in older patients discharged from acute care hospitals. *JAMA Internal Medicine*, *173*(7), 518–523.

Mangialasche, F., Solomon, A., Kåreholt, I., Hooshmand, B., Cecchetti, R., Fratiglioni, L., … Kivipelto, M. (2013). Serum levels of vitamin E forms and risk of cognitive impairment in a Finnish cohort of older adults. *Experimental Gerontology, 48*(12), 1428–1435. doi: 10.1016/j. exger.2013.09.006.

Mangialasche, F., Xu, W., Kivipelto, M., Costanzi, E., Ercolani, S., Pigliautile, M., ... Mecocci, P. (2012). Tocopherols and tocotrienols plasma levels are associated with cognitive impairment. *Neurobiology of Aging, 33*(10), 2282–2290.

Marriage,

Marx, C. E. (2009, December). *Abstract P-805.* Presented at the American College of Neuropsychopharmacology (ACNP) 48th annual meeting, Hollywood, FL.

Marx, C. E., Bradford, D. W., Hamer, R. M., Naylor, J. C., Allen, T. B., Lieberman, J. A., ... Kiltsa, J. D. (2011). Pregnenolone as a novel therapeutic candidate in schizophrenia: Emerging preclinical and clinical evidence. *Neuroscience, 191*(15), 78–90.

Massey, P. B. (2007). Reduction of fibromyalgia symptoms through intravenous nutrient therapy: Results of a pilot clinical trial. *Alternative Therapies in Health and Medicine, 13*(3), 32–34.

Matthews, L. R., Danner, O. K., Ahmed, Y. A., Dennis-Griggs, D. M., Frederick, A., Clark, C., ... Wilson, K. L. (2012). Combination therapy with vitamin d_3, progesterone, omega 3-fatty acids and glutamine reverses coma and improves clinical outcomes in patients with severe traumatic brain injuries: A case series. *International Journal of Case Reports and Images, 4*(3), 143–149.

Mato, J. M., Cámara, J., Fernández de Paz, J., Caballería, L., Coll, S., Caballero, A., ... Rodés, J. (1999). S-adenosylmethionine in alcoholic liver cirrhosis: A randomized, placebo-controlled, double-blind, multicenter clinical trial. *Journal of Hepatology, 30*(6), 1081–1089.

Maurer, I. C., Schippel, P., & Volz, H. P. (2009). Lithium-induced enhancement of mitochondrial oxidative phosphorylation in human brain tissue. *Bipolar Disorder, 11*(5), 515–522. doi: 10.1111/j.1399-5618.2009.00729.x.

May, J., Andrade, J., Kavanagh, D. J., & Hetherington, M. (2007). Elaborated intrusion theory: A cognitive-emotional theory of food craving. *Current Obesity Reports, 1*(2), 114–121.

Maylor, E. A., Simpson, E. E., Secker, D. L., Meunier, N., Andriollo-Sanchez, M., Polito, A., ... Coudray, C. (2006). Effects of zinc supplementation on cognitive function in healthy middle-aged and older adults: The ZENITH study. *British Journal of Nutrition, 96*(4), 752–760.

McNamara, D. J. (2014). Dietary cholesterol, heart disease risk and cognitive dissonance. *Proceedings of the Nutrition Society, 73*(2), 161–166. doi: 10.1017/S0029665113003844.

McPartland, J. M., Guy, G. W., & Di Marzo, V. (2014). Care and feeding of the endocannabinoid system: A systematic review of potential clinical interventions that upregulate the endocannabinoid system. *PLoS One, 9*(3), e89566. doi: 10.1371/journal.pone.0089566.

Mendle, J., Turkheimer, E., & Emery, R. E. (2007). Detrimental psychological outcomes associated with early pubertal timing in adolescent girls. *Development Review, 27*(2), 151–171.

Meskanen, K., Ekelund, H., Laitinen, J., Neuvonen, P. J., Haukka, J., Panula, P., & Ekelund, J. (2013). A randomized clinical trial of histamine 2 receptor antagonism in treatment-resistant schizophrenia. *Journal of Clinical Psychopharmacology, 33*(4), 472–478.

Messaoudi, M., Lefranc-Millot, C., Desor, D., Demagny, B., & Bourdon, L. (2005). Effects of a tryptic hydrolysate from bovine milk alphaS1-casein on hemodynamic responses in healthy human volunteers facing successive mental and physical stress situations. *European Journal of Nutrition, 44*(2), 128–132.

Miller, W. R., & Rollnick, S. (2012). *Motivational interviewing: Helping people change.* New York: Guilford Press.

Mitchell, C., Hobcraft, J., McLanahan, S. S., Siegel, S. R., Berg, A., Brooks-Gunn, J., ... Notterman, D. (2014). Social disadvantage, genetic sensitivity, and children's telomere length. *Proceedings of the National Academy of Sciences USA, 111*(16), 5944-5949.

Mitchell, J. E., & de Zwaan, M. (Eds.). (2011). *Psychosocial assessment and treatment of bariatric surgery patients*. New York: Routledge.

Monteleone, P., Catapano, F., Tortorella, A., Di Martino, S., & Maj, M. (1995). Plasma melatonin and cortisol circadian patterns in patients with obsessive-compulsive disorder before and after fluoxetine treatment. *Psychoneuroendocrinology, 20*(7), 763–770.

Morgan, C. J., & Curran, H. V. (2008). Effects of cannabidiol on schizophrenia-like symptoms in people who use cannabis. *British Journal of Psychiatry, 192*(4), 306–307. doi: 10.1192/bjp.bp.107.046649.

Morgan, C. J. A., Das, R. K., Joye, A., Curran, H. V., & Kamboj, S. K. (2013). Cannabidiol reduces cigarette consumption in tobacco smokers: Preliminary findings. *Addictive Behaviors, 38*(9), 2433–2436. doi: 10.1016/j.addbeh.2013.03.011.

Mori, K., Inatomi, S., Ouchi, K., Azumi, Y., & Tuchida, T. (2009). Improving effects of the mushroom Yamabushitake (Hericium erinaceus) on mild cognitive impairment: A double-blind placebo-controlled clinical trial. *Phytotherapy Research, 23*(3), 367–372. doi: 10.1002/ptr.2634.

Muraki, M., Fujiwara, Y., Machida, H., Okazaki, H., Sogawa, M., Yamagami, H., … Arakawa, T. (2014). Role of small intestinal bacterial overgrowth in severe small intestinal damage in chronic nonsteroidal anti-inflammatory drug users. *Scandinavian Journal of Gastroenterology, 49*(3), 267–273. doi: 10.3109/00365521.2014.880182.

Mysels, D. J., & Sullivan, M. A. (2010). The relationship between opioid and sugar intake: Review of evidence and clinical applications. *Journal of Opioid Management, 6*(6), 445–452.

Nakano, M., Ubukata, K., Yamamoto, T., & Yamaguchi, H. (2009). Effect of pyrroloquinoline quinone (PQQ) on mental status of middle-aged and elderly persons. *FOOD Style, 13*(7), 50–53.

Nimmrich, V., & Eckert, A. (2013). Calcium channel blockers and dementia. *British Journal of Pharmacology, 169*(6), 1203–1210. doi: 10.1111/bph.12240.

Norton, D., Angerman, S., Istfan, N., Lopes, S. M., Babayan, V. K., Putz, S. N., … Blackburn, G. L. (2004). Comparative study of coconut oil, soybean oil, and hydrogenated soybean oil. *Philippine Journal of Coconut Studies, 29*(1&2), 1–5.

Nunes, M. A., Viel, T. A., & Buck, H. S. (2013). Microdose lithium treatment stabilized cognitive impairment in patients with Alzheimer's disease. *Current Alzheimer Research, 10*(1), 104–107.

Oliveira, A. M., & Bading, H. (2011). Calcium signaling in cognition and aging-dependent cognitive decline. *Biofactors, 37*(3), 168–174. doi: 10.1002/biof.148.

O'Neil, A., Quirk, S. E., Housden, S., Brennan, S. L., Williams, L. J., Pasco, J. A., … Jacka, F. N. (2014). Relationship between diet and mental health in children and adolescents: A systematic review. *American Journal of Public Health, 104*(10), e31–e42. doi: 10.2105/AJPH.2014.302110.

O'Reardon, J. P., Peshek, A., & Allison, K. C. (2005). Night eating syndrome: Diagnosis, epidemiology and management. *CNS Drugs, 19*(12), 997–1008.

Owen, G. N., Parnell, H., De Bruin, E. A., & Rycroft, J. A. (2008). The combined effects of L-theanine and caffeine on cognitive performance and mood. *Nutritional Neuroscience, 11*(4), 193–198.

Oxford Biomedical Technologies. (2013). *What food sensitivities are*. Retrieved May 2015, from http://nowleap.com/food-sensitivity/what-they-are/

Parker, G., Gibson, N. A., Brotchie, H., Heruc, G., Rees, A-M., & Hadzi-Pavlovic, D. (2006). Omega-3 fatty acids and mood disorders. *American Journal of Psychiatry, 163*(6), 969–978.

Pase, M. P., Scholey, A. B., Pipingas, A., Kras, M., Nolidin, K., Gibbs, A., … Stough, C. (2013). Cocoa polyphenols enhance positive mood states but not cognitive performance: A randomized, placebo-controlled trial. *Journal of Psychopharmacology, 27*(5), 451–458. doi: 10.1177/0269881112473791.

Pasula, M. J. (2014, January). The patented mediator release test (MRT): A comprehensive blood test for inflammation caused by food and food-chemical sensitivities. *Townsend Letter.*

Pedersen, L., Parlar, S., Kvist, K., Whiteley, P., & Shattock, P. (2014). Data mining the ScanBrit study of a gluten- and casein-free dietary intervention for children with autism spectrum disorders: Behavioural and psychometric measures of dietary response. *Nutritional Neuroscience, 17*(5), 207–213. doi: 10.1179/1476830513Y.0000000082.

Penland, J. G. (1994). Dietary boron, brain function, and cognitive performance. *Environmental Health Perspectives, 102*(Suppl 7), 65–72.

Percy, M. E., Kruck, T. P. A., Pogue, A. I., & Lukiw, W. J. (2011). Towards the prevention of potential aluminum toxic effects and an effective treatment for Alzheimer's disease. *Journal of Inorganic Biochemistry, 105*(11), 1505–1512.

Perez-Rodriguez, M. M., Baca-Garcia, E., Diaz-Sastre, C., Garcia-Resa, E., Ceverino, A., Saiz-Ruiz, J., …de Leon, J. (2008). Low serum cholesterol may be associated with suicide attempt history. *Journal of Clinical Psychiatry, 69*(12), 1920–1927.

Perlmutter, D. (2014). Rethinking dietary approaches for brain health. *Alternative and Complementary Therapies, 20*(2), 1–3.

Petursson, H., Sigurdsson, J. A., Bengtsson, C., Nilsen, T. I., & Getz, L. (2012). Is the use of cholesterol in mortality risk algorithms in clinical guidelines valid? Ten years prospective data from the Norwegian HUNT 2 study. *Journal of Evaluation in Clinical Practice, 18*(1), 159–168.

Pfeiffer, C. C. (1988). *Nutrition and mental illness: An orthomolecular approach to balancing body chemistry.* Rochester, VT: Healing Arts Press.

Picard, M., Juster, R-P., & McEwen, B. S. (2014). Mitochondrial allostatic load puts the 'gluc' back in glucocorticoids. *Nature Reviews Endocrinology, 10,* 303–310. doi:10.1038/nrendo.2014.22.

Pigeon, W. R., Carr, M., Gorman, C., & Perlis, M. L. (2010). Effects of a tart cherry juice beverage on the sleep of older adults with insomnia: A pilot study. *Journal of Medicinal Food, 13*(3), 579–583.

Pope, H. G., Cohane, G. H., Kanayama, G., Siegel, A. J., & Hudson, J. I. (2003). Testosterone gel supplementation for men with refractory depression: A randomized, placebo-controlled trial. *American Journal of Psychiatry, 160*(1), 105–111. doi:10.1176/appi.ajp.160.1.105.

Pottala, J. V., Yaffe, K., Robinson, J. G., Espeland, M. A., Wallace, R., & Harris, W. S. (2014). Higher RBC EPA + DHA corresponds with larger total brain and hippocampal volumes: WHIMS-MRI study. *Neurology, 82*(5), 435–442.

Presse, N., Belleville, S., Gaudreau, P., Greenwood, C. E., Kergoat, M. J., Morais, J. A.,… Ferland, G. (2013). Vitamin K status and cognitive function in healthy older adults. *Neurobiology of Aging, 34*(12), 2777–2783. doi: 10.1016/j.neurobiolaging.2013.05.031.

Preston, A. M. (1991). Cigarette smoking-nutritional implications. *Progress in Food and Nutrition Science, 15*(4), 183–217.

Prousky, J. E. (2005). Orthomolecular treatment of anxiety disorders. *Townsend Letter for Doctors and Patients, 259/260,* 82–87.

Prousky, J. (2007). *Anxiety: Orthomolecular diagnosis and treatment.* Toronto, ON: CCNM Press.

Prousky, J. E. (2014). The treatment of alcoholism with vitamin b3. *Journal of Orthomolecular Medicine, 29*(3), 1–9.

Quinesa, C. B., Rosaa, S. G., Da Rochaa, J. T., Gaia, B. M., Bortolattoa, C. F., Duarteb, M. M., & Nogueira, C. W. (2014). Monosodium glutamate, a food additive, induces depressive-like and anxiogenic-like behaviors in young rats. *Life Sciences, 107*(1–2), 27–31.

Rajindrajith, S., Devanarayana, N. M., Lakmini, C., Subasinghe, V., de Silva, D. G., & Benninga, M. A. (2014). Association between child maltreatment and constipation: A school-based survey using Rome III criteria. *Journal of Pediatric Gastroenterology and Nutrition, 58*(4), 486–490.

Rao, A. V., Bested, A. C., Beaulne, T. M., Katzman, M. A., Iorio, C., Berardi, J. M., & Logan, A. C. (2009). A randomized, double-blind, placebo-controlled pilot study of a probiotic in emotional symptoms of chronic fatigue syndrome. *Gut Pathogens, 1,* 6. doi:10.1186/1757 -4749-1-6.

Rapkin, A. J., Mikacich, J. A., Moatakef-Imani, B., & Rasgon, N. (2002). The clinical nature and formal diagnosis of premenstrual, postpartum, and perimenopausal affective disorders. *Current Psychiatry Reports, 4*(6), 419–428.

Renshaw, P. F., Daniels, S., Lundahl, L. H., Rogers, V., & Lukas, S. E. (1999). Short-term treatment with citicoline (CDP-choline) attenuates some measures of craving in cocaine-dependent subjects: A preliminary report. *Psychopharmacology (Berl), 142*(2), 132–138.

Ricci, A., Bronzetti, E., Vega, J. A., & Amenta, F. (1992). Oral choline alfoscerate counteracts age-dependent loss of mossy fibres in the rat hippocampus. *Mechanisms of Ageing and Development, 66*(1), 81–91.

Roberts, A. L., Lyall, K., Hart, J. E., Laden, F., Just, A. C., Bobb, J. F., … Weisskopf, M. G. (2014). Perinatal air pollutant exposures and autism spectrum disorder in the children of nurses' health study II participants. *Environmental Health Perspectives, 121*(8), A152.

Robson, P. J., Guy, G. W., & Di Marzo, V. (2014). Cannabinoids and schizophrenia: Therapeutic prospects. *Current Pharmaceutical Design, 20*(13), 2194–2204.

Rogers, M. A. M., Greene, M. T., Young, V. B., Saint, S., Langa, K. M., Kao, J. Y., & Aronoff, D. M. (2013). Depression, antidepressant medications, and risk of *clostridium difficile* infection. *BMC Medicine, 11,* 121.

Rosenthal, N. E. (2009). Issues for DSM-V: Seasonal affective disorder and seasonality. *American Journal of Psychiatry, 166*(8), 852–853.

Rosenthal, N. E., Bradt, G. H., & Wehr, T. A. (1984). *Seasonal pattern assessment questionnaire.* Bethesda, MD: National Institute of Mental Health.

Ross, C. C. (2012). Bariatric surgery: A realistic look at the risks and rewards. *Psychology Today.* Retrieved May 2015, from http://www.psychologytoday.com/blog/real-healing/201205/ bariatric-surgery-realistic-look-the-risks-and-rewards

Rubey, R. N. (2010). Could lysine supplementation prevent Alzheimer's dementia? A novel hypothesis. *Neuropsychiatric Disease and Treatment, 6,* 707–710. doi: 10.2147/NDT.S14338.

Ruetsch, O., Viala, A., Bardou, H., Martin, P., & Vacheron, M. N. (2005). Psychotropic drugs induced weight gain: A review of the literature concerning epidemiological data, mechanisms and management. *Encephale, 31*(4 Pt 1), 507–516.

Rush, A. J., Trivedi, M. H., Wisniewski, S. R., Nierenberg, A. A., Stewart, J. W., Warden, D., … Fava, M. (2006). Acute and longer-term outcomes in depressed outpatients requiring one or several treatment steps: A STAR*D report. *American Journal of Psychiatry, 163*(11), 1905–1917.

Russo, E. B. (2004). Clinical endocannabinoid deficiency (CECD): Can this concept explain therapeutic benefits of cannabis in migraine, fibromyalgia, irritable bowel syndrome and other treatment-resistant conditions? *Neuro Endocrinology Letters, 25*(1–2), 31–39.

Sakamoto, T., Cansev, M., & Wurtman, R. J. (2007). Oral supplementation with docosahexaenoic acid and uridine-5'-monophosphate increases dendritic spine density in adult gerbil hippocampus. *Brain Research, 1182,* 50–59.

Salonoja, M., Salminen, M., Vahlberg, T., Aarnio, P., & Kivelä, S-L. (2012). Withdrawal of psychotropic drugs decreases the risk of falls requiring treatment. *Archives of Gerontology and Geriatrics, 54*(1), 160–167.

Samaroo, D., Dickerson, F., Kasarda, D. D., Green, P. H. R., Briani, C., Yolken, R. H., & Alaedini, A. (2010). Novel immune response to gluten in individuals with schizophrenia. *Schizophrenia Research, 118*(1–3), 248–255. doi: 10.1016/j.schres.2009.08.009.

Sartori, H. E. (1986). Lithium orotate in the treatment of alcoholism and related conditions. *Alcohol*, *3*(2), 97–100.

Sartori, S. B., Whittle, N., Hetzenauer, A., & Singewald, N. (2012). Magnesium deficiency induces anxiety and HPA axis dysregulation: Modulation by therapeutic drug treatment. *Neuropharmacology*, *62*(1), 304–312.

Schmidt, A., Hammann, F., Wölnerhanssen, B., Meyer-Gerspach, A. C., Drewe, J., Beglinger, C., & Borgwardt, S. (2014). Green tea extract enhances parieto-frontal connectivity during working memory processing. *Psychopharmacology*, *231*(19), 3879–3888.

Schrauzer, G. N., & de Vroey, E. (1994). Effects of nutritional lithium supplementation on mood: A placebo-controlled study with former drug users. *Biological Trace Element Research*, *40*(1), 89–101.

Secades, J. J., & Frontera, G. (1995). CDP-choline: Pharmacological and clinical review. *Methods and Findings in Experimental and Clinical Pharmacology*, *17*(Suppl B), 1–54.

Seneff, S., Wainwright, G., & Mascitelliemail, L. (2011). Nutrition and Alzheimer's disease: The detrimental role of a high carbohydrate diet. *European Journal of Internal Medicine*, *22*(2), 134–140.

Sharp, W. G., Berry, R. C., McCracken, C., Nuhu, N. N., Marvel, E., Saulnier, C. E., … Jaquess, D. L. (2013). Feeding problems and nutrient intake in children with autism spectrum disorders: A meta-analysis and comprehensive review of the literature. *Journal of Autism and Developmental Disorders*, *43*(9), 2159–2173.

Shaw, W. (2011, Fall). Usefulness of HPHPA marker in a wide range of neurological, gastrointestinal, and psychiatric disorders. *BioMed Today*. Retrieved May 2015, from http://integrativeme dicineformentalhealth.com/ articles/shaw_hphpa.html

Shaw W. (2013a). Evidence that increased acetaminophen use in genetically vulnerable children appears to be a major cause of the epidemics of autism, attention deficit with hyperactivity, and asthma. *Journal of Restorative Medicine*, *2*, 1–16.

Shaw, W. (2013b). *Oxalates: Test implications for yeast and heavy metals.* Retrieved May 2015, from http://www.greatplainslaboratory.com/home/span/oxalates.asp

Shealy, C. N. (2006). *Life beyond 100.* New York: Tarcher.

Shen, J., Gammon, M. D., Terry, M. B., Wang, Q., Bradshaw, P., Teitelbaum, S. L., … Santella, R. M. (2009). Telomere length, oxidative damage, antioxidants and breast cancer risk. *International Journal of Cancer*, *124*(7), 1637–43. doi: 10.1002/ijc.24105.

Siebecker, A. (2005). Traditional bone broth in modern health and disease. *Townsend Letter.* Retrieved May 2015, from http://www.townsendletter.com/FebMarch2005/broth0205.htm

Singh, K., Connors, S. L., Macklin, E. A., Smith, K. D., Fahey, J. W., Talalay, P., & Zimmerman, A. W. (2014). Sulforaphane treatment of autism spectrum disorder (ASD). *Proceedings of the National Academy of Sciences USA*, *111*(43), 15550–15555. doi: 10.1073/pnas.1416940111.

Slutsky, I., Abumaria, N., Wu, L-J., Huang, C., Zhang, L., Li, B., … Liu, G. (2010). Enhancement of learning and memory by elevating brain magnesium. *Neuron*, *65*(2), 165–177.

Söderpalm, A. H., Lindsey, S., Purdy, R. H., Hauger, R., & de Wit, H. (2004). Administration of progesterone produces mild sedative-like effects in men and women. *Psychoneuroendocrinology*, *29*(3), 339–354.

Soffritti, M., Padovani, M., Tibaldi, E., Falcioni, L., Manservisi, F., & Belpoggi, F. (2014). The carcinogenic effects of aspartame: The urgent need for regulatory re-evaluation. *American Journal of Industrial Medicine*, *57*(4), 383–397.

Sogg, S., & Mori, D. L. (2009). Psychosocial evaluation for bariatric surgery: The Boston interview and opportunities for intervention. *Obesity Surgery*, *19*(3), 369–377.

Stanley, D., & Tunnicliffe, W. (2008). Management of life-threatening asthma in adults. *British Journal of Anaesthesia: Continuing Education in Anaesthesia, Critical Care and Pain, 8*(3), 95–99.

Stevens, L. J., Kuczek T., Burgess J. R., Hurt, E., & Arnold, L. E. (2010). Dietary sensitivities and ADHD symptoms: Thirty-five years of research. *Clinical Pediatrics, 50*(4), 279–293.

Stork, C., & Renshaw, P. F. (2005). Mitochondrial dysfunction in bipolar disorder: Evidence from magnetic resonance spectroscopy research. *Molecular Psychiatry, 10*(10), 900–919. doi:10.1038/sj.mp.4001711.

Stoschitzky, K., Sakotnik, A., Lercher, P., Zweiker, R., Maier, R., Liebmann, P., & Lindner, W. (1999). Influence of beta-blockers on melatonin release. *European Journal of Clinical Pharmacology, 55*(2), 111–115.

Suez, J., Korem, T., Zeevi, D., Zilberman-Schapira, G., Thaiss, C. A., Maza, O., … Elinav, E. (2014). Artificial sweeteners induce glucose intolerance by altering the gut microbiota. *Nature, 514*(7521), 181–186.

Sundqvist, T., Lindström, F., Magnusson, K. E., Sköldstam, L., Stjernström, I., & Tagesson, C. (1982). Influence of fasting on intestinal permeability and disease activity in patients with rheumatoid arthritis. *Scandinavian Journal of Rheumatology, 11*(1), 33–38.

Tawfik, M. S., & Al-Badr, N. (2012). Adverse effects of monosodium glutamate on liver and kidney functions in adult rats and potential protective effect of vitamins C and E. *Food and Nutrition Sciences, 3*(5), 651–659.

Underwood, M., Sivesind, P., & Gabourie, T. (2011). Effect of apoaequorin on cognitive function. *Alzheimer's and Dementia, 7*(4), e65.

Unlu, N. Z., Bohn, T., Clinton, S. K., & Schwartz, S. J. (2005). Carotenoid absorption from salad and salsa by humans is enhanced by the addition of avocado or avocado oil. *Journal of Nutrition, 135*(3), 431–436.

Vallée, M., Vitiello, S., Bellocchio, L., Hébert-Chatelain, E., Monlezun, S., Martin-Garcia, E., … Piazza, P. V. (2014). Pregnenolone can protect the brain from cannabis intoxication. *Science, 343*(6166), 94–98. doi: 10.1126/science.1243985.

Vancassel, S., Durand, G., Barthélémy, C., Lejeune, B., Martineau, J., Guilloteau, D., … Chalon S. (2001). Plasma fatty acid levels in autistic children. *Prostaglandins, Leukotrienes and Essential Fatty Acids, 65*(1), 1–7.

van Elst, K., Bruining, H., Birtoli, B., Terreaux, C., Buitelaar, J. K., & Kas, M. J. (2014). Food for thought: Dietary changes in essential fatty acid ratios and the increase in autism spectrum disorders. *Neuroscience and Biobehavioral Reviews, 45*, 369–378.

van De Sande, M. M., van Buul, V. J., & Brouns, F. J. (2014). Autism and nutrition: The role of the gut-brain axis. *Nutrition Research Reviews, 27*(2), 199–214.

van Dixhoorn, J., & Duivenvoorden, H. J. (1985). Efficacy of Nijmegen questionnaire in recognition of the hyperventilation syndrome. *Journal of Psychosomatic Research, 29*(2), 199–206.

Van Ittersum, K., & Wansink, B. (2012). Plate size and color suggestibility: The Delboeuf illusion's bias on serving and eating behavior. *Journal of Consumer Research, 39*(2), 215–228.

Vasquez, A. (2004). *Inflammation mastery.* Retrieved May 2015, from http://www.inflammationmastery.com

Vasquez, A., Manso, G., & Cannell, J. (2004). The clinical importance of vitamin D (cholecalciferol): A paradigm shift with implications for all healthcare providers. *Alternative Therapies in Health and Medicine, 10*(5), 28–36.

Vukadin, K. T. (2014, Fall). Failure to warn: Facing up to the real impact of pharmaceutical marketing on the physician's decision to prescribe. *Tulsa Law Review*, pp. 1–52.

Vuksan-Ćusa, B., Marcinko,, D., Nać, S., & Jakovljević, M. (2009). Differences in cholesterol and metabolic syndrome between bipolar disorder men with and without suicide attempts. *Progress in Neuro-Psychopharmacology and Biological Psychiatry, 33*(1), 109–112.

Wadden, T. A., & Foster, G. D. (2006). The weight and lifestyle inventory (WALI). *Obesity, 14*(Suppl 2), 99S–118S.

Walton, R. G., Hudak, R., & Green-Waite, R. J. (1993). Adverse reactions to aspartame: Double blind challenge in patients from a vulnerable population. *Biological Psychiatry, 34*(1–2), 13–17.

Wang, H-X., Wahlin, Å., Basun, H., Fastbom, J., Winblad, B., Fratiglioni L. (2001). Vitamin B12 and folate in relation to the development of Alzheimer's disease. *Neurology, 56*(9), 1188–1194.

Wansink, B., & van Kleef, E. (2013). Dinner rituals that correlate with child and adult BMI. *Obesity, 22*(5), E91–E95. doi: 10.1002/oby.20629

Warrington, T. P., & Bostwick, J. M. (2006). Psychiatric adverse effects of corticosteroids. *Mayo Clinic Proceedings, 1*(10), 1361–1367.

Watts, D. L. (2006). *Trace elements and other essential nutrients: Clinical application of tissue mineral analysis.* Provo, UT: Writer's B-L-O-C-K.

Wei, J., & Xiao, G-M. (2013). The neuroprotective effects of progesterone on traumatic brain injury current: status and future prospects. *Acta Pharmacologica Sinica, 34,* 1485–1490.

Weinberg, B. A., & Bealer, B. K. (2002). *The world of caffeine: The science and culture of the world's most popular drug.* New York: Routledge.

Westmark, C. J., Westmark, P. R., & Malter, J. S. (2013). Soy-based diet exacerbates seizures in mouse models of neurological disease. *Journal of Alzheimer's Disease, 33*(3), 797–805.

Whitaker, R. (2010). *Anatomy of an epidemic: Magic bullets, psychiatric drugs, and the astonishing rise of mental illness in America.* New York: Broadway Books.

Whiteley, P. (2014). Nutritional management of (some) autism: A case for gluten- and casein-free diets? *Proceedings of the Nutrition Society, 14,* 1–6.

Whiteley, P., Shattock, P., Knivsberg, A-M., Seim, A., Reichelt, K. L., Todd, L., … Hooper, M. (2013). Gluten- and casein-free dietary intervention for autism spectrum conditions. *Frontiers in Human Neuroscience, 6,* 344.

Williams, R. (1998). *Biochemical individuality.* New York: McGraw-Hill.

Wilson, R. S., Barnes, L. L., Aggarwal, N. T., Boyle, P. A., Hebert, L. E., Mendes de Leon, C. F., & Evans, D. A. (2010). Cognitive activity and the cognitive morbidity of Alzheimer disease. *Neurology, 75*(11), 990. doi: 10.1212/WNL.0b013e3181f25b5e.

Wollschlaeger, B. (2003). Zinc-carnosine for the management of gastric ulcers: Clinical application and literature review. *Journal of the American Nutraceutical Association, 6*(2), 33.

Yokogoshi, H., Kobayashi, M., Mochizuki, M., & Terashima, T. (1998). Effect of the- anine, yl-glutamylethylamide, on brain monoamines and striatal dopamine release in conscious rats. *Neurochemical Research, 23*(5), 667–673.

Zuardi, A. W., Crippa, J. A., Hallak, J. E., Moreira, F. A., & Guimarães, F. S. (2006). Cannabidiol, a Cannabis sativa constituent, as an antipsychotic drug. *Brazilian Journal of Medical and Biological Research, 39*(4), 421–429.

Index